CURING EVERYDAY AILMENTS

the Natural Way

CURING EVERYDAY AILMENTS
the Natural Way

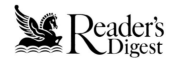

Reader's Digest

THE READER'S DIGEST ASSOCIATION, INC.
Pleasantville, New York/Montreal

Note to readers
The information in this book should not be substituted for, or used to alter,
medical therapy without your doctor's advice. For a specific health problem,
consult your physician for guidance.

Address any comments about *Curing Everyday Ailments the Natural Way* to
Reader's Digest, Editor-in-Chief, U.S. Illustrated Reference Books,
Reader's Digest Road, Pleasantville, NY 10570.

To order additional copies of *Curing Everyday Ailments the Natural Way* call
1–800–846–2100.

You can also visit us on the World Wide Web at http://www.readersdigest.com

Library of Congress Cataloging in Publication Data

Curing everyday ailments the natural way.

    p.   cm.
  ISBN 0-7621-0240-3
  1. Alternative medicine Handbooks, manuals, etc. 2. Self-care,
Health Handbooks, manuals, etc. I. Reader's Digest Association.
R733.C865   2000
615.5—dc21   99-21950

Curing Everyday Ailments the Natural Way

READER'S DIGEST PROJECT STAFF

Editor: Mary Lyn Maiscott

Design Director: Barbara Rietschel

Contributing Editor: Marianne Wait

Contributing Researchers: Deirdre van Dyk, Claudia Kaplan

Administrative Assistant: Donna Gataletto

Technology Manager: Douglas A. Croll

READER'S DIGEST HEALTH AND SCIENCE BOOKS
Group Editorial Director: Wayne Kalyn

READER'S DIGEST ILLUSTRATED REFERENCE BOOKS
Editor-in-Chief: Christopher Cavanaugh

Art Director: Joan Mazzeo

Operations Manager: William J. Cassidy

Consultant:
Woodson C. Merrell, M.D.
Executive Director, Center for Health and Healing, Beth Israel Medical Center, New York; Assistant Clinical Professor of Medicine, Columbia University, College of Physicians and Surgeons, New York.

CREATED BY GAIA BOOKS LTD.

Project Manager: Cathy Meeus

Art Editor: Malcolm Smythe

Copy Editors: Lynn Bresler, Sarah Chapman

Proofreader: Deirdre Clark

Designers: Phil Gamble, Ann Thomson

Illustrators: Hayward Art Group, Karen Hiscock, Aziz Khan, Ruth Lindsay, Sheilagh Noble, James G. Robins, Harry Titcombe

Photographic Direction: Tania Volhard, Sara Mathews, Matt Moate

Photographers: Ray Moller, Paul Forrester

Picture Researcher: Jan Croot

Indexer: Jill Ford

Production: Lyn Kirby, Kate Gaudern

Managing Editor: Pip Morgan

Direction: Joss Pearson, Patrick Nugent

Chief Medical Editor: Dr. Penny Stanway MB BS

Consultants: Stefan Ball (Flower Essences), Ann Gillanders (Reflexology), Robin Hayfield (Homeopathy), Paul Lundberg (Acupressure and Shiatsu), Robin Monro (Yoga), Roger Newman Turner (Naturopathy), Jane Rieck (Massage), Robert Stephen (Aromatherapy), Christine Steward (Herbalism)

Writers: Jane Alexander, Chris McLaughlin, Ricki Ostrov, Anna Selby, Wendy Teasdill, Philip Wilkinson

About This Book

What can you do when you wake up in the middle of the night with a headache? How can you relieve pain or fever without prescription and over-the-counter drugs? What foods can you eat to reduce the level of cholesterol in your blood? To these and a whole host of other questions, *Curing Everyday Ailments the Natural Way* provides you with authoritative yet easy-to-apply answers you can trust.

THE BASICS OF NATURAL HEALTH

In the introductory chapter, "Maintaining Health the Natural Way," you will find important information about the kind of diet, lifestyle, and home environment you need to become healthy and to stay healthy. General advice about safely using natural therapies culminates in practical advice about creating your own natural medicine cabinet. This way, you will have on hand the main remedies you need to treat common minor ailments at home.

ABOUT THE THERAPIES

Part One: The Therapies familiarizes you with the various types of treatments recommended in this book. It describes the theories behind 10 major therapies that you can use at home, along with instructions in basic techniques and important general cautions. A range of additional therapies that cannot properly be undertaken without the help of a qualified therapist are described more concisely in the "Glossary of Therapies."

TREATING AILMENTS NATURALLY

The heart of the book is *Part Two: Symptoms and Ailments*, arranged for easy reference in A-to-Z order. If you don't find a specific problem in the table of contents, check the general index, which will guide you to the appropriate article. In Part Two, you will discover the nature and possible causes of your disorder, how you can prevent it, and which natural treatments can be used for it. With this information, you can make up your own mind about which therapies to choose, according to your preferences and symptoms. Always check the general instructions and cautions on using a particular therapy in Part One of the book before embarking on that form of treatment.

GETTING MEDICAL HELP

At the end of each article you will find advice about when you should consult a doctor instead of treating a disorder at home with natural therapies. In some cases, certain symptoms are noted as requiring medical help right away—for example, by calling 911 or going to the emergency room. Otherwise, make an appointment with your health-care provider at the earliest opportunity. Because it is impossible to address every possible combination of symptoms, readers should also use their own judgment and always seek their doctor's guidance for unexplained or worrisome symptoms.

EXTENDING YOUR UNDERSTANDING

Cross-references appear in the text where appropriate to guide you to further explanations elsewhere in the book. A box at the end of each article notes related topics. Unfamiliar terms used in the text can be looked up in the "Glossary of Terms." Organizations that you may want to contact for more detailed information about natural therapies are listed, along with their addresses, telephone numbers, and web sites, where available, in the "Resource Guide."

Contents

Maintaining Health the Natural Way

The various forms of natural medicine provide a gentle kind of health care that is becoming increasingly popular, though most people expect to combine it with orthodox medicine. Natural medicine offers long-term well-being because it acknowledges a person's lifestyle and treats the whole person—body, mind, and spirit—not just the symptoms of ill health.

Natural medicine is attracting increasing numbers of people. One recent survey showed that 34 percent of Americans had tried at least one nonorthodox therapy in the previous year, mostly for chronic problems, such as arthritis and insomnia. The use of herbal remedies in the United States increased by an astounding 380 percent between 1990 and 1997. This evidence suggests that while orthodox medicine is claiming more and more success in tackling major health problems, such as cancer and heart disease, it is not meeting other needs that natural medicine is better able to satisfy.

Why choose the natural way?

Healing based on natural remedies, home treatments, and lifestyle measures is considerably gentler and more user-friendly than taking potent medications. It is also empowering, enabling you to take responsibility for your everyday well-being while being free to consult a doctor or other health-care professional when appropriate. Perhaps most important, it acknowledges the good sense of maintaining the health of the entire person, rather than focusing only on symptoms of disease, and it attempts to prevent, rather than simply treat, sickness.

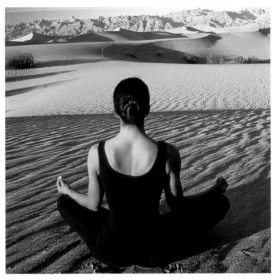

Harnessing your own healing power
Natural therapies, from acupressure to yoga, aim to utilize the body's inherent power of self-healing.

Natural approaches to health recognize the body's own healing power and try to maximize or enhance it. They are also less likely than orthodox treatments to cause troublesome side effects. Each herbal remedy, for example, contains small amounts of several active ingredients, each of which tends to balance the actions of the others. This is in contrast to most prescription drugs, which typically contain a powerful dose of a single substance and therefore have the potential to unbalance the body chemistry and create new problems that may in turn necessitate further treatment.

Natural medicine places great emphasis on the important links between the body and mind. Scientific research provides an ever-increasing volume of evidence to substantiate this approach. A wealth of studies shows that patients who think positively and address any emotional problems tend to have improved outcomes in diseases ranging from arthritis to cancer. Brain and body are intimately linked by hormones, neurotransmitters (substances that help transmit messages between nerve cells), and other chemicals. Mood changes can affect the functioning of your immune system, your cardiovascular health, and the quality of your sleep. On the other hand,

physical problems affect your happiness, alertness, and anxiety level. This explains why physical illness can lead to mental distress and vice versa, and why physical therapies can alleviate mental illness and mind therapies may indeed encourage physical healing. A good example is laughter therapy (see p. 63). Seeing the funny side of life promotes chemical changes in the body that help keep you well.

CHOICES FOR HEALTH

It is tempting, perhaps, to see conventional and natural medicine as irreconcilable opposites. But the reality is that many mainstream physicians are happy for patients to include natural approaches in their treatment. Similarly, reputable practitioners of alternative therapies recognize the importance of obtaining orthodox medical advice for all but minor ailments. Trying natural therapies does not have to imply excluding yourself from the undisputed benefits of "high-tech" medicine; instead it's a way of extending your treatment options. This "integrated" approach to health is discussed further on page 17.

THE KEYS TO HEALTHY LIVING

A good diet, regular exercise, and using strategies for managing stress are the main ways to maintain health naturally. Other important aids include fostering your relationships, making your home a healthful place in which to live, and avoiding damaging practices, such as smoking. Looking after yourself in this way encourages mental well-being and helps you protect every part of your body, from arteries to nerves, intestines to hormone-producing glands. It can also bolster your immune system, helping protect you from infections, allergies, and even cancer.

This introduction contains information about all these essential aspects of health maintenance. It also contains guidelines about selecting the natural therapies that will work the best for you.

Eat well, be well

The food you eat is the source of the energy you need to fuel the activity of every cell in your body. It also provides the nutrients required for physical growth and repair and enables the body to produce the variety of substances, such as hormones, enzymes, and neurotransmitters, that are essential for normal body functioning.

Ideas about food have changed in recent years. Not so long ago, a widespread belief was that avoiding certain foods, such as fats, ensured a healthy diet. While reducing the excessive consumption of fats is still seen as important, greater emphasis is now placed on following a diet that contains a good balance of nutrient-rich foods. The "Healthy Eating Pyramid" on page 10 shows the proportions of different types of foods that most people need to achieve this balance.

BUYING AND PREPARING FOOD

When you buy food, think about which items are best for your health. For example, choose poultry and fish over red meat, because red meat contains more saturated fat. Use cold-pressed oils that contain beneficial monounsaturated and polyunsaturated fats, rather than butter or other solid fats, which contain saturated fats. Select low-fat dairy products whenever you can. If available, choose organic foods, which are grown without pesticides, antibiotics, or growth-promoting hormones. Such foods are cultivated in ways that promote healthy growth and development, as well as disease resistance. Maximize nourishment by eating a high proportion of foods that have been processed as little as possible, such as whole grains and fresh fruits and vegetables.

Preserve the nutritional value of fresh foods by preparing them just before mealtimes. With organic foods, you should generally discard as little vegetable and fruit rind as possible. But if you eat nonorganic fruits and vegetables, remember that any traces of insecticides, fungicides, or herbicides used by the grower are most likely to be found in the rind or

Healthy eating pyramid

This illustrates the relative amount of each food group you should include in your daily diet. Make the foods at the base of the pyramid your staples and include only small quantities of the foods shown at the apex.

Sweets: *Add sweetness to food, if necessary, with a little honey, maple syrup, or sugar. But try to make these ingredients only an occasional treat. Sweet foods provide quick energy and, sometimes, trace amounts of minerals.*

Fats: *Restrict your fat intake to no more than 30 percent of total calories. This includes fats "hidden" in other foods and used for cooking. Favor vegetable fats (in nuts, seeds, whole grains, vegetables, cold-pressed vegetable oils) and fats from oily fish over fats in meat, eggs, and dairy products. Fats provide fatty acids that are vital for cell structure and contain fat-soluble vitamins.*

Protein-rich foods: *Eat four to six daily servings. These foods include poultry, fish, eggs, low-fat dairy products, lean meat, nuts, beans, and bean products, such as tofu. Proteins are needed for cell growth and repair and for the production of antibodies, hormones, and enzymes.*

Vegetables and fruits: *Eat at least three to five daily servings of vegetables and two to four of fruits. Include a variety of roots, tubers, stems, leaves, fruits, and seed pods. Choose fruits and vegetables of a range of colors (because different plant pigments offer different health benefits). These foods supply fiber, vitamins, minerals, and some essential fatty acids.*

Complex carbohydrates: *Eat 6 to 11 servings of unrefined starchy foods, such as rice, beans, root vegetables, bananas, and whole grains, or foods made from them (such as whole-grain bread, breakfast cereal, and pasta). Complex carbohydrates are a ready source of energy and contain vitamins and minerals.*

Serving size

Protein
2–3 ounces of meat, fish, and poultry
1 egg
1 cup of milk or yogurt
1 1/2 ounces of hard cheese
1/2 cup of nuts or cooked beans or lentils

Vegetables and fruit
1/2 cup of non-leafy vegetables
1 cup of leafy vegetables
1 medium apple, orange, or pear
1/2 grapefruit or cantaloupe
1/2 cup of canned or stewed fruit

Carbohydrates
1 slice of bread
1 ounce of uncooked cereal
1/2 cup of cooked root vegetable, pasta, cereal, or rice

outer leaves. Clean produce carefully. Cook fruits and vegetables lightly to retain vitamins and minerals. If you fry, do so quickly, without burning, using fresh oil each time.

SUPPLEMENTING YOUR DIET

Supplements are no substitute for eating well, and most of the time a healthy diet provides all the nutrients you need. Your body builds reserves of some nutrients. Body fat, for example, stores fat-soluble vitamins (vitamins A, D, E, and K). Calcium and many other minerals can move from your bones to wherever else they are needed in your body. This means that you need a certain amount of these nutrients over a period of some weeks or months, but a daily variation in intake does no harm. Some other nutrients, such as water-soluble vitamins (vitamins B and C), are not stored, so you need to replenish them every day. Several conditions make supplements advisable, either to keep you well or to treat illness. For example, supplements can:

■ Provide nutrients that may be needed to maintain optimum health at such times as pregnancy and later life.

■ Help prevent ill health from a lack of nutrients in the diet.
■ Help treat illnesses, such as infections, that increase the rate at which the body uses certain nutrients.
■ Help treat illnesses, such as arthritis, that respond to increased levels of particular nutrients.
■ Help prevent cardiovascular disease and diabetes or assist in their treatment.

Product packaging suggests doses and indicates the percentage of the "Daily Value" or the RDA—Recommended Dietary Allowance (see box below)—per capsule or tablet. The best choice is often a general-purpose multiple vitamin and mineral supplement, or one devised for a particular problem or time of life, though sometimes supplements of individual nutrients are advisable. Some formulations are more efficiently utilized than others. Look for the following:

■ Calcium—with magnesium, zinc, and vitamin D
■ Iron—with vitamin C and copper
■ Magnesium—with calcium, phosphorus, and vitamin B_6
■ Selenium—yeast-based selenium with vitamins A, C, and E
■ Zinc—zinc gluconate (if for colds and flu) with vitamin A and copper
■ Vitamin A—as mixed carotenoids
■ Vitamin B—as vitamin B complex
■ Vitamin C—in a preparation with flavonoids (sometimes called bioflavonoids)
■ Vitamin E—with mixed tocopherols

The average healthy person converts linoleic and alpha-linolenic acids, known as essential fatty acids (see "Key Nutrients and Foods," p. 12), into such important body chemicals as prostaglandins, which regulate a number of body processes. Some people cannot convert essential fatty acids properly, and nutritionists may recommend for them supplements of evening primrose oil, flaxseed oil, or fish oil.

Another group of supplements that is gaining in popularity comprises those containing one or more essential amino acids (the molecules that make up proteins). There are many

---

Recommended Dietary Allowance (RDA)

Supplement labels sometimes give the percentage of the RDA for each nutrient in the product. More often, they list percentages of "Daily Values," which are indirectly based on RDAs. The RDA is the amount of a nutrient generally thought adequate to prevent deficiency in a normal, healthy adult. These figures do not allow for variations in requirements resulting from illness or body size, and may vary for smokers or people taking medication. RDAs are meant to provide general guidelines rather than hard-and-fast rules. A therapist may therefore advise you to eat more than the RDA of some nutrients. Another measure often used by nutritionists is the optimum daily allowance. This is the amount of a nutrient needed to keep the body functioning at its best, which may be more than the RDA.

Key nutrients and foods

Nutrient and its role	Common food sources
Beta-carotene *Antioxidant*	Yellow and orange vegetables and fruits, green leafy vegetables
Calcium *Bone and tooth maintenance, muscle and nerve function*	Milk and cheese, fish with edible bones, whole-grain cereals, legumes, nuts, green cabbage
Chromium *Blood-sugar regulation*	Cheese, whole-grain cereals
Copper *Iron absorption, energy utilization, nerve function*	Fish, legumes, green leafy vegetables, mushrooms, avocados, garlic, seaweed, nuts, cocoa
Essential fatty acids *Blood-fat regulation, hormone production*	Whole-grain cereals, legumes, nuts, seeds, cold-pressed vegetable oils (especially flaxseed and safflower oils), dark green leafy vegetables
Fiber *Bowel function*	Whole-grain cereals, vegetables and legumes, fruits, nuts, seeds
Flavonoids *Antioxidant*	Whole-grain cereals, brightly colored vegetables and fruits
Folic acid *Red blood cell formation, healthy cell division*	Liver, whole-grain cereals, green leafy vegetables, fruits, nuts, yeast
Iodine *Thyroid hormone formation*	Fish, shellfish, meat, whole-grain cereals, green leafy vegetables, peppers, seaweed, iodized salt
Iron *Oxygen transport*	Eggs, shellfish, meat, whole-grain cereals, legumes, peanuts, green leafy vegetables, seaweed, dates, figs, raisins, seeds, molasses, cocoa

Nutrient and its role	Common food sources
Magnesium *Energy production, nerve function, insulin regulation*	Fish, shellfish, meat, whole-grain cereals, nuts, green leafy vegetables, mushrooms, seaweed, seeds, cocoa
Phosphorus *Bone and tooth formation and maintenance*	Egg yolks, fish, shellfish, meat, whole-grain cereals, legumes, milk products
Potassium *Fluid balance, muscle function*	Whole-grain cereals, nuts, seeds, vegetables, fruits, molasses, cocoa
Selenium *Antioxidant*	Milk products, fish, meat, whole-grain cereals, legumes, green leafy vegetables, mushrooms, garlic
Zinc *Growth and reproduction, enzyme action, immune function*	Milk products, fish, shellfish, meat, whole-grain cereals, legumes, root vegetables, garlic, sprouted seeds
Vitamin A *Skin, hair, and eye maintenance, immune function*	Milk products, eggs, fish, legumes, cold-pressed vegetable oils
Vitamin B complex *Healthy metabolism, nerve function*	Milk products, fish, meat, legumes, whole-grain cereals, green leafy vegetables, seeds, nuts, molasses
Vitamin C *Blood-vessel strength, wound healing, antioxidant*	Citrus and most other fruits, broccoli, peppers, and most other vegetables
Vitamin D *Bone and tooth maintenance*	Milk products, egg yolks, seaweed, nuts, oily fish, fish-liver oils
Vitamin E *Antioxidant, muscle function, red blood cell formation*	Vegetable oils, eggs, fish, whole-grain cereals, lentils, beans, nuts, seeds

different types of amino acids, and these play an important role in building and repairing body tissues. They are normally obtained from protein-rich foods in your diet. But as with other nutrients, a number of conditions may impair the body's ability to absorb or utilize them. People whose diet may contain a limited range of proteins, such as vegans, should consider taking a supplement that supplies a wide range of amino acids. Supplements of individual amino acids should not be taken for more than a few weeks without medical supervision. Amino acids should not be given to children without medical advice.

Get active, get fit

Getting active helps keep your bones, joints, and muscles in good condition. It can also boost your metabolism, counter stress, and help fight depression. To maintain good health, get the three types of exercise described on pages 13–14. Exercise regularly. Aim for a half hour of aerobic exercise, whether you do it all at once or in five- to ten-minute sessions throughout the day, for three to five days a week. If you no longer exercise, try to determine why you have become inactive and choose a new program of exercise that more closely meets your needs and preferences. Consider all your

---

Exercising safely

- Choose an activity of suitable intensity for you.
- Stay within the target heart rate guidelines for your age (see box, p. 14).
- Warm up and cool down for 10 minutes before and after exercise.
- Consult your doctor if you are new to exercise, have an existing medical condition or back problem, are pregnant, or if you don't feel well after exercise.
- Get expert advice from a doctor or physical therapist after any exercise-induced injury.

---

personal circumstances: your ability, whether you like competition, whether you prefer to be alone or in a group, at home or away, indoors or outside. If motivation is a problem, consider consulting a professional trainer, who can tailor exercises to your needs and help you achieve your goals.

AEROBIC EXERCISE

This type of exercise works large groups of muscles. If it is sufficiently intense, it raises your heart rate enough to build cardiovascular fitness. Examples include walking fast enough to make you warm, running, swimming, and playing tennis. Aerobic exercise also raises the blood levels of natural, hormone-like chemicals called endorphins, inducing a feeling of well-being; it speeds up circulation, helping keep the arteries, veins, and heart healthy; and it raises the body's metabolic rate (the rate at which cells burn energy), which helps prevent you from putting on weight. In summary, aerobic exercise improves lung capacity and circulation, promotes heart health, boosts immunity, benefits digestion, helps maintain joint health, fosters weight control, and lifts the spirits.

Exercise that raises the heart rate to 50 to 75 percent of your maximum rate (approximately 220 minus your age) is classified as moderate intensity, and that which raises the heart rate to a higher level is considered high intensity. For most people, regular moderate-intensity exercise provides all the health benefits they need. High-intensity exercise is mainly for serious athletes and those who wish to achieve above-average levels of fitness. It should not be attempted by those who are new to exercise.

Check your pulse periodically during exercise sessions. Unless you're more advanced, don't let your pulse rise above the moderate-intensity limit for your age (see box, p. 14). If you have trouble taking your pulse, use this rule of thumb for gentler forms of exercise, such as walking: If you can talk while exercising, you're not overdoing it; if you can sing, you may need to exert more effort.

Your target heart rate

When starting exercise, aim to keep your pulse at the lower end of the moderate-intensity range, indicated below. Build up to a higher level gradually. (These figures are based on average maximum heart rates; they may vary.)

Age	Lower rate	Upper rate
	(beats per minute)	
20	100	150
30	95	142
40	90	135
50	85	127
60	80	120
70	75	112

STRENGTH TRAINING

This type of exercise involves working individual muscles or muscle groups. Strength training can be done with or without weights or other loads. Examples include carrying around an infant, lifting weights in a gym, and any repeated muscle work, such as rowing or cycling (which also provides aerobic exercise). Strengthening your muscles can prevent lower back pain, ease osteoarthritis pain, increase bone density, encourage weight loss, foster agility and balance, and lessen the risk of muscle injury.

STRETCHING

This type of exercise lengthens muscles to their full natural extent, promoting flexibility.

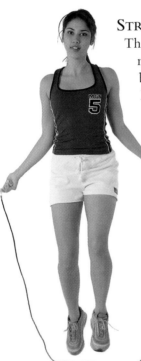

Fat-burning exercise
Aerobic exercise helps you get rid of excess fat.

Whether you stretch before aerobic exercise or strength training, or perform yoga or another activity that limbers the muscles and joints, you'll help prepare muscles for activity, prevent and relieve muscle stiffness after exercise, reduce the risk of muscle injury, and prevent or ease back pain and repetitive strain injury.

Health hazards

A good diet, regular exercise, and stress management are at the core of any disease prevention program. Nevertheless, many other areas of life under your control have an impact on health. For instance, it is important to not smoke—or at least cut down—and to consume only moderate amounts of alcohol. Also, make sure you protect yourself against the sun's ultraviolet rays, while also getting sufficient exposure to natural light. In addition, eliminate or reduce toxins, allergens, and contaminants in your home.

CIGARETTES AND ALCOHOL

Many people enjoy smoking or drinking, but both can adversely affect health—and the more you indulge in either habit, the riskier it becomes.

Smoking: The addictive nature of nicotine encourages ongoing exposure to the harmful tars and gases in tobacco smoke. Breathing the smoke from other people's cigarettes or cigars—passive smoking—also carries risks, although of a lower order. Health problems linked to smoking include the following:

Common threats
Smoking and excessive drinking are standard practice in some social situations. However, they carry many health risks.

- The destruction of 25 milligrams of vitamin C per cigarette
- Poor wound healing and premature skin aging
- Asthma, bronchitis, and emphysema
- Mouth, lung, and other cancers
- Rheumatoid arthritis
- Anxiety and depression
- Deafness
- Ulcerative colitis
- Arterial disease
- Osteoporosis

In addition, smoking or passive smoking by a pregnant woman can lead to low birth weight in the baby. Parental smoking before and after the birth increases the risk of sudden infant death syndrome (SIDS, or crib death).

Alcohol: Drinking in moderation and at appropriate times has little or no negative effect and may even be beneficial to your heart, perhaps because it raises the levels of HDL—good—cholesterol. However:

- Driving or undertaking other potentially hazardous operations after drinking alcohol increases the risk of accidents.
- Overindulgence can cause a hangover.
- Drinking too much in any one session intensifies your current mood and in the long run has a depressant effect.
- Alcohol consumption disrupts normal sleep patterns.
- Addiction can lead to social problems (including violence), malnutrition, high blood pressure, gastritis, liver damage and reduced liver function, and mouth and other cancers.
- Drinking alcohol during pregnancy can affect the health of the unborn baby.

Once consumed, alcohol is absorbed into the bloodstream. The liver gradually breaks down the circulating alcohol into other substances and eventually clears alcohol from the blood completely—unless you have drunk more alcohol in the meantime. The more alcohol you drink, the longer it takes for the liver to clear it from your bloodstream.

Drinking one unit of alcohol (a glass of wine, a glass of average-strength beer, or a single measure of spirits) raises the blood alcohol level by 15 milligrams per 100 milliliters. It takes an hour for the average person's body to clear a drink containing one unit of alcohol. Women are more susceptible than men to the damaging effects of alcohol because they absorb it faster and develop higher levels in their blood.

Giving up or cutting down: If you want to smoke or drink less or stop completely:

- Acknowledge the pros and cons of both your habit and being a nonsmoker or nondrinker.
- Look at alternative, nondamaging ways of enjoying yourself and managing stress.
- Forgive yourself for any lapses, then resume abstinence.
- Accept any need for support, then find that help.

For further advice on conquering your habit, see "Addictions," pp. 76–77.

LIGHT EXPOSURE

Growing scientific evidence indicates that good health depends partially on adequate exposure to the various wavelengths of electromagnetic radiation in natural light. Daily exposure to bright light affects the pineal gland and hypothalamus and alters the levels of various hormones and neurotransmitters. Too little exposure can lead to seasonal affective disorder (SAD) and symptoms of jet lag.

The proportions of the different wavelengths in light form its "spectral balance." The spectral balance of sunlight changes with the time, season, weather, and distance from the equator, as well as the level of air pollution and any passage through glass (in windows or eyeglasses), both of which reduce the concentration of ultraviolet light. Different types of electric light have different spectral balances, and these can affect physical and mental health. Full-spectrum bulbs are available that mimic the afternoon sun; these may be worth

investing in for some of your light fixtures, especially if you suffer from SAD. Exposing your skin to a certain amount (15 or 20 minutes) of direct sunlight boosts your production of vitamin D and the "feel-good" chemicals called endorphins.

Be very careful, however, not to overdo it. Too much of the sun's ultraviolet light can cause skin cancer, including malignant melanoma, and increases the likelihood of cataracts. To protect yourself, follow the advice on page 350, and also wear sunglasses in strong sun.

Making your home a healthy place

Some home comforts can be hazardous to your health. Wall-to-wall carpets, for example, harbor dust mites, which can trigger asthma and eczema in some people. Dust mites also flourish in the warm, still air encouraged by central heating and well-insulated homes. Electrical gadgets create electromagnetic fields, which at close range may increase the risk of cancer. Make your home safer by adopting as many as possible of the following strategies:

- Introduce enough fresh air (especially if someone smokes).
- Avoid extremes of temperature and humidity.
- Keep some houseplants to freshen the air. Plants can absorb certain potentially toxic chemicals. Among the most efficient plants are spider plants, chrysanthemums, coconut palms, weeping figs, gerberas, and dracaenas.
- Do not use household cleaners and other chemicals in spray form; these encourage asthma in susceptible people.
- Whenever possible, substitute such substances as baking soda and vinegar for harsh household cleansers.
- Have adequate lighting.
- Keep sound levels within reasonable limits.
- Do not sit close to the sides or back of a television or computer for long periods.
- Carefully follow instructions when using potentially poisonous household chemicals (including solvents, glues, drain openers, and pesticides).

- Get expert advice when removing old lead paint.
- Take care of such hazards as loose stair carpeting and trailing electrical cords.
- Do not turn up your boiler thermostat too high.
- Minimize formaldehyde exposure by avoiding pressed-wood furniture (coating all exposed surfaces with varnish or polyurethane) and by painting pressed-wood paneled walls with paint designed to absorb formaldehyde emissions.
- Install smoke detectors and consider a carbon-monoxide detector, especially if you have a gas stove or a garage attached to your home.
- Have your home checked for radon gas.

Using natural therapies

Many people already treat ailments with natural remedies and therapies, and a lot more are interested in finding out what to use and how. Turning to natural therapies is not a substitute for a doctor. Most people who use alternative therapies, such as homeopathy, rely on their regular doctor for diagnosis and for health care in cases of serious illness. But increasing numbers of mainstream doctors are recognizing that certain complementary therapies have much to offer in treating specific ailments (for example, osteopathy or chiropractic for back pain), and they are likely to refer their patients to the appropriate complementary practitioner.

Home use

The natural approach often works well for common, everyday ailments, from coughs and colds to upset stomachs. There are so many therapies available that the choice can seem baffling. Use Part One of this book to find out about specific therapies, and consult the ailment entries in Part Two to learn which therapies are best for your problem.

Some therapies are especially well suited to specific types of ailments. Posture and movement training, for example, often improves such problems as back pain and tension

headaches, while breathing exercises may shorten panic attacks and prevent asthma. But many therapies, from massage to herbal medicine, can be used to treat a wide variety of conditions.

You should also be guided by your personal preferences when selecting a natural therapy. Some people prefer therapies based on exercise; others favor those based on medicines. A therapy is more likely to work for you if you are comfortable with it. Remember that caring for yourself in a kind and thoughtful way is often the most important form of therapy.

HEALTH PROFESSIONALS:
AN INTEGRATED APPROACH

Consider yourself and your doctor or other health-care provider as a team. Play your part by

Consultation
Natural therapists usually allow plenty of time to discuss your medical history and specific health problems.

Choosing a natural therapist

Look in the ailment section in Part Two of this book to find out which therapies are recommended for your complaint, then read about the therapies in Part One to see if you find them appealing.

Finding a therapist
Once you have decided on a therapy, select a therapist by:
- Asking your doctor, friends, or neighbors for their recommendations.
- Scanning the register of therapists compiled by that therapy's national or local professional association.
- Checking with hospital-based referral lines.

Interviewing a therapist
Your first visit should be an exploratory one in which you:
- Ask the therapist about his or her treatments and personal approach.
- Ask about the therapist's training and qualifications.
- See if you feel comfortable with the person.
- Enquire about the therapist's experience, professional support, and indemnity.
- Afterward, check his or her credentials with the relevant professional association.

Working with your therapist
- Aim to work as a team with your therapist for the good of your health by sharing all relevant information and following a sensible program of treatment.
- Be aware that your therapist may one day want to discuss your ailment with your doctor. However, he or she will seek your permission first.

When to beware
- Do not continue with a course of treatment if you feel uneasy or doubt the person's skill.
- Be suspicious of any therapist who promises a complete cure, emphasizes unusual or expensive testing, or promotes the sale of large amounts of costly supplements or equipment.

maintaining a healthy lifestyle and treating yourself with natural remedies and therapies when appropriate. In the past, many doctors based most of their treatments on drugs and ignored traditional therapies. However, attitudes are now changing, with more and more doctors regaining an interest in older, natural healing methods. Preventive lifestyle measures, such as regular exercise, stress management, and a good diet, are well accepted, as are some complementary therapies.

Nowadays doctors work in conjunction with other health providers. These include nurse practitioners and physician's assistants. These health professionals are not medical doctors, but they are licensed to provide primary care and to carry out certain procedures and tests, such as monitoring long-term conditions. They are becoming increasingly popular as a source of sound advice on problems that are not life-threatening, and will know when to advise you to consult a physician for further evaluation.

Physicians and other health providers also work with complementary or alternative therapists, such as naturopaths, aromatherapists, and reflexologists. Some medical centers offer a blend of orthodox and complementary medicine known as integrated health care. This allows doctors and complementary practitioners to work alongside each other and so provide access to a greater variety of healing skills and to in-depth knowledge of more specialized areas, such as nutrition and stress counseling. As communication and co-operation increase, the exchange of ideas can enrich both practitioners and patients.

Tell your doctor if you are undergoing other therapy at the same time as medical treatment, in case the two types of treatment might interact. See your doctor for:

■ Screening tests, routine checkups, immunizations, guidance on diet and lifestyle, and contraception.

■ Prenatal care.

■ Advice on ailments. See individual entries in this book for guidance on when to ask for help.

The natural remedy cabinet

On the following pages you will find lists of natural health products—food supplements, medicines, and basic equipment—that you may want to keep at home. Some of these items you may already have on hand; others you will have to buy. Resist the temptation to purchase large numbers of natural medicines. Most of these products have a limited shelf life, so keep only those supplements and remedies you will use every day and those that you think will be helpful for common ailments or first aid. Buy or make anything else only when you need it, so you won't have to discard expired products. Make sure that remedies remain clearly labeled and that implements are cleaned after each use. Purchase replacements before they are needed.

The uses described for the remedies in this section are for general reference only. Refer to the appropriate section in Part One of this book for cautions concerning each type of natural therapy. Check the appropriate entry in Part Two for more detailed guidance on using natural remedies for specific ailments.

Safe storage
Natural remedies should be kept in the same way as other kinds of medicines: in a cool place (or the refrigerator, when indicated) and away from children, sunlight, and humidity.

Vitamin, mineral, and other supplements

Keep your basic stock to a minimum. The following products are useful for many families:

- **Multiple vitamin and mineral supplement:** Particularly helpful if your eating habits are poor. Special vitamin and mineral supplements are available for certain times of life (as for pregnancy).
- **Borage (starflower) or evening primrose oil:** A good source of omega-6 fatty acids if your diet or digestion is poor. Also recommended if you suffer from premenstrual syndrome.
- **Fish-oil capsules:** An alternative source of fatty acids.
- **Vitamin C:** 500-milligram vitamin C tablets with flavonoids (as vitamin C complex or as separate items) can help at the first sign of a viral or bacterial infection, for inflammatory conditions, for daily use if you are a smoker, or if your diet is lacking in vitamin C.
- **Vitamin E:** Helps protect against heart disease; enhances the immune system; aids in skin healing. Especially good for people with circulatory disorders.

Flower essences

If you are frequently affected by mental or physical distress and you find that flower remedies help, stock those that most closely match your emotions. The following are good standbys for most people:

- **Olive:** For stress.
- **Rescue Remedy:** For emotional shock or physical trauma, such as may follow a fall or other injury.

Herbal remedies

Select those remedies that you consider appropriate for your family's needs. For safety concerns, see pp. 34–37.

- **Aloe vera gel:** For burns or to soothe irritated skin (use a leaf from a houseplant or a commercial preparation).
- **Arnica cream:** For bruises, sprains, and chilblains (distinct from the homeopathic cream of the same name).
- **Black cohosh or dong quai:** For menstrual and menopausal problems.
- **Chamomile leaves or teabags:** For anxiety; anxiety-provoked gas, nausea, indigestion, diarrhea, and sleep problems; itching; menstrual pain; and infections.
- **Comfrey ointment:** For sprains and strains when skin is not broken.
- **Cramp bark tincture or dried bark:** For menstrual pain and leg cramps.
- **Echinacea tincture:** For boosting resistance to infection and to counter allergic reactions and inflammation.
- **Elderberry extract:** For colds and influenza.
- **Elderflowers:** For fevers and allergic rhinitis.
- **Fennel seeds:** For gas and indigestion.
- **Ginger (dried):** For nausea, gas, and cold extremities.
- **Myrrh tincture:** For mouth ulcers, gum disease, and sore throat.
- **Slippery elm:** For indigestion and splinters.
- **Willow bark:** For inflammation.
- **Witch hazel liquid:** For cuts, scrapes, bruises, insect bites, varicose veins, and hemorrhoids.

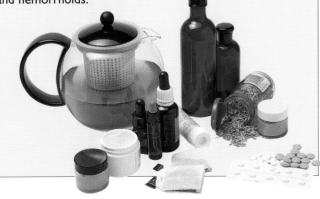

Aromatherapy oils

Select from the following list the essential oils that you think will be most useful. You will also need cold-pressed vegetable, nut, or seed oil for diluting essential oils other than lavender, tea tree, and clove (see p. 29).

- **Clove:** For toothache.
- **Eucalyptus:** For respiratory infections and fungal skin infections.
- **Lavender:** For burns, insect bites, cold sores, aching muscles, weakness, anxiety, headaches, depression, sleep problems, and splinters.
- **Peppermint:** For upper respiratory infections, fever, irritable bowel syndrome, and cuts and scrapes.
- **Roman chamomile:** For fever, insomnia, and inflammatory conditions.
- **Tea tree oil:** For bacterial and fungal skin infections, and vaginal yeast infections.

Homeopathic remedies

These remedies need to be selected according to the precise nature of your symptoms. However, the following are applicable to a wide range of conditions and are good to have on hand. Choose 12c potency (see "Less is More," p. 39) for remedies taken by mouth.

- **Aconite:** For sudden onset of high fever.
- **Arnica tablets or cream:** For bruising (the homeopathic cream is distinct from herbal arnica cream).
- **Belladonna:** For headache.
- **Coffea:** For insomnia.
- **Hypercal (St. John's wort and calendula):** As cream or topical solution for chilblains and other skin problems.
- **Ipecacuanha:** For nausea.
- **Ledum:** For puncture wounds.
- **Nux vomica:** For nausea.
- **Rhus toxicodendron:** For sprains and strains.

Useful items

- **Glass droppers:** For measuring essential oils.
- **Skin brush or loofah:** For boosting circulation if you have cold hands and feet or varicose veins.
- **Hot-water bottle or heatable pad:** For relieving muscle aches and abdominal cramps.
- **Thermometer:** For measuring temperature (the ear type is the most accurate and easy to use).
- **Ice pack:** For bruises and sprains.

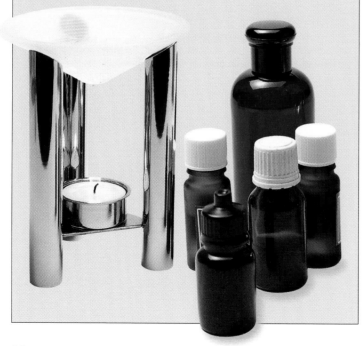

Kitchen cabinet basics

Many foods, herbs, and other products normally kept in the kitchen can also be used to treat common ailments. The following examples are helpful for a variety of illnesses. Check appropriate articles in Part Two for advice on correct usage.

- **Apple-cider vinegar:** For arthritis, colds, fungal skin infections, hair and scalp problems, indigestion, insect bites and stings, itching.
- **Baking soda:** For allergic skin reactions (including poison ivy), cuts and scrapes, gum disease, insect bites.
- **Carrots:** For appetite loss, coughs, weak nails, pinworms. As a broth, for dermatitis and dry or chapped skin (apply cooled carrot broth to the skin).
- **Bag of frozen peas:** To use as an ice pack.
- **Extra-virgin olive oil:** For diluting essential oils and for treating earwax, earache, dermatitis, indigestion, sore lips.
- **Garlic (fresh):** For cold hands and feet, earache, fungal skin infections, bacterial and viral infections, urinary-tract infections, pinworms, warts.

- **Ginger (fresh):** For colds, fever, indigestion, nausea, menstrual cramps, poor circulation (cold hands and feet).
- **Honey:** For colds, coughs, fever, allergic rhinitis, splinters (in a poultice), skin infections, and for sweetening herbal teas.
- **Lemons:** For corns, fever, indigestion, infections, sore throat.
- **Mustard seeds or powder:** For cold hands and feet and to make warming footbaths to treat colds.
- **Onions:** For upper respiratory-tract infections, gas, insect bites and stings, warts.
- **Prunes or figs:** For constipation.
- **Salt:** For diarrhea (to make a sugar-salt mixture, see p. 290), earache, gum disease, mouth ulcers, sore throat.

First-aid kit

Gather the following items for first aid and keep them all in one place, such as a suitably marked box or closet, so that you know where to find what you need in an emergency.

- **Sterile cotton:** For cleaning wounds.
- **Clean cotton fabric:** For making compresses.
- **Stretch bandages and safety pins:** For supporting sprained muscles.
- **Gauze bandages:** For holding dressings in place.
- **Surgical adhesive tape:** For securing gauze bandages or holding dressings in place.
- **Large triangular piece of cotton fabric:** For making a sling.
- **Nonadherent sterile dressings:** For cuts and burns.
- **Adhesive bandages:** For minor cuts and scrapes.
- **Scissors**
- **Eye bath:** For bathing irritated or infected eyes.

- **Sterile eye-pad with ties:** For eye injuries.
- **Tweezers:** For removing splinters, insect stingers, and ticks.

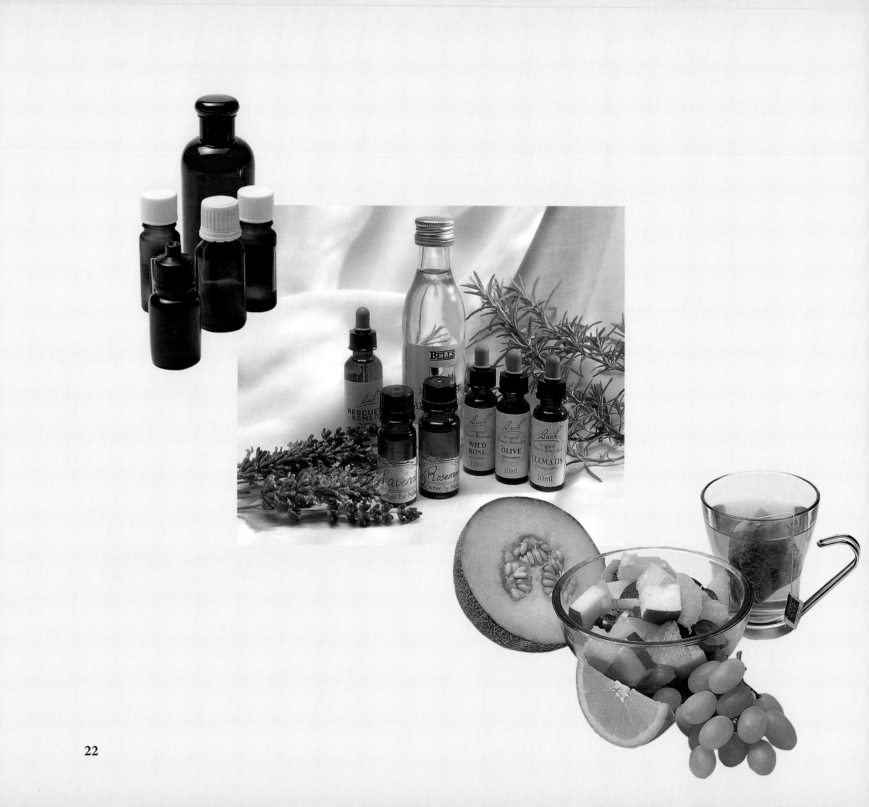

1 *The Therapies*

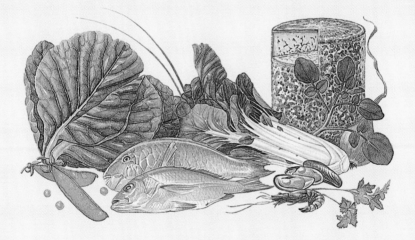

In this part of the book you will find information on the general principles behind a wide range of popular natural therapies. These remedies may serve as a gentle adjunct to the treatment and advice provided by your doctor and other health-care professionals. However, before using any of the therapies at home or consulting a natural therapist, be sure to familiarize yourself with the basic techniques and, above all, take note of any special precautions.

ACUPRESSURE AND SHIATSU

These two therapies are based on the theory that a form of energy flows through the body along channels called meridians. Pressing key points on the meridians is believed to regulate the flow of energy, thereby improving health. Acupressure is the technique for applying pressure to these points. Shiatsu uses acupressure together with a range of other methods to affect the energy flow.

Acupressure has its roots in ancient Chinese medicine, which views the health of the body in terms of the level and flow of energy along the meridians, said to run up and down the body from head to toe. In Chinese medicine, this vital energy is called *qi* (pronounced "chee" and sometimes written "chi"). Imbalances or blockages in the flow of qi around the body are said to lead to ill health, so Chinese physicians may treat disease by regulating the flow of qi. One way in which they do this is by pressing on certain points on the body where the meridians are said to come close to the skin. Pressing on these points is believed to strengthen or disperse qi, according to the condition being treated and the type of pressure used.

Palm pressure
With shiatsu, before working specific points, you may move along the limbs, pressing with your whole hand.

Practitioners in China have been working with pressure points for thousands of years, using acupuncture (see p. 58) as well as acupressure to affect the flow of qi. During the sixth century, Buddhist monks took this form of therapy to Japan, where it also became popular. Much more recently, in the 1920s, Japanese physicians developed shiatsu, a therapy that combines finger pressure on the pressure points (known by shiatsu practitioners as *tsubos*) with such techniques as palm pressure and muscle stretches.

CONSULTING A PROFESSIONAL

A professional shiatsu or acupressure practitioner will first assess your state of health. Besides examining you and asking you questions about your medical history, lifestyle, and diet, he or she will study your muscle and skin tone and listen to your voice and breathing.

For treatment, you usually lie on a mat on the floor. The therapist will apply pressure to certain points on your body and may also perform massage or muscle stretches. As the therapist works, he or she uses the sense of touch to

Meridians and pressure points

The meridians are invisible pathways along which energy is said to flow around the body. Pressing points along them is thought to regulate energy. There are corresponding meridians and therefore acupressure points on both sides of the body (right). The illustrations at right show points on one side of the body. Two meridians, called the Governing and Conception Vessels, lie along the body's midline.

Although practitioners work with several hundred points, the figures here show only the main points used in this book. Their technical names are included so that you can relate them to the instructions given for specific ailments. While some points have Chinese names, most consist simply of a letter or letters, which refer to the organ or system that the point is thought to affect, and a number indicating its position on the meridian. In Chinese medicine the functions of the organs are viewed very differently from the way they are in Western medicine. For example, the point LI (Large Intestine) 4 is used not only to regulate the intestine, but also to treat headaches, colds, and sinus trouble. The Heart Protector, linked to the pericardium, has a wide influence on all the chest organs. The Triple Heater is an "organ" that has a function— distributing energy—but no physical form.

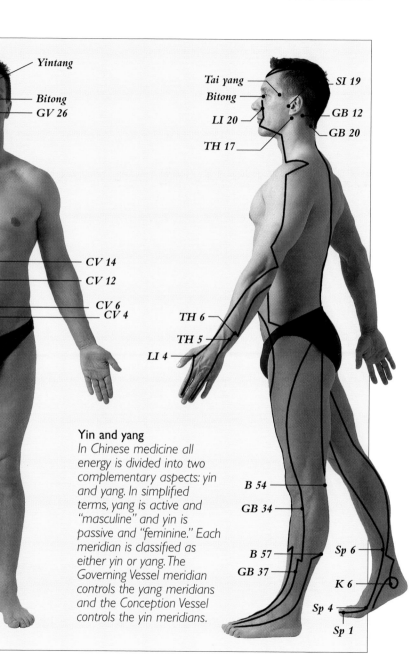

Yin and yang

In Chinese medicine all energy is divided into two complementary aspects: yin and yang. In simplified terms, yang is active and "masculine" and yin is passive and "feminine." Each meridian is classified as either yin or yang. The Governing Vessel meridian controls the yang meridians and the Conception Vessel controls the yin meridians.

Key			
B	= **Bladder**	**K**	= **Kidney**
CV	= **Conception Vessel**	**Liv**	= **Liver**
GB	= **Gallbladder**	**LI**	= **Large Intestine**
GV	= **Governing Vessel**	**SI**	= **Small Intestine**
H	= **Heart**	**Sp**	= **Spleen**
HP	= **Heart Protector**	**St**	= **Stomach**
		TH	= **Triple Heater**

"read" your body, finding out more about the flow of energy and how it is affecting your health. Most people feel both refreshed and relaxed at the end of such a session. However, occasionally a patient may feel slightly worse before feeling better, with fatigue, headaches, or flulike symptoms. These symptoms, thought to be caused by the release of pent-up energy from the acupressure points, should not be severe or last longer than one or two days.

USING THE THERAPY AT HOME

Self-treatment with acupressure may provide relief from a variety of common ailments, but you can undertake a much wider range of treatments with the help of a partner.

To use acupressure effectively, you first need to find the required pressure point by carefully following the instructions given for the specific ailment. Then apply the correct type of pressure

---

Special precautions

Acupressure is generally safe, provided that the person who is giving the treatment is not too forceful. Do not use acupressure directly over inflamed, swollen, very tender, or recently injured areas; treat only points above or below such areas, or points on the opposite side of the body. Always consult your doctor first if you have a high fever or severe pain, if you have had an accident or injury and suspect that there might be broken bones or a concussion, or if you are unsure of the cause of your symptoms.

Pregnancy
With a pregnant woman, avoid strong downward pressure anywhere along the tops of the shoulders. The following acupressure points must not be treated during pregnancy, since it is believed that doing so may cause miscarriage:
- The point (LI 4) in the web between the thumb and index finger on the back of the hand.
- The point (Sp 6) four finger-widths above the inside ankle bone, just behind the tibia.
- All bladder (B) points below the chest and upper back (see p. 25).

Children and the elderly
Be careful if treating a child or an elderly person. The bones may be somewhat fragile, so press gently on points.

The right touch
The thumb is the perfect tool for acupressure. Use the rest of the hand to steady your thumb as you press.

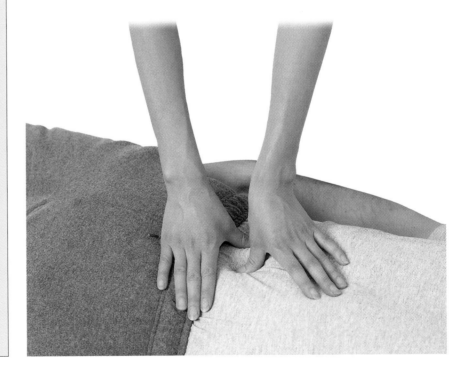

to the point. By using acupressure on yourself, you will learn what it feels like and how to provide the right amount of pressure. If you are ill, certain points may become tender, and pressure may make the point hurt a bit. However, any slight pain should ease after a few moments if you stay relaxed during your treatment. If a minor ailment is not better within two or three days following acupressure, or if your condition seems serious or worsens, consult your doctor.

TREATMENT BY A PARTNER

Lie on a blanket or a rug on the floor. Do not start until you feel comfortable—your treatments will be more effective if you are relaxed. Your partner should sit or kneel by your side and lean toward you, using his or her weight to apply gentle pressure to the appropriate points. The instructions that follow are for your partner.

Thumb technique: Use the pad of your thumb, which you should keep straight. Rest your extended fingers on an adjacent part of the person's body to give you support as you press.

- Feel for the pressure point, which is a hollow under the skin. Once you feel the bottom of the hollow, release your pressure slightly; this will encourage the qi to respond.
- Press firmly, but do not use too much force.
- Use the rhythm of your breathing to time the treatment. As you press, count two or three breaths before gently releasing and then repeating the pressure for two or three more breaths.
- Press and release several times for each point, remaining aware of your own breath to help you maintain the rhythm and to keep relaxed.

Self-treatment techniques

If you are treating yourself, sit in an upright chair or on pillows. Do not start until you feel comfortable, and make especially sure that the part of the body you are working on is well supported and relaxed. Do not lean your head too close to the area on which you are working. Work at arm's length, with your thumb held straight, so that it feels like an extension of your arm. To work on your arm, rest the hand of that arm on your lap. If you are working on your head or face, practice letting the weight of your head relax down onto your fingertips rather than applying pressure upward or inward with your arm. It may help to rest your elbows on a table when you are treating yourself in this way.

Types of pressure: You can use three types of pressure, to regulate the flow of energy in different ways. "Tonifying" stimulates a weak flow of energy; "dispersing" releases blocked energy, restoring the flow along the meridian; "calming" slows down the flow of overactive energy.

- To tonify, keep your thumb stationary as you press, and hold the pressure steadily for about two minutes.
- To disperse energy, move your thumb in a circular motion as you press. Continue for about two minutes.
- For a calming effect, cover the point with your palm or stroke the point gently for about two minutes.

AROMATHERAPY

Each plant contains a unique combination of oils in its roots, stems, leaves, seeds, and flowers that is known as its essential oil. The essential oils of selected plants are used in aromatherapy to foster balance and harmony of the body, mind, and spirit. Their therapeutic benefit may result from their effect on hormones and other chemical messengers in the body and brain.

The use of essential oils goes back to at least 4500 B.C., when the Egyptians created perfumes and medicines from them. The Egyptians linked perfumery to religion, assigning a particular fragrance to each of their many deities. Their priests also included essential oils in the embalming process, and traces of these substances can still be detected on 3,000-year-old mummies.

This ancient knowledge was preserved by Greek, Roman, and Arab physicians, whose work was influential for centuries. Even as recently as the 18th century, essential oils were widely used in medicines. But by the late 19th century, many of these extracts could be produced synthetically. This was a cheaper, easier process than obtaining these substances from plants, and the use of natural medicines began to decline.

Modern aromatherapy began with the work of the French chemist René-Maurice Gattefossé, who discovered the healing properties of lavender oil in the 1920s. This encouraged him to investigate the antiseptic properties of essential oils, and in 1937 he published the first modern book on aromatherapy.

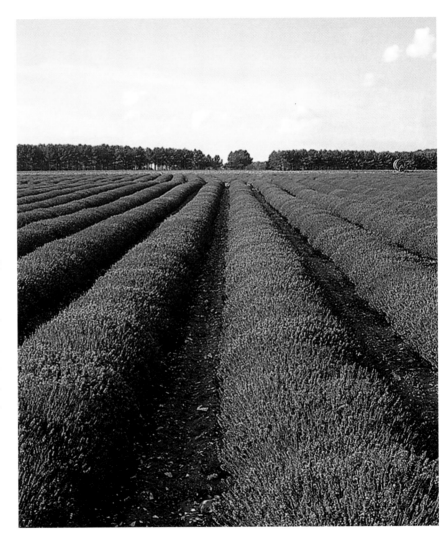

Fields of flowers
Lavender (right), which contains the first essential oil to be investigated in modern times, is grown abundantly in the south of France.

CONSULTING A PROFESSIONAL

An aromatherapist will begin by asking you about your health, your stress levels, and your current mood. There will also be questions about any other remedies you are taking, since the action of certain medicines, especially homeopathic treatments, may be affected by the powerful smell of many aromatherapy oils.

When the aromatherapist has chosen the best oils for you, he or she will decide how to administer the treatment. There are several ways in which a professional therapist can do this, but the most common form of treatment is to give a relaxing, full-body massage with the oils.

After the massage, you will have some time to relax quietly. The therapist may advise you not to bathe for several hours after the massage, so that all the oil is absorbed into your body. You may then be given some oils for home use. The full session, including both consultation and massage, will probably last between 60 and 90 minutes.

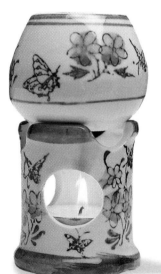

Relaxing fragrance
A vaporizer offers a means of releasing essential oils into the atmosphere. Place a few drops of oil in the water-filled top section and light the candle beneath (don't leave unattended).

Basic mixing of lotions and oils

Before using an essential oil for massage or bathing, you should dilute the oil in a suitable substance, known as a carrier. For massage, use a good quality, cold-pressed plant oil, such as sweet-almond, grapeseed, or sunflower oil, as a carrier. For bathing, mix the oils in an unscented white lotion or bubble bath base and then add the mixture to the water. Mix the oils and carrier in the proportions shown below. Do not add more than the specified amount of essential oil; it will not increase the benefit.

Standard mix for bathing	30 drops of essential oil in 20 teaspoons of carrier
Bathing mix for the young, elderly, and those in poor health	16 drops of essential oil in 20 teaspoons of carrier
Bathing mix for babies under 2 years old	8 drops of essential oil in 20 teaspoons of carrier
Massage oil	8–12 drops of essential oil in 6–8 teaspoons of carrier

---

USING THIS THERAPY AT HOME

It is important to obtain a reliable medical diagnosis before using aromatherapy to treat symptoms for which you would normally consult your doctor. Essential oils are widely available, and such treatments as inhalation, massage, and bathing are simple to carry out at home. But the oils will be effective only if they have been extracted carefully and stored correctly.

The best oils are sold in dark glass bottles with labels showing the Latin name of the plant, instructions for use, and precautions listed clearly. Quality oils are usually labeled "true" or "pure" essential oil, and are produced by steam distillation or expression from natural, usually organic, plant material.

Buy from a reputable source (ask an aromatherapist for advice) and keep your oils in a cool place in tightly sealed, dark glass bottles. Choose the oils you need by listing those that are effective for your particular ailments and then selecting the most appropriate. Before using an essential oil for massage or bathing, you should dilute it in a suitable substance, known as a carrier (see box, page 29). Mix the oils and carrier oil or lotion in the proportions recommended. You can prepare enough for several uses in advance. If the oil or blend of oils you have chosen does not improve your condition, consider consulting a suitably qualified therapist for advice.

Inhaling: This is the quickest way to get an essential oil into the bloodstream. There are two simple ways of inhaling oils:
- Place a few drops of the volatile oil on a tissue, put the tissue to your nose, and inhale.
- Add one or two drops of essential oil to a bowl of hot water, place a towel around your head and over the bowl, and inhale the vapor for up to five minutes.

You can repeat either treatment up to three times daily, as required. Or use your chosen oils in a vaporizer (see photograph, p. 29). Be aware, however, that this method provides a less concentrated dose and is therefore more suitable for mild mood-lifting or soothing effects.

Bathing: Soaking in water to which you have added essential oils is one of the simplest ways of absorbing oils into your body.
- Use about 10 teaspoons of carrier to which you have added essential oils in the proportions recommended in the box on page 29. (If you add oils to a bath without a carrier, they will float on the top of the water and the therapeutic benefits may be reduced.)
- Swirl the water around so that the oil disperses.
- Close the door and windows and relax in the bath for 10 minutes.

Special precautions

Although pure essential oils can help skin problems and can be absorbed into the bloodstream to spread their benefits around the body, some synthetic oils may cause skin reactions or trigger asthma attacks. Use the purest essential oils available to ensure maximum benefit and reduce risks.

If you have sensitive skin, epilepsy, high blood pressure, or have recently had an operation, you should consult a qualified practitioner before using essential oils.

If you are or might be pregnant, you should avoid certain essential oils, such as those listed below. If in doubt, consult a qualified aromatherapist.

Oils to be avoided in the first 20 weeks of pregnancy

- Basil (Ocimum basilicum)
- Cajuput (Melaleuca leucadendron)
- Cedarwood (Cedrus atlantica)
- Clary sage (Salvia sclarea)
- Cypress (Cupressus sempervirens)
- Myrrh (Commiphora myrrha)
- Niaouli (Melaleuca viridiflora)
- Rosemary (Rosmarinus officinalis)

Oils to be avoided throughout pregnancy

- Angelica (Angelica archangelica)
- Aniseed (Pimpinella anisum)
- Camphor (Cinnamomum camphora)
- Caraway (Carum carvi)
- Clove (Eugenia caryophyllata)
- Cinnamon (Cinnamomum zeylanicum)
- Fennel (Foeniculum vulgare)
- Hyssop (Hyssopus officinalis)
- Juniper berry (Juniperus communis)
- Lemongrass (Cymbopogon citratus)
- Nutmeg (Myristica fragrans)
- Oregano (Origanum vulgare)
- Parsley (Petroselinum crispum)
- Pennyroyal (Mentha pulegium)
- Savory (Satureia montana)
- Tarragon (Artemisia dracunculus)
- Thyme, red (Thymus vulgaris, chemotype—or ct—thymol or carvacrol)

Popular aromatherapy oils

Oil	Possible benefits: mental	Possible benefits: physical
Eucalyptus *Eucalyptus globulus*	Promotes alertness; clears the mind	Helps fight colds and congestion; soothes dry coughs; combats skin infections, such as boils and pimples; reduces swellings and muscle aches and pains
Geranium *Pelargonium graveolens*	Helps reduce mental stress and anxiety	Tones and cleanses the skin; fights throat and mouth infections; stimulates the liver and cleanses the digestive system; helps the body remove waste products; combats fluid retention
Lavender *Lavandula officinalis*	Combats anxiety, stress, and depression	Stimulates renewal of skin cells; reduces skin inflammation; helps heal mouth ulcers; reduces bad breath and nausea
Peppermint *Mentha piperita*	Uplifting; useful in treatment of emotional shock	Helps reduce coughs and throat infections; soothes intestinal cramps and heartburn; alleviates motion sickness
Roman chamomile *Chamaemelum nobile*	Relaxing; reduces anxiety; often effective for calming children's tantrums	Helps clear acne, rashes, and skin inflammation; reduces muscle inflammation; stimulates appetite; combats diarrhea
Rosemary *Rosmarinus officinalis*	Stimulates the memory	Relieves indigestion and flatulence; helps circulation; alleviates muscular aches; cleanses and stimulates the skin; counters infection
Sandalwood *Santalum album*	Sedative and relaxing; good remedy for insomnia	Soothes throat irritation, bronchitis, and asthma; softens dry skin; combats dandruff; alleviates vomiting and diarrhea
Sweet marjoram *Origanum marjorana*	Calms and comforts in cases of grief, loneliness, and loss	Eases respiratory problems, such as bronchitis and asthma; helps relieve constipation; relaxes muscle cramps
Tea tree *Melaleuca alternifolia*	No special benefits	Works as antiseptic against bacterial infections, particularly of the skin; used for cleaning cuts and surface wounds

FLOWER ESSENCES

Made from the blossoms of plants and trees, flower essences are prepared in water and preserved in alcohol. They are used for their possible impact on the mind and the spirit, to reverse negative mental states and rebalance the emotions. Their gentle action—there are no known adverse effects—makes them an ideal complement to other treatments.

The first person to prepare flower essences was Dr. Edward Bach, a bacteriologist and pathologist working in Wales in the 1930s. Bach became convinced that human illnesses were often symptoms of basic imbalances in the personality and the emotional life. He believed that flowers had the power to ease mental stress, and he used intuition and self-testing to investigate the therapeutic effects of a variety of flowers. To begin with, he prepared a dozen flower essences and called them the "Twelve Healers"

Healing holly
A flower essence derived from this plant is said to counteract envy and hatred.

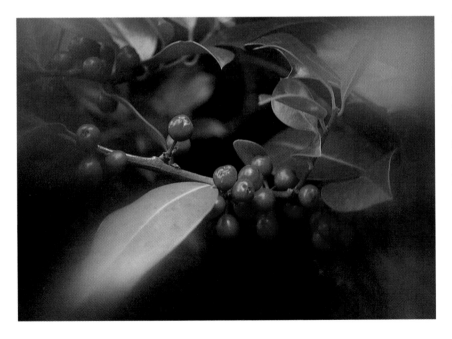

(see facing page). These were followed by another 26 remedies, making a total of 38. Each essence is said to help dissipate a particular unpleasant emotion, such as fear, impatience, or worry. Bach prepared his remedies as liquids so that they would be easy to mix together to create personalized treatments. In recent decades, people all over the world have borrowed Bach's ideas to make new flower-based preparations, adding further to the number of essences and combination remedies available for use.

CONSULTING A PROFESSIONAL

A practitioner will draw upon two kinds of flower essences to arrive at a personalized mix for a client. Those that describe someone's personality are known as "type" essences, while those that describe a mood are called "mood" or "helper" essences. The practitioner usually prescribes a blend that includes both kinds of essences. For example, a normally authoritarian person who is anxious about having to make a speech at a wedding might be given Vine as a type essence and Mimulus as a helper for his fear. Simple problems may require only one essence.

Flower-essence practitioners do not delve too deeply into the underlying causes of psychological states. Instead, troublesome emotions that have accumulated over years are resolved slowly, layer by layer. Most practitioners stick to what is

An all-purpose elixir

Dr. Edward Bach called his most famous flower essence the Rescue Remedy. This is a mix of five different essences selected to help people through crises and emergencies of all kinds. Take four drops in a glass of water, or put the drops straight onto your tongue if no water is readily available.

on the surface and give the essences time to work on a person's most obvious problems as they arise. Always seek your doctor's advice about any worrisome symptoms. More than most other therapies, flower essences are meant to be a complementary treatment. They do not take the place of conventional care for medical conditions, but rather are intended to help you deal with underlying emotional problems that may have caused or are complicating your current condition.

USING THIS THERAPY AT HOME

You can experiment with flower essences secure in the knowledge that selecting the wrong essence will not do you any harm. If you feel stuck, or if you have taken your own carefully selected essences for three weeks with no improvement, consult a professional.

When selecting flower essences for yourself, take the time to think about how you feel, and match your feelings to the essences. You can take up to seven essences at one time. If you intend to use flower essences on a regular basis, consider investing in a reference book that gives full details about each remedy.

Making a personal mixture

- Put two drops of each of your chosen essences into an empty one-fluid-ounce dropper bottle.
- Add a teaspoon of brandy and top off the bottle with uncarbonated mineral water. Use glycerin instead of brandy if you prefer to avoid alcohol.
- Take four drops four times a day, or more frequently if you feel the need.
- The treatment bottle will last two to three weeks if you take the essence regularly. When you have used it up, take a fresh look at your emotions. If you need to, make up another bottle with the same or different essences.
- For passing moods, simply add two drops of the essences you need to a glass of water, or drop the essence directly onto your tongue.

Special precautions

Flower essences are safe—even for babies and pregnant women. However, alcohol is generally used to preserve them. If this may be a problem, make your own with glycerin instead of alcohol or consult a qualified practitioner. The essences do not react with other medicines.

The Twelve Healers

Essence	Principal symptoms
Agrimony	Concealed anxiety
Centaury	Excessive desire to please, lack of assertiveness
Cerato	Doubting your own judgment and decision-making
Chicory	Excessive interference in the concerns of others
Clematis	Absent-mindedness, dreaminess
Gentian	Despondency
Impatiens	Impatience
Mimulus	Shyness, anxiety, everyday fears
Rock Rose	Terror
Scleranthus	Indecision, mood swings
Vervain	Extremes of energy and enthusiasm
Water Violet	Excessive self-sufficiency, aloofness

HERBAL MEDICINE

The use of plant remedies to strengthen weakened body systems, control symptoms, and boost the body's own healing powers is perhaps the oldest form of medicine. Herbalists maintain that the natural balance of compounds in plants provides a more effective means of restoring health than synthesized, single-ingredient drugs, as prescribed in orthodox modern medicine.

No one knows how or when people realized that plants could be used to treat disease, but herbal medicine probably developed from the use of plants as foods, partly by a system of trial and error, and partly from knowledge gained by people living close to nature that has been handed down through the generations.

Buying and using herbs safely

- Make sure that your ailment is diagnosed correctly before you use herbal medicines.
- Use only herbs specifically recommended in this book or by a doctor.
- Tell your doctor about any herbs you plan to take.
- Buy herbs from a well-established company. Choose a brand with an address and telephone number on the packaging, so that you can ask questions about the herb.
- Be aware that the U.S. Food and Drug Administration (FDA) prohibits manufacturers from making therapeutic claims for herbal products. However, the agency is currently working on ways to improve information to consumers.
- Avoid bulk herbs (sold loose) that may have been exposed to light and air for long periods.
- Choose products with evidence of quality control testing, especially the herbs standardized for one or more of the active ingredients.
- Be aware that herbal tinctures are often prepared in a base of water and alcohol. If you want to avoid alcohol, buy tinctures in a glycerin base.
- Bear in mind the shelf lives of different forms of herbs. Bulk herbs can last from three months (for leaves and flowers) to a year (for roots and bark); tinctures about a year; capsules and tablets one to two years.
- If you are interested in using herbal remedies on a regular basis, invest in a sound reference book that gives full information about specific herbs.

With the development of science, it became possible to isolate plant compounds and to find out which chemicals in a plant have particular actions. These chemicals were duplicated in laboratories to produce what we now regard as orthodox medicines. Work by medical researchers has given herbalists a wider understanding of why herbs have particular effects on the body. But this insight has not changed the way herbalists work.

Herbalists have always believed, and continue to believe, that using whole plants, which contain a huge variety of compounds, is the ideal way to help strengthen the body's healing powers and to help restore any imbalances within the body. Although a plant may be chosen primarily for the action of one ingredient, the other compounds in the plant—or in several plants in a combination remedy—may limit or enhance the main action, prevent side effects, or act in a generally nutritive way. Some herbal products contain several active compounds in an extract from the whole plant. Others contain only one or two compounds that have been isolated from the plant. A standardized extract contains known amounts of one or more active compounds.

CONSULTING A PROFESSIONAL

Herbal remedies can be used to treat many common ailments, as well as to enhance immunity

Special precautions

- Herbal remedies contain active constituents that can be harmful if taken in excess. Keep to recommended strengths and doses, and if in any doubt, consult a doctor familiar with herbal medicines.
- With remedies bought over the counter, keep to the dose recommended on the label.
- Do not take herbal remedies in combination with orthodox medicines without the approval of your physician.
- Always check with your doctor before taking herbal medicines if you are or might be pregnant or you are breast-feeding, if you have any medical condition, or if you are over 70 and in poor health.
- Do not give herbal medicines to children under 16 without first checking with your doctor. Expert advice is needed to determine the correct dosage.

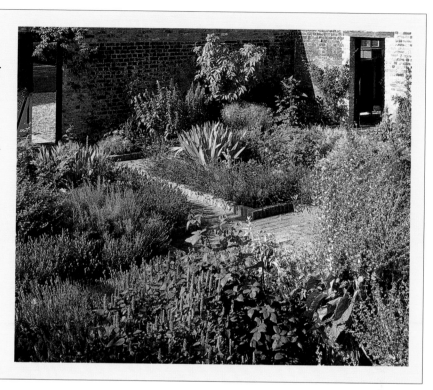

A healing garden
In times gone by, many hospitals, often run by religious orders, maintained their own herb gardens to ensure a constant supply of herbal medicines.

and energy. Although they are suitable for self-treatment of many minor conditions, it is often best to seek advice from a professional practitioner of herbal medicine (see "Special Precautions," above). Some fully qualified doctors (M.D.s) have also studied herbal medicine. Naturopathic doctors (N.D.s) are not medically qualified, but have undergone extensive training. You should make sure that any practitioner you consult has qualifications from the American Herbalists Guild.

When you visit an herbalist, he or she will ask about your medical history, paying especially close attention to your diet and lifestyle. If necessary, the therapist will perform a physical examination. Having assessed your condition, the herbalist then looks for the root cause of the problem, trying to find out where any imbalance in your health could have occurred. The practitioner believes that until this is addressed, the underlying problem will not be resolved, although it may be possible to alleviate or suppress the symptoms.

The herbalist will give dietary advice, suggesting changes that may help the patient better deal with the stresses of life. He or she may then

Strain well
Use a fine strainer to remove the coarse, woody pieces of plant material that remain after you have simmered an herb for a decoction.

recommend a blend of herbal remedies specially suited to your individual needs. The initial consultation usually takes about one hour. Subsequent sessions, when the herbalist may suggest adjustments, take about half an hour.

USING THIS THERAPY AT HOME

Medicinal herbs lend themselves well to home use, and many of them are easy and fun to grow in your backyard or window box. However, it is important to recognize that they *are* medicines —some can be taken safely in large amounts; others cannot. It is also very important to be certain, if collecting herbs yourself, that you collect the right plants. The best way is to learn this from an expert. Never consume an herb unless you are absolutely sure that you have identified it correctly.

Herbal remedies should generally be taken until symptoms disappear. If this does not happen within two weeks, if the condition worsens, or if any other unexpected effects occur, stop taking the preparation and seek medical help.

TAKING HERBS BY MOUTH

Many herbs are available from health-food stores as tablets, capsules, or tinctures (extracts in alcohol). Follow the dosage instructions on the package, starting with the lowest dose.

The traditional way to take herbs by mouth is in the form of teas. There are two kinds of herbal teas. The type of tea made with the flowers or leaves of a plant is called an infusion. It is made by pouring boiling water over the herb to release the active ingredients. The hard or woody parts of an herb, such as the roots, bark, seeds, or berries, need to be simmered in water for some time to bring out the healing constituents. This is known as a decoction. In Part Two of this book, the term *tea* has been used to describe both forms of preparation. Herbal teas may be drunk hot or cold.

Dosages for teas vary according to your age and health, but the usual amount for adults is one cup three times a day. Elderly people should take half this dose. Seek professional advice before giving herbs to children under 16 years old.

How to make an infusion: This type of herbal preparation is made rather like ordinary tea. You can make either a whole pot to provide several doses or a single cup for one dose.
- To make a pot, pour one pint of boiling water over one ounce of dried herb (or two ounces of fresh). Cover, and leave to infuse for 5 to 10 minutes. Strain, and pour into a cup.
- To make a single cup, put one teaspoon of dried herb (or two teaspoons of fresh) into a cup, pour on boiling water, and leave covered for five minutes. Strain, then use.

How to make a decoction: This type of herbal preparation is made by simmering hard plant material over low heat.

- Gently simmer one ounce of the herb in one pint of water for at least 15 minutes.
- Strain to remove the plant material.
- Some of the liquid will have evaporated, so add more water until you have one pint again.

USING HERBS EXTERNALLY

You can buy a wide variety of herbal creams, lotions, and other products for external use. These can be convenient when you need a remedy for immediate use, as for first aid. However, preparing your own can give greater control over the ingredients. Some herbal applications are not available commercially.

Herbal baths: These provide an easy and pleasant way of gaining benefit from herbs.

- Hang a calico bag containing the chosen dried or fresh herbs under the hot faucet when running the bath.
- Prepare an herbal hand or foot bath by adding a strong infusion or decoction of the herb(s) to a bowl of hot water. Soak your hands or feet in the mixture until the water cools.

Steam inhalations: You can use fresh or dried herbs. Make a strong infusion of the herb in a ceramic or glass bowl. Place your face over the bowl with a towel over your head, and breathe in the steam.

Compresses: Herbal compresses are helpful in the treatment of sprains and bruises, to cool fevers or inflammation, and to soothe headaches.

- Soak a clean cloth in a strong infusion or decoction (used hot or cold as recommended), or in a diluted tincture.
- After wringing excess liquid from the cloth, wrap it around the affected area.
- Repeat as necessary.

Poultices: Commonly used to draw pus from ulcers or boils, herbal poultices can also ease nerve or muscle pain. Make a poultice from fresh or dried herbs.

- Chop the herbs finely, cover with water, and heat to boiling.
- Put the resultant paste of hot herbs between two pieces of gauze, and apply to the affected area while still hot.
- Secure the poultice (see photograph, right).
- Use a hot-water bottle to keep the poultice warm.
- Replace the poultice when it has cooled.

Kept in place
Bind an herbal poultice to the affected area with a cotton bandage secured with tape or a safety pin.

37

HOMEOPATHY

The word homeopathy, *derived from the Greek, means "similar suffering." The therapy is based on the principle that "like cures like." Homeopaths believe that if a substance can produce the symptoms of illness when taken in a large dose, it has the potential to heal the same symptoms when taken in an infinitesimally small dose. And it does this without causing any harm.*

The concept of "like curing like" has been around for thousands of years, but the development of homeopathy as a medical system took place only relatively recently, with the work of the German doctor, chemist, and linguist Samuel Hahnemann (1755–1843).

With homeopathy, Hahnemann developed a system that embraces a natural form of healing that treats the whole person, not just the symptoms. He "proved," or tested, about 100 remedies, almost all of which are regularly used today. Many more remedies have been discovered since Hahnemann's time. Remedies are prepared from many sources (plants, minerals, even venoms) but are given in such small amounts that they are gentle and safe. The full name of a homeopathic remedy is usually the Latin for the plant or other source material, for example, *Arsenicum album*. However, most homeopaths use abbreviated forms, either the first word of the Latin name (the form used in this book)—in this example, Arsenicum—or a short form of both words—Ars. alb.

CONSULTING A PROFESSIONAL

The first time you visit a qualified practitioner, he or she will ask you about your medical history, lifestyle, diet, likes, dislikes, and personality, as well as your illness, to help determine your physical and emotional type. Hardly any physical examination is needed—the key is listening and understanding.

Homeopaths believe that, as a rule, people are self-healing, provided that they are properly fed and cared for. So a homeopath treats the symptoms of illness as signs that the body is fighting disease, and he or she will prescribe a remedy that, in a larger dose, would produce similar symptoms. The purpose of homeopathic treatment is to stimulate your powers of self-healing. The practitioner therefore usually seeks a remedy that suits you as a whole person, rather than one that simply addresses your symptoms, although symptomatic remedies are sometimes used. Generally, only one remedy at a time is prescribed. Shorter return visits, three or four weeks apart, are usually necessary.

It is advisable to seek out an expert practitioner if you have a long-term disease, if you are

Taking the remedy
Handle only the pill you are taking. You may find it easier to shake the pill onto a spoon first.

very worried by your illness, or if you have tried several remedies without success—all of these circumstances also necessitate seeing a medical doctor. When treating children or the elderly, it is a good idea to consult a professional first.

USING THE THERAPY AT HOME

Always obtain a medical diagnosis for symptoms for which you would normally seek your doctor's advice before attempting home treatment. Most homeopathic remedies are readily available, usually in the form of pills. For injuries, a topical cream, which you apply liberally and rub in gently, may be used. Choose homeopathic Arnica cream for bruises and Calendula (marigold) cream for minor cuts and sores.

Less is more

Turning a substance into a homeopathic remedy is a process called potentization. This involves alternately diluting and shaking the substance, often until no physical molecules of the original substance remain. Homeopaths believe that the more times this is carried out, the more powerful the remedy becomes. In other words, the more dilute the solution, the stronger its effect. Remedies are normally given a number and a letter—for example, 30c. This means that the process of diluting and shaking has been carried out 30 times, starting with a dilution of one part in 100 each time. For home use, the twelfth potency (12c) is ideal.

Constitutional remedies

When you visit a professional homeopath, he or she may seem just as interested in your medical history, character, and likes and dislikes as in your current illness. This is because the practitioner is trying to build up a picture of your whole nature, or constitution. He or she may then try to find a remedy that suits your constitution, rather than just your specific ailment. A constitutional remedy is often considered especially effective for a chronic condition, such as arthritis.

Throughout this book, you will find instructions on which remedies to use for particular ailments. But you should always bear in mind that, when prescribing, homeopaths take into account not only your symptoms but also your mood, personality, and constitutional type.

Taking homeopathic pills: The pills are sweet because they contain milk sugar (lactose).

- Dosage intervals vary from once an hour to once a day, according to your condition.
- Take the pills on a clean tongue, preferably allowing a 15-minute gap after meals or after cleaning your teeth.
- Some practitioners recommend that you avoid caffeine while you are having homeopathic treatments, as it may reduce their effectiveness.
- Suck the pill for about 30 seconds before chewing and swallowing.
- When your symptoms begin to subside, stop taking the remedy. If they return, start again. If there is no improvement in an acute illness within 24 hours, choose another remedy.

➤ continued, p. 40

Special precautions

Because homeopathic remedies are used in such minute dilutions, there is little chance of any harm arising from overprescribing. However, a remedy may cause a temporary worsening of symptoms before it starts to relieve them. Remedies from the twelfth (12c) to thirtieth (30c) potency are safe for people of all ages, including pregnant women. For babies and young children, crush each pill to a fine powder.

Common homeopathic remedies

This chart correlates symptoms with 18 of the most widely used homeopathic remedies (with alternative abbreviated names in parentheses). Refer to the appropriate article in Part Two of this book for advice on treating specific ailments.

Remedy	Origin	Symptoms
Aconite	The monkshood plant, *Aconitum napellus*	• High fever, often coming suddenly in the night • Extreme thirst and perspiration • Symptoms that may arise from a chill or fright • Dry coughs in children • Fear or extreme anxiety along with other symptoms
Apis	The honeybee, *Apis mellifica*	• Swelling in which the affected area is red and puffy or seems fluid-filled • Burning and stinging pains • Irritability and restlessness • Symptoms that are relieved by cool air or cold compresses
Arnica	A perennial herb of mountainous regions, *Arnica montana*	• Shock from injury • Muscle strain, jet lag, post-operative recovery • Bruising where skin is not broken
Arsenicum album (Ars. alb.)	Arsenic trioxide, a poisonous white powder that is safe in homeopathic doses	• Vomiting, diarrhea, abdominal and stomach cramps, such as might arise after food poisoning • Head colds with runny nose • Symptoms relieved by warmth and sips of cold water • Anxiety, chilliness, restlessness, and weakness along with symptoms
Belladonna	The deadly nightshade plant, *Atropa belladonna*	• High fever, perhaps with delirium, which comes on suddenly • Burning dry skin, red face, and little thirst with the fever • Throbbing pains, especially in the head area • Dilated pupils and oversensitivity to light
Bryonia (Bry.)	The bryony plant, *Bryonia alba*	• Slowly developing fever • Dry, painful coughs relieved by holding the chest • Extreme thirst for large amounts of cold water • Symptoms that are worse for slight motion • Irritability, desire to be left alone
Chamomilla (Cham.)	German or wild chamomile, *Matricaria chamomilla*	• Any illness, especially in children, that includes bad temper and irritability • Teething and colic, with irritability
Gelsemium (Gels.)	The yellow jasmine of North America, *Gelsemium sempervirens*	• Flu—with weak, achy muscles, tiredness, weakness, shivering, fever, little thirst • Anxiety that includes trembling

Remedy	Origin	Symptoms
Hepar sulphuris calcareum (Hepar sulph.)	A compound of calcium and sulfur made by heating oyster shells and calcium sulfide together	● Sore throat that feels as though something is stuck in your throat ● Harsh, dry cough with yellow mucus ● Boils and abscesses that will not heal ● Extreme irritability, coldness, and sour-smelling perspiration
Hypericum (Hyper.)	The European herb St. John's wort, *Hypericum perforatum*	● Bruising of very sensitive areas, such as fingers, toes, lips, ears, eyes, and coccyx ● Shooting pains along nerve pathways
Ignatia (Ign.)	St. Ignatius' bean, a tree that grows in China	● Sadness and grief following emotional loss ● "Locked-up" grief, in which the tears will not flow ● Mood swings
Ipecacuanha (Ipecac.)	The dried root of the South American shrub, *Cephaëlis ipecacuanha*	● Nausea and vomiting, whether or not accompanied by other symptoms, such as coughing, wheezing, headache, or diarrhea ● Morning sickness
Ledum (Led.)	The small shrub known as marsh tea, *Ledum palustre*	● Puncture wounds, as from splinters, nails, or stings, that look puffy and feel cold ● Pain eased by cold compresses ● Eye injuries that look puffy and bloodshot and that feel cold to touch
Mercurius (Merc.)	The metal mercury	● Swollen glands, coated tongue, profuse sweating, increased thirst ● Offensive breath and perspiration ● Feeling alternately hot and cold ● Irritability and restlessness along with other symptoms
Nux vomica (Nux vom.)	The poison nut tree, *Strychnos nux vomica,* native to eastern Asia	● Gastrointestinal upset, especially after a rich meal ● Undigested food lying like a weight in the stomach ● Feeling of nausea, but inability to vomit ● Feeling that bowel movements are incomplete ● Heartburn
Pulsatilla (Puls.)	The pasqueflower *Pulsatilla nigricans,* a member of the anemone family	● Conditions in which such emotional symptoms as weepiness, clinginess, and changeable moods predominate, especially in children ● Yellow-green discharges, as from nose or eyes ● Menstrual problems ● Symptoms that are helped by sympathy and hugs, as well as fresh, cool air
Rhus toxico-dendron (Rhus tox.)	The North American poison ivy	● Sprains and stiffness in the joints that are eased by gentle motion ● Symptoms that are better for warmth and worse for cold and damp, or are accompanied by extreme restlessness ● Red, itchy, painful rashes
Ruta	The herb rue, *Ruta graveolens*	● Bruises near the bones, as from a kick on the shin ● Strains to joints, especially ankles and wrists ● Symptoms that are better for warmth and worse for cold and damp ● Eyestrain from overwork

MASSAGE

The use of touch to promote a sense of physical and emotional well-being is one of the oldest of all natural therapies. Massage employs many different strokes that can stimulate or relax muscles, improve circulation, and encourage healing of a wide variety of complaints. It can be used in conjunction with aromatherapy to achieve a broad range of therapeutic benefits.

Touch is one of the most basic of the senses, experienced even by babies still in the uterus. Chinese physicians have made use of this knowledge for thousands of years. In China, massage is part of the system of traditional medicine that also includes acupuncture. The doctors of ancient Greece and Rome recommended massage, but the therapy disappeared from the West during the Middle Ages. Massage became popular again largely due to the work of a Swede, Per Henrik Ling, who developed Swedish movement treatment, also known as Swedish massage, in the early part of the 19th century.

During the 20th century, many types of massage have developed. Some derive from Ling's work; others are influenced by Chinese and Japanese medicine. They are all beneficial to the muscular system, relaxing tight muscles and toning loose ones. There are, in addition, more wide-reaching effects, because massage helps the circulation of the blood and lymph.

Gliding hands
Masseurs use a lubricating oil or lotion to help the hands move smoothly across the skin. One who is also familiar with aromatherapy will choose a blend of essential oils that is appropriate for your problem, warming the oil on the hands before rubbing it into your skin.

According to Chinese practitioners, massage also promotes the flow of vital energy, or *qi*, along a network of channels, or meridians, to all parts of the body, and so can be used in the treatment of many ailments. One specialized therapy, shiatsu, is based on a form of massage developed in Japan that works specifically on points where meridians (or energy channels) are thought to be near the surface of the skin. This is believed to regulate the flow of energy (see p. 24).

CONSULTING A PROFESSIONAL

When you make a call for a professional massage, you will probably be advised to avoid drinking alcohol on the day of the appointment and to abstain from eating for about two hours before the massage.

The massage itself will vary according to your problem. The therapist may concentrate on one area or work on your whole body. The treatment should not be painful, although stiff muscles may feel uncomfortable during massage. At the end of the session, the therapist may "ground" you by holding your feet for 20 seconds or so. You will then be given some time on your own to lie still.

After the massage, you may feel either relaxed or full of energy. Your muscles may be a little stiff for a while afterward, especially if they have been causing you pain. If muscle stiffness is likely, the therapist may advise you to lie for 30 minutes in

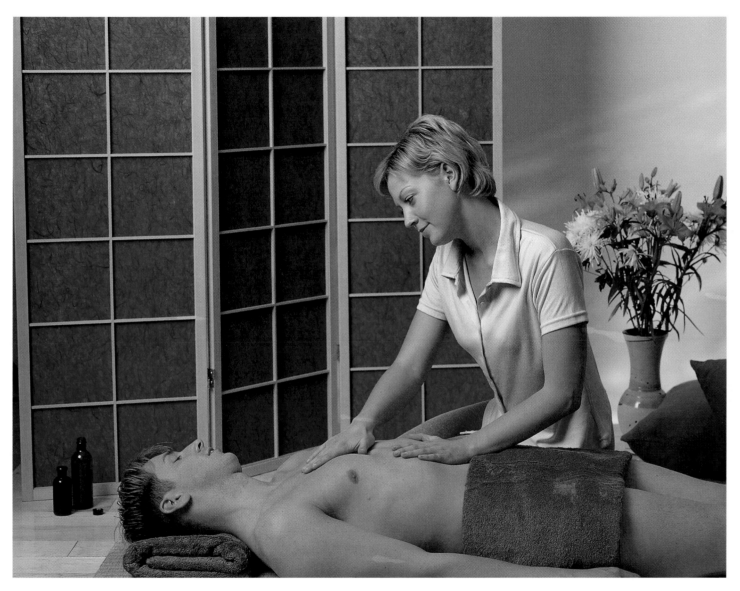

A healing experience
An effective massage depends on the sense of ease engendered by comfortable surroundings and trust in the masseur, as well as the technical expertise with which the strokes are carried out.

43

Strokes for folks: the basics of massage

There are three main massage strokes: effleurage, pettrissage, and friction. Use these to relax and tone the muscles. (Be sure your fingernails are trimmed before giving a massage.)

Effleurage

This gentle stroke is a good one to use at the beginning of a massage, because it helps you distribute the massage oil across the person's skin. It is a good stroke for general relaxation, but you can also use it for very sore muscles, since it stretches the muscle fibers.

- Hold your hands side by side, with the fingers together; your hands should be relaxed, but not limp.
- Glide your hands along the whole length of the muscles, moving toward the head; on this stroke, keep your palms and fingers in contact with the person's skin, letting your hands feel the contours of the body.
- Make a lighter return stroke, using only your fingertips.

Pettrissage

Use this kneading stroke after effleurage. The best places for pettrissage are the back, upper chest, legs, and buttocks. The stroke separates tight muscle fibers and helps rid muscles of waste products.

- With your fingers outstretched, put the heels of your hands in the middle of the area on which you are going to work.
- Push with the heel of each hand in turn. Press quite hard, but not so hard that you hurt the person.
- Do not use this stroke for too long on any one area.

Friction

Apply friction massage to a series of specific points or in any place on the back where the muscles are stiff. Use little or no oil; otherwise, you may slip away from the point you are massaging. The main direction of movement should be downward and circular. Avoid pressing directly on the spine.

- Slowly apply pressure to the point, using the pad of your thumb or index finger. Increase the pressure gradually.
- Rotate very slightly for about 10 to 15 seconds.
- Release the pressure very gradually.
- Repeat once or twice.
- Use effleurage to relax the muscles.

a warm bath when you get home. Towel yourself down briskly afterward.

USING THE THERAPY AT HOME

Massage is easy to perform. You can do some types on yourself—for example, on the hands, arms, legs, and shoulders. However, the result is generally better if you perform the massage, following the instructions in this book, on someone else and vice versa.

The only equipment you need to perform a massage is your hands. The kind of massage table used by a professional is helpful, but not necessary. The person can lie on a mattress or the floor, covering it with foam or a thick blanket and a large towel. When you are working on the shoulders, the person should sit on a stool and lean forward onto the back of an armchair.

Support: Depending on which part of the body you are working on, you may have to provide some additional support.
- If you are massaging someone's back and he or she is lying face down, place a pillow under the head and a rolled towel under the knees.
- If you are massaging the calves, support the ankles with a pillow.
- If you are working on the fronts of the legs, place a pillow under the knees.
- If you are massaging the back and shoulders of someone lying face down, put a pillow under the chest.

Oils and lotions: Many different massage oils are available. One of the best for general use is sweet almond oil, but you can also use any cream that is not highly scented and is not absorbed into the skin too quickly. If a person has very oily skin, use powder or cornstarch instead of oil.

Warmth: Massage is most effective in a relaxed atmosphere, so keep the room warm and quiet. For extra heat and comfort, keep the parts of the body not being massaged covered with a towel.

Pressure: Whichever kind of stroke you are using, this rule applies: the longer the stroke, the lighter it should be, and the shorter the stroke, the deeper it should be. Faster strokes are energizing, slower strokes more sedating. Different people feel comfortable with different levels of pressure, so be guided by the person you are massaging. At the same time, consider your own well-being. Leaning over to give a massage can strain your back, so adopt a comfortable position in which to work and stay as relaxed as you can.

Special precautions

- Do not have a massage if you have a fever.
- If you have recently had surgery, do not have a massage on or near the affected area.
- Do not have a massage if you have just eaten a meal or if you have drunk alcohol on the same day.
- Do not allow massage of bruised or inflamed areas, and avoid pressure on the backs of the knees or on bony areas.
- If you are or might be pregnant, permit only gentle strokes, and do not have massage on the lower back or abdomen. Consider consulting a masseur trained in pregnancy massage.
- If you are undergoing medical treatment, first ask your doctor whether it is safe to have massage.
- If you have unexplained pain, swelling, or illness, consult your doctor before trying a massage.

MEDITATION

The art of stilling the mind, or meditation, is a remarkably simple, straightforward technique. Many people find it easy to fit it into their daily lives. In recent years, an increasing number of scientific studies have recognized it as highly effective in treating a range of problems, both physical and psychological, that can result from stress or a low energy level.

Meditation helps you train your mind to filter out the unwanted distractions of life—the odd worries, concerns, and seemingly random images that spring to mind during the course of our everyday lives. Meditation techniques can induce a serene state, sometimes akin to deep sleep. Mind and body can relax fully, and many people find that just 20 minutes of meditation is as refreshing as several hours of sleep.

People in many parts of the world have been using various forms of meditation for millennia. The ancient yogis (yoga practitioners) described the practice as a powerful tonic that increases energy, rejuvenates cells, and holds back the ravages of time. Science is now confirming that meditation is a powerful healer. Researchers have found that it can help reduce the symptoms of high blood pressure, angina, allergies, diabetes, chronic headaches, and bronchial asthma; it can also help reduce dependence on alcohol and cigarettes. Those who meditate see their doctors less and spend 70 percent fewer days in the hospital. Anxiety and depression decrease, while memory improves. Meditation appears to give us more stamina, a happier disposition, and in some cases even better relationships.

JOINING A MEDITATION CLASS

The easiest way to start meditating is to join a class. There are classes available in all types of

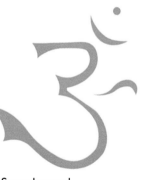

Sacred sound
The Hindu sacred syllable ohm, shown above as written in Sanskrit, is often used by practitioners of yoga and other Hindu-based forms of meditation as a "mantra," or sound on which to focus.

meditation. Also, many yoga teachers incorporate meditation into their work, using sound or breathing to focus the mind. You can even learn to chant—a form of sound meditation—choosing among Eastern mantras or Western forms, such as the Gregorian chant developed by medieval monks.

USING MEDITATION AT HOME

Meditation is very simple to practice. Find a quiet, warm place where you will not be disturbed. It is usually best to sit down, adopting whatever position you find comfortable. You may want to sit cross-legged, either directly on the floor or on a firm cushion, three to six inches thick. Or you may prefer to sit in a supportive, straight-backed chair, with your hands resting gently on your knees and your feet flat on the floor. It is not usually a good idea to meditate lying down, because you may fall asleep.

Basic meditation exercise: There are many different ways of meditating. Try this basic technique, which suits many people, first. If it does not suit you, consider the variations suggested on the facing page.
- Sit comfortably upright, so that you are alert but not tense.
- Keep your back straight, aligned with your head and neck, and relax your body.

- Breathe steadily and deeply. Concentrate on your breath as it flows in and out, and be aware of your abdomen falling and rising. Give your full attention to your breathing.
- If your attention starts to wander, gently bring your thoughts back to your breathing and to the rising and falling of your stomach.
- It is usual to keep eyes gently closed, to help you concentrate.
- Many people find it helpful to repeat a special word or sound, such as *ohm* (see illustration, facing page), the Hebrew word *shalom* (meaning "peace"), or another sound or phrase that has special meaning.
- Continue for about 20 minutes.
- Bring yourself slowly back to normal consciousness. Do not jump up quickly. Become aware of your surroundings; stretch gently. Stand up and move around, slowly at first.

Counting meditation: Sitting comfortably, slowly count from one to ten in your head, keeping your attention on each number. If you feel your attention wandering (as undoubtedly it will), simply go back to one and start again.

Candle meditation: Sit in front of a lighted candle. Focus your eyes on the flame and keep your attention there.

Visualization/imagery: A relaxation technique related to meditation, visualization, or guided imagery, can help focus your mind on positive images to overcome negative emotions and manage stress. Sit or lie in a relaxed position and focus on your breathing, as for the basic meditation exercise. Then conjure up a peaceful and happy scene in your mind, visualizing yourself as part of it. Maintain a steady breathing rhythm and use your imagination to fill in as many details as you can of this tranquil scene.

Special precautions

Meditation occasionally produces negative effects. For example, the act of stilling the mind can sometimes bring up old, repressed memories. If you are already seeing a therapist, you may want to consult him or her before beginning meditation. If you have any frightening or disturbing experiences as a result of meditation, consult a trained counselor or psychotherapist.

Position for meditation
The lotus and half-lotus yoga poses are popular for meditation because they provide a well-balanced, steady posture, but you should choose the position that is most comfortable for you.

47

NATUROPATHY

This system of medicine emphasizes the value of restoring and promoting the human body's own self-healing processes. Naturopaths use a wide range of natural treatments, the most important of which are dietary management, herbal remedies, and a variety of physical therapies, selected according to the individual needs of the patient.

Beginning with the earliest civilizations, healers have made careful observations of the body in sickness and in wellness and used natural resources—food, water, air, and herbs—to help in the healing process. In the 19th century, a group of doctors began to develop this way of treating people into the science of naturopathy. The movement began in Europe and involved fasts, dietary regimes, baths, sprays, and compresses. As word of their success spread, these techniques were refined; in the early 20th century, they were introduced to America.

The healing crisis

When you adopt a healthier lifestyle, eating more fresh natural foods, getting more exercise, and learning methods of relaxation, you may experience an improvement in general well-being. But after a few days or weeks, you may find that some of your old problems, such as colds or fatigue, return. Dr. Henry Lindlahr, the pioneering American naturopathic physician, called this worsening of symptoms the healing crisis. He viewed it as a sign of the body increasing its normal ability to deal with toxins, infections, and waste products as it gains vitality. The symptoms usually clear in a few days with the help of appropriate naturopathic treatments.

The naturopathic pioneers made many recommendations—such as the medicinal use of botanicals and the consumption of more fresh vegetables, fruits, and whole-grain cereals—that have been borne out by modern research. The diets they designed are intended to rest the body from unhealthy foods, which increase the burden on the digestive processes and the body's detoxification and elimination systems, and to substitute foods that are easily processed and that strengthen the immune system. Today's naturopaths also often use water treatments and physical therapies to help the skin, lungs, intestines, and kidneys eliminate waste products that might otherwise hamper the healthy functioning of the body. Cold-water therapies are considered especially beneficial for boosting the effectiveness of the immune system.

Life force
Most naturopathic physicians place emphasis on the therapeutic power of water, in the form of hot or cold baths, compresses, and spray treatments.

Special precautions

If you are elderly, frail, or chronically sick, you may need to build up your vitality before being able to cope with the acute symptoms of a healing crisis (see facing page). In this case, consult a naturopath before trying any treatments on your own. Do not undertake naturopathic treatments without first seeking medical advice if you have epilepsy, diabetes, anemia, unexplained weight loss, a psychiatric illness, or are pregnant or caring for a young child.

CONSULTING A PROFESSIONAL

The naturopath gives you a thorough examination and asks you questions about your health, diet, lifestyle, likes, and dislikes. The purpose is to find out about your level of vitality and general health, as much as to diagnose any disease.

The practitioner may use laboratory tests, such as measuring mineral levels in your sweat or hair, essential fatty acids in your blood, or stress hormones in your saliva. He or she may also test the working of organs, such as your liver or pancreas, and check the permeability (leakiness) of the intestines. This will help build up a picture of the underlying causes of such problems as allergies, digestive disorders, headaches, chronic fatigue, hormone imbalances, and skin diseases. The naturopath may then recommend dietary changes, nutritional supplements, herbal treatments, or preparations that supplement digestive enzymes, such as pancreatin. Some practitioners are also trained in homeopathy (see pp. 38–41) and may prescribe remedies of this type. Many naturopaths are also qualified in some form of

bodywork, such as osteopathy, and may use special soft-tissue massage techniques and gentle mobilization of joints—for example, to ease arthritic pain or improve breathing in people with asthma.

The practitioner may also prescribe some hydrotherapy treatments. Hydrotherapy involves a wide range of techniques that utilize water, from cold compresses to sitz baths (see below), showers, and sprays. These treatments are used for

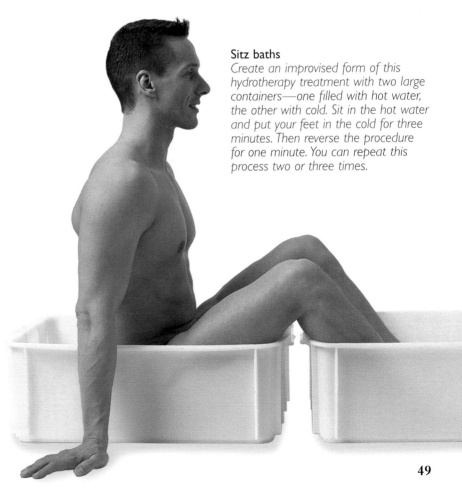

Sitz baths
Create an improvised form of this hydrotherapy treatment with two large containers—one filled with hot water, the other with cold. Sit in the hot water and put your feet in the cold for three minutes. Then reverse the procedure for one minute. You can repeat this process two or three times.

many disorders, from painful joints and menstrual problems to sore throats and feverish illnesses.

USING THE THERAPY AT HOME

Common ailments in people of any age respond very well to naturopathic medicine, and many of its treatments are easy to carry out at home. A major advantage of naturopathy is that its range of dietary and other remedies enables you to take more responsibility for your own health.

Naturopaths regard most acute symptoms—such as fevers, rashes, and diarrhea—as positive signs of the body's defenses at work (see box, p. 48). These symptoms generally need not be suppressed, but if you wish, you can help your body heal itself more quickly. Check the relevant article in Part Two for specific advice on treating a particular ailment.

Cold compress: Used to treat a wide variety of disorders, from joint strains and pains to headaches and bronchitis, cold compresses are generally applied to the affected area. Alternate hot and cold compresses are recommended for certain conditions (see Part Two). You will need a cotton handkerchief or piece of cloth for the compress itself; a towel, scarf, or bandage for the outer layer; and safety pins or bandage clips to keep the compress in place.

- Select a piece of compress fabric of appropriate size—for throat, knee, wrist, or ankle, use a handkerchief; for the abdomen or torso, use a sheet (see box, left).
- Soak the cloth in cold water, then wring it out and shake well.
- Fold the material lengthwise and apply to the appropriate area.
- Wrap the towel or other outer layer around the material and secure it in place with the safety pins or clips.
- Keep the compress on for up to three hours or overnight. It should warm up within about 10 minutes; if it remains cold, it may have been too

---

Body wrap

Use this treatment for colds and fevers. This type of compress should start to warm up within about 10 minutes. Test by putting your hand between the compress and the skin. If the compress is still cold, remove it and rub yourself vigorously with a dry towel.

1 Lay a towel on your bed or a mat on the floor. Place a folded sheet that has been wrung out in cold water over the towel, and lie on it.

2 Wrap the sheet around your abdomen, followed by the towel, and pin at the side.

wet, or your body may be too weak to respond satisfactorily, in which case the compress should be removed.

- When you take off the compress, sponge the area with cool or lukewarm water to remove any perspiration.
- You can use a similar technique to make a large compress to cover your waist or torso (see facing page).

Hot or lukewarm baths: For this type of treatment, you can add healing ingredients to your bathwater, such as:

- Two heaping tablespoons of Epsom salts (do not use if you have high blood pressure)
- One heaping tablespoon of baking soda
- Hayflowers (a bag of mixed, dried herbs, available from stores that stock herbs)
- Aromatherapy oils (see pp. 28–31)

Cleansing diets: These short-term diets can help your body rid itself of waste products and environmental toxins. They eschew highly processed foods, which place a burden on the digestive system, and instead focus on raw foods. Naturopaths use cleansing diets (see box) for acute illnesses—such as colds, flu, bronchitis, gastroenteritis (for which soups and steamed vegetables may need to be used in place of raw salads)—and inflammatory disorders, such as skin rashes. Individual variations may need to be determined by a naturopathic physician. You should always consult a professional practitioner before beginning a cleansing diet. Some diets are unsuitable for children, the elderly, or those in poor health.

Three-day cleansing diet

Healthy people of most ages can follow this simple regimen for a limited period, but check with a health professional first.

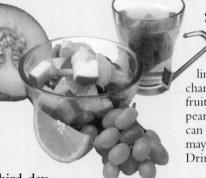

First day
Consume only pure fruit or vegetable juice. Use freshly extracted juices or canned or bottled unsweetened juices of apple, pear, grape, or pineapple (dilute 50 percent with water). Drink one glass four or five times daily. At other times drink pure spring water or boiled water with a teaspoon of lemon juice or apple-cider vinegar.

Second day
On rising and retiring or between meals, drink fruit juice or herbal tea (for example, lime tree flower, peppermint, chamomile). At meals eat fresh raw fruits (for example, grapes, apples, pears, peaches, melon, oranges). You can grate or cube hard fruits, and all may be mixed to make a fruit salad. Drink as much water as you like.

Third day
For breakfast have fresh or puréed fruit with goat's or sheep's milk yogurt with live cultures.

For lunch fix a raw salad with a selection of leafy and grated root vegetables. Garnish with raisins and sunflower seeds. Eat fresh fruit for dessert.

For dinner eat vegetable soup or steamed vegetables flavored with miso or soy sauce. Drink water when thirsty.

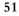

REFLEXOLOGY

This therapy is based on the theory that there are "reflex points" on the hands and feet that correspond to the organs, functions, and parts of the body. Applying pressure to these places is said to stimulate the flow of energy through the body, improve nerve function and blood supply, release tension, and encourage the organs of the body to work properly.

Reflexology has been practiced for millennia in Western Asia, Japan, and China. In Egypt, drawings in the tomb of Ankamahor at Saqqara—known as the Physician's Tomb—show the therapy being performed on the feet and hands. These pictures date back to 2330 B.C.

In the West, reflexology dates from the early 20th century. American physician William Fitzgerald described 10 channels of communication, running vertically through the body from the feet and hands to the brain. Fitzgerald found that he could anesthetize the face, head, and neck by means of pressure applied to the fingers. Fitzgerald's follower Eunice Ingham developed his work, performing reflexology on thousands of pairs of feet and finding out which parts of the feet correspond to which organs of the body.

Today foot reflexology is one of the most popular forms of complementary medicine, though its healing powers are not scientifically proven. Many people report it to be of benefit in a host of common everyday ailments—from sinusitis to irritable bowel syndrome, menstrual problems to back pain—and believe that it has powerful effects in relieving tension in the body.

CONSULTING A PROFESSIONAL
The reflexologist will work on each foot, paying special attention to areas that are tender or painful (this is believed to indicate a blockage of

Giving treatment

The person receiving treatment should be seated on a comfortable chair with the leg of the foot being treated supported on a stool or a large pillow. To administer the therapy, either kneel on the floor or sit on a low chair or stool. Work across the sole, front, and sides of the feet using your thumb or index finger. Because you are contacting tiny reflex points, move your thumb or finger forward slowly, using controlled, deep pressure. The forward movement should be like the creeping motion of a caterpillar.

The thumb technique
Use your thumb for the soles and sides of the feet. Wrap one hand around the toes and apply controlled, deep pressure using the inside edge of the thumb of the other hand. Bend the thumb joint slightly and "walk" the thumb forward by bending and straightening the joint.

The index finger technique
Use your index finger for the tops and sides of the feet. Press with the index finger, again "walking" it forward by alternately bending and unbending the first joint. Use your thumb and other three fingers for support.

Special precautions

Reflexology is generally safe for all age groups, but do not use it if the feet have open sores or signs of infection, inflammation, or athlete's foot. Also avoid reflexology if you have diabetes or varicose veins or if you are or might be pregnant.

energy in the corresponding part of the body). He or she will apply pressure to the relevant reflex points to free congestion and aid healing.

USING THIS THERAPY AT HOME

Be sure to seek medical advice for symptoms of unknown cause before trying reflexology. You can treat yourself, but practitioners believe that having someone else work on your reflex points greatly expands the range of benefits. If problems continue after treatment, consult your doctor.

The right position
The person giving reflexology supports the heel in his free hand while working on the underside of the foot.

Reflexology foot maps

The reflexes on the left and right soles are similar, with points for many parts of the body appearing on both feet (indicated with an asterisk in the illustration below). But some organs have points on one sole only, usually reflecting the side of the body on which the organ is situated.

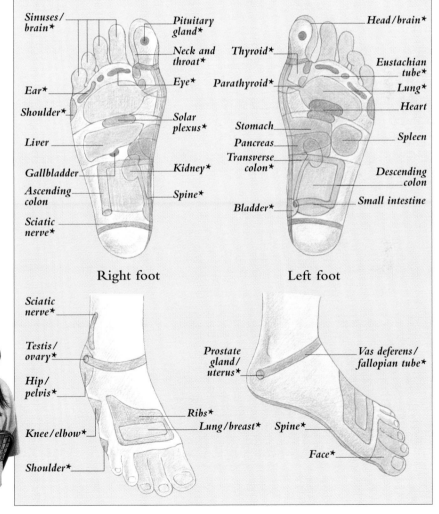

Right foot

Left foot

YOGA

The ancient Indian tradition of yoga involves a wide variety of mind-body exercises, ranging from postural and breathing exercises to deep relaxation and meditation. Yoga therapy tailors these exercises to the needs of individuals with health problems. Besides helping particular disorders, regular yoga practice also boosts energy levels and improves all-round well-being.

Yoga therapy springs from the rich, age-old tradition of yoga, which emerged on the Indian subcontinent thousands of years ago. The philosophy behind yoga encompasses every level of existence, from the physical to the spiritual. However, it is possible to work with only the aspects that appeal to you. Some people seek improvements to their physical and mental health, others something more.

Indian physicians have long relied on yoga. But today's yoga therapy, pioneered by Swami Kuvalayananda in Bombay during the early 1920s, is a relatively new discipline, marrying traditional yoga and modern medicine. In the decades following its inception, the therapy spread to other parts of India. Today, many of the country's yoga therapy clinics are associated with hospitals.

In the West, psychologists and doctors now widely use relaxation techniques derived from

Ultimate relaxation
The Sanskrit name for the yoga position shown below is savasana, meaning "corpse pose." It provides physical stillness, which encourages mental peace. Lie down on your back. Place your feet a little apart, allowing them to roll outward. Rest your arms, hands palms-up, away from your sides. Close your eyes and feel tension ebb away.

Breathing awareness

Breathing is one of the few bodily processes that are governed by both the central and autonomic nervous systems. In other words, it is controlled automatically, so that you can continously breathe without thinking about it, but you can also intervene consciously in your breathing patterns. This provides a very important link between mind and body. Yoga uses exercises to correct poor breathing patterns, which can have profound effects on general health and on particular disorders, such as asthma and anxiety. Try the following basic breathing exercise:

1 Lie down in the corpse pose (see photograph), with folded blankets placed under your head and back.

2 Close your eyes, but keep your gaze turned downward toward your chest. Relax and notice how your breathing slows.

3 Be aware of your breath entering and leaving your body. Notice the changing temperature of the air and feel how it passes into your body.

4 Listen to the soft sounds of your breathing. Notice the differences between the inhalation and the exhalation.

yoga for the treatment of anxiety and stress. They are also beginning to recognize the value of yoga's postural, breathing, relaxation, and meditation exercises for the treatment of many other common conditions, such as arthritis, heart disease, high blood pressure, migraine, obesity, and premenstrual syndrome.

CONSULTING A PROFESSIONAL

A yoga therapist assesses your health problems together with your constitution, lifestyle, stress level, and other general health factors. He or she then selects yoga techniques that are most suited to your condition and teaches them to you either individually or in a small, specialized class. At the same time, the therapist devises a yoga session for your daily practice at home. He or she will revise this regimen as your skills develop and your condition responds.

Because yoga therapy seeks to establish harmony between mind, body, and spirit, your regimen should include a balanced set of practices that calm and vitalize you both mentally and physically, as well as working on specific ailments. The yoga techniques used in therapy work are often surprisingly simple, and a skilled therapist will be able to devise a program that you can start to put into practice without difficulty, whatever your condition.

USING THE THERAPY AT HOME

Yoga's effectiveness depends on frequent, regular practice, even if only for a short period each day. You should therefore develop a yoga routine that suits your lifestyle as well as your particular health problems. This basic yoga session should not be

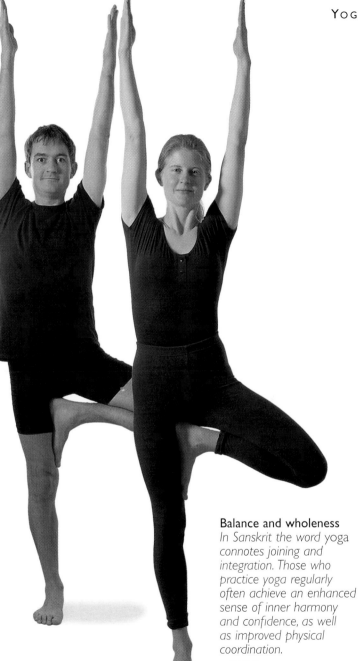

Balance and wholeness
In Sanskrit the word yoga *connotes joining and integration. Those who practice yoga regularly often achieve an enhanced sense of inner harmony and confidence, as well as improved physical coordination.*

too long, so that you can easily integrate it into your daily life.

The best way to create your yoga program is to consult a qualified yoga therapist, or a yoga teacher if no therapist is available locally. Books and videos can help you to learn yoga, but they are no substitute for a good teacher. There are many subtle aspects of yoga practice that cannot be adequately learned without an expert to observe and advise you. Specific postures to address specific health needs are even more helpful when integrated into a structured session of yoga exercises, which may include a variety of postures, breathing exercises, and relaxation and meditation techniques.

Practice tips
- Find a quiet place in an uncluttered, well-ventilated room.
- Wear nonrestrictive clothing, and place a nonslip mat or a blanket on the floor to make yourself more comfortable.
- Use folded blankets as padding for your head and back when doing postures that require lying down.
- Avoid bright lights, distractions, and interruptions.

Serene moments
One of the goals of yoga is to allow life energy, or prana, to flow freely through body and mind.

- Establish a regular time for your session before breakfast, lunch, or dinner. If this is not possible, do your yoga practice at least one hour after a snack or three and a half hours after a main meal.

Although such mild ailments as aching shoulders may be resolved by just a few minutes of daily practice, more entrenched conditions, such as asthma, usually require longer sessions. You may have to continue these for many months. However, even short-term practice will often yield significant improvements.

Postures: Yoga positions (or *asanas*) work to relax, strengthen, and vitalize every part of your body. They often target the spine, bending it forward, backward, and sideways, and rotating it in both directions. They work the body's joints through their full range of motion, thus helping to maintain flexibility. And they improve breathing by releasing tension in the muscles of the rib cage. Because of the close interrelation between body and mind, these actions on the body also affect the mind, helping to reduce the effects of stress and emotional discord.

Relaxation: Deep relaxation can dispel states of stress and fatigue within minutes. It can also benefit a wide range of disorders, such as migraine and irritable

bowel syndrome, that may be triggered by the release of chemicals in the body in response to anxiety. Yoga relaxation is usually carried out lying motionless on your back (see p. 54). A variety of techniques are used. In most cases these involve focusing your awareness on parts of the body, on your breathing, or on mental images.

Meditation, a technique related to yoga, involves slowing down your thoughts and enhancing awareness (see p. 46).

Special precautions

You should always practice yoga in a gentle manner. It should not cause pain or discomfort. When practiced in this way, yoga is very safe. However, there are a number of ailments for which particular yoga postures may be unsuitable or even dangerous. When in doubt, consult your doctor. Examples of these conditions are listed below.

- **Abdominal hernia:** Avoid postures (for example, prone postures) that increase pressure in the abdomen.
- **Arthritis:** Avoid exercising inflamed joints.
- **Back or neck pain:** Avoid any posture that increases the pain, either during the yoga session or afterward.
- **Chronic bronchitis and emphysema:** Avoid strenuous exercises.
- **Depression:** Deep relaxation and meditation can help in some cases but may exacerbate the condition in others.
- **Epilepsy:** Avoid breathing techniques that may increase the aeration of the lungs, for example, rapid abdominal breathing or deep breathing, unless practiced under expert supervision.
- **High blood pressure (hypertension):** Avoid inverted postures, strenuous exercises, and any exercise involving breath-holding.
- **Heart disease:** Seek advice from a qualified yoga therapist.
- **Obesity:** Avoid inverted postures and the plow.

Using a mat
A yoga mat provides a safe, non-slip surface on which to practice. Ask your teacher for advice on where to buy one.

GLOSSARY OF THERAPIES

This glossary lists the most popular natural therapies that cannot generally be undertaken without the help of an expert therapist. (For advice on finding a suitable therapist, see p. 17.) They vary widely in their acceptance by orthodox doctors, so each therapy is given a star rating as a rough guide to how it is valued by the medical profession.

> ### Medical Rating Key
>
> Very high ★★★★   Average ★★
> High ★★★   Low ★

ACUPUNCTURE ★★★★

Part of the system of traditional Chinese medicine, acupuncture aims to restore the body to a state of health and balance by regulating the flow of energy (known as *qi*, pronounced "chee") along a series of lines, called meridians, that are believed to run through the body. Acupuncturists do this mainly by inserting fine needles into the skin at certain points on the meridians. Each point is thought to affect a particular organ or function. Acupuncturists claim to be able to

> ### Auricular therapy
>
> In this branch of acupuncture, needles are inserted into points on the ear. Therapists see the ear as a mirror of the whole body, with acupuncture points relating to each organ and function. Some therapists also use light, small electrical charges, or magnetic ball bearings to stimulate the points.

treat a wide variety of diseases, including anxiety and depression, musculoskeletal problems, high blood pressure and circulation problems, menstrual and menopausal symptoms, headaches, allergic rhinitis, and back pain.

Professional consultation

On your first visit, the therapist takes a detailed medical history and asks you questions about your lifestyle. He or she examines your tongue and skin tone and takes your 12 meridian pulses—6 on each wrist. Most people need further visits, the number depending on the particular problem.

The most common form of treatment is insertion of needles. This is usually painless, although you may feel a slight tingle. The needles are left in place for a time ranging from a few minutes to a half hour. You may also be given other treatments, such as acupressure (see pp. 24–27) and moxibustion (the burning of an herb called moxa over an acupuncture point).

ALEXANDER TECHNIQUE ★★★

The aim of Alexander technique is to improve your posture and the way you move and carry out everyday actions in order to reduce effort and muscle tension and improve overall health. The technique was devised by an Australian actor, Frederick Matthias Alexander (1869–1955).

Professional consultation

When you begin a series of Alexander lessons, the teacher assesses the way you stand, sit, and move. He or she then uses gentle manipulation to show you what your best posture and body movements feel like.

You are also told how to encourage good posture and movement and how to discourage tension between lessons.

Many Alexander students feel better after their first lesson, but most need about 25 lessons before they achieve lasting results. Teachers have reported benefits to people who suffer from a range of disorders, including digestive problems, heart and circulation disorders, breathing difficulties, gynecological conditions, and back pain.

ANTHROPOSOPHICAL MEDICINE ★★

This form of medicine relies on the theory that each person has four systems that must be kept in balance: the physical body, the astral body (said to control the senses and emotional life), the etheric body (responsible for growth), and the ego (a person's consciousness of self).

Anthroposophical physicians are qualified in orthodox medicine but prefer to draw on a range of treatments, including herbal and homeopathic medicines, massage, and creative therapies, whenever possible. With this broad approach, anthroposophical medicine claims to be able to deal with all types of ailments.

AUTOGENIC TRAINING ★★★

This system provides a highly effective way of relaxing and of surviving stress. It can help prevent stress-related illnesses of many kinds, as well as being beneficial in treating different types of addiction.

A qualified practitioner leads you through exercises designed to induce different physiological states that bring about relaxation. These states include feelings of warmth, sensations of heaviness, concentration on the

heartbeat, calm breathing, and sensations of cold on the forehead.

AYURVEDIC MEDICINE ★★★

The traditional Indian form of healing is called Ayurvedic medicine. Its basic premise is that health depends on a balance between the five basic elements, known as the *doshas*, each of which governs five body systems: ether (networks and channels within the body), earth (solid parts, such as bones), water (soft tissue and fluids), fire (the digestive system), air (the nervous system and senses). The energy (*prana*) that connects them is also very important.

Professional consultation

The therapist aims to find out about as many as possible of the factors that can affect your health, from your lifestyle and medical history to your astrological chart. Once the practitioner has examined you, taken your pulse, and asked you about your health, he or she may prescribe such treatments as detoxification (using steam, baths, and essential oils), massage, and herbal medicines. You will also be given advice about your diet, and the therapist may recommend yoga or some other suitable form of exercise. Ayurvedic physicians look on the therapy as a system of medicine that can be used for any complaint. You may need a number of return visits, especially if you have a long-standing illness or health problem.

BATES METHOD ★

This system of exercises, devised by Dr. William H. Bates (1860–1931), is designed to improve poor eyesight. The exercises are based on the idea that eyesight problems are often the result of the poor functioning of muscles around the eyes. Such eye disorders as far- and nearsightedness, squinting, and astigmatism may respond to regular practice of Bates method exercises.

BIOCHEMIC TISSUE SALTS ★

Therapy with biochemic tissue salts is based on treatment with pills containing minerals in highly dilute form. The minute amounts of minerals contained in these pills makes many orthodox doctors skeptical of the effectiveness of this form of therapy.

BIOENERGETICS ★

This therapy relies on the idea that a "life force" flows through the body and mind. If the flow is interrupted, illness can result. Therapists aim to unblock the flow of life energy, relieving tension and bringing emotional release. Practitioners claim success with anxiety and depression and with those affected by Down's syndrome and autism.

Professional consultation

Bioenergetics begins with a one-to-one consultation with your practitioner. He or she assesses your problem and recommends a series of exercises designed to unblock your energy. Later, you may join a group session in which you can practice the exercises.

BIOFEEDBACK ★★★★

This technique provides a way of measuring changes in the body, such as skin temperature and muscle tension. It is possible to use the power of thought to alter some of these changes, and this becomes easier when you can see the results on a meter or screen. Since many physical changes are related to illness, it

> ### Biodynamics
>
> Biodynamics works in a similar way to bioenergetics but is based on the idea that the digestive system reacts to your moods and emotions. Therapists use massage to treat the digestive system, and look on a rumbling stomach as a sign that treatment is working.

is sometimes possible to treat the disease as well. For example, some people have been able to ease the pain of migraine by imagining the head getting cooler. Biofeedback can also be effective against stress-related problems like asthma, high-blood pressure, insomnia, and anxiety.

Professional consultation

After instructing you in a specific relaxation technique, such as focusing on your health, the therapist shows you how to read the meters and how to recognize changes in your nervous system. The goal is to help you bring on a state of relaxation yourself.

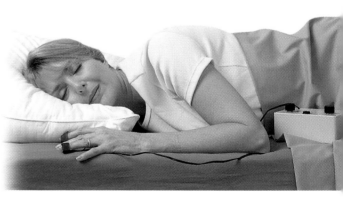

BIORHYTHMS ★

The theory behind biorhythms is that there are three fixed-length cycles that affect your health and performance in different areas of life. The physical cycle lasts 23 days and governs such areas as vitality, the immune system, confidence, and sex drive. The emotional cycle lasts 28 days and affects creativity and moods. The intellectual cycle lasts 33 days and influences mental function.

Advocates of this theory believe it is possible to plot the biorhythms for your entire life, starting with your birth, as a series of graphs. Special computer programs are available to do this. When a particular cycle is at its peak, your performance and energy in that area are said to be at their highest; troughs indicate passive periods. You can use biorhythms to plan events in your life, scheduling important events that require high performance on days when one or more of your rhythms is high.

BUTEYKO BREATHING ★★

This therapy is based on the work of Konstantin Buteyko, a Russian scientist. Its premise is that breathing too rapidly can cause chemical changes in the blood that result in various health problems, including anxiety, muscle tension, headaches, dizziness, and asthma. When you attend a Buteyko breathing course, you perform exercises in breathing slowly and holding your breath. Some asthma sufferers have been able to reduce their need for drug treatment after learning Buteyko breathing, but the therapy should be undertaken only in consultation with your doctor. People with asthma should not adjust their medication except on the advice of a medical practitioner.

CHI KUNG (QI GONG) ★★★

The term chi kung means "internal energy exercise." An ancient Chinese system of exercises, chi kung aims to stimulate the flow of energy, which Chinese physicians believe travels around the body along channels known as meridians. The therapy concentrates on your posture and breathing and teaches you how to focus your mind. There are also chi kung healers who try to use the energy to cure illnesses.

Many different forms of chi kung exist, but, in contrast to some Western exercise regimes, they are all gentle. Tai chi chuan (see p. 65) is one well-known form of chi kung.

CHINESE MEDICINE ★★★

Traditional Chinese physicians use herbs along with such techniques as acupuncture, diet, and exercise to provide a complete system of medical treatment. The goal is to regulate the flow through the body of the vital energy called qi. The therapist examines you as a whole person (taking into account the health of your mind, body, and spirit)— examining your hair, eyes, skin, and tongue, as well as taking your pulse.

The practitioner will recommend a treatment program to suit your particular symptoms rather than to cure a specific ailment. Chinese physicians prescribe from a wide variety of herbs, including some, such as ginseng and ginkgo, that are now well-known in the West. They are selected for such properties as their ability to warm, cool, affect specific organs of the body, and regulate the flow of *qi*. For example, cooling herbs might be prescribed if you have a high temperature. You will usually be asked to make several return visits so that the therapist can review the treatment. As Chinese herbalism is part of a complete medical system, practitioners claim to be able to treat a wide range of disorders.

CHIROPRACTIC ★★★

Chiropractic is a manipulative therapy, primarily designed to treat disorders of the muscles and bones, especially the joints. The therapy began as a way of treating diseases by manipulating the bones of the spine, but modern chiropractors treat a wide range of musculo-skeletal problems. People with joint problems, especially back

Zhan zhuang

A powerful and popular form of chi kung is called zhan zhuang (which means "standing like a tree"). To do zhan zhuang exercises, you adopt a series of different stationary positions, which may involve lying down, sitting, or standing.

pain, often report good results from chiropractic treatment. Other conditions—such as arthritis, rheumatism, migraine, and asthma—have also responded well to this form of therapy.

Professional consultation

When you first visit a chiropractor, he or she examines you thoroughly, feels your spine, and tests the mobility of your joints. The practitioner may also take X rays of your spine and check your blood pressure. He or she may then use gentle manipulative techniques on your joints and may also massage your muscles. The chiropractor may give you advice about exercises to help the mobility of your joints.

CLINICAL ECOLOGY ★★★

Also known as environmental medicine, clinical ecology attempts to heal illnesses that result from our surroundings. Clinical ecologists treat people who suffer from allergies to foods and those who are adversely affected by chemicals in the environment, such as pesticides and gasoline fumes.

A range of disorders may be caused by allergies and similar reactions. Clinical ecologists claim to be able to help people with asthma, headaches, psoriasis and eczema, repeated stomach upsets, long-standing fatigue, and rheumatoid arthritis.

Professional consultation

The therapist may test blood, urine, and, occasionally, hair—to detect your responses to different substances. For food allergies the simplest method of diagnosis is an exclusion diet, in which you eat only a small number of different foods, gradually adding others until

you find one that causes an adverse reaction (see also "Food Sensitivity," pp. 212–215). With the information from the various methods of analysis, the clinical ecologist recommends a diet or lifestyle that helps you avoid foods or substances that make you ill.

COLOR THERAPY ★

This therapy involves treatment with particular colors of light, applied in a variety of ways. It is based on the idea that certain wavelengths of light have healing effects on specific parts of the body or on the mind. Therapists claim to be able to treat many disorders, including depression, stress, learning difficulties, and skin problems.

The therapist takes your medical history and asks you about your color preferences. He or she then suggests treatment. This may involve basking in colored lights, wearing clothes of certain colors, eating foods of a particular color, or drinking water that has been treated with colored light.

CRANIAL OSTEOPATHY ★★

This branch of osteopathy involves gentle manipulation of the bones of the skull (cranium). A cranial osteopath may also work on your shoulders and spine to help the joints and tissues to move freely. Cranial osteopaths believe that if these bones or the nearby tissues are shifted even slightly out of place—for example, by an injury—health problems may develop throughout the body. Cranial osteopaths therefore claim to be able to provide benefit not only for head and spinal injuries, mouth and jaw pain, and sinusitis, but also for ailments affecting other parts of the body, such as arthritis, constipation, menstrual problems, and migraine.

CREATIVE THERAPIES ★★★

The use of the arts—such as painting, drawing, music, and dance—can have powerful healing effects. Emotions that are too deep for words can come to the surface through such expression, helping people overcome difficult feelings, aiding relaxation, and ideally leading to greater physical well-being. Creative therapies have been found especially effective for people with emotional problems, particularly those who find it difficult to communicate their feelings to others. Dance therapy has the additional benefit of providing physical exercise.

CRYSTAL THERAPY ★

Practitioners of this therapy believe that crystals and gemstones produce different types of healing energy. Crystal therapists arrange crystals around you or place them on your body, choosing stones that are thought to be effective for your problem.

FELDENKRAIS METHOD ★★

This is a technique—influenced by yoga, martial arts, and the Alexander technique—that aims to help you move with ease, using minimal effort and maximum efficiency. Teachers of the Feldenkrais method try to make you more aware of your body movements, recognizing any tensions and correcting them by changing the way you move. They do this by teaching you simple exercises to change your habitual patterns of movement, and by using touch to direct you toward less stressful, and therefore less damaging, ways of moving your body. Teachers of the method claim that it can help people suffering from back pain, paralysis, and the aftereffects of stroke.

FENG SHUI ★★

The ancient Chinese art of placement, or feng shui, relies on the theory that, like the human body, the earth is crisscrossed by a series of channels, along which flows vital energy, or *qi*. Practitioners of feng shui believe that the design and position of a building and the way its contents are chosen and arranged can affect the flow of *qi*, and thus make the building a more auspicious and healthier place in which to live. If you consult a feng shui practitioner, he or she will take readings with a special compass and assess the rooms of your home using Chinese astrology and the ancient *I Ching* ("Book of Changes"). The practitioner may then recommend alterations, such as moving mirrors and other items and rearranging the furnishings. Exponents claim such changes may improve psychological and physical well-being.

FLOTATION THERAPY ★★

A method of relaxation, flotation therapy involves floating in a large tank filled with water containing a high concentration of Epsom salts. You wear earplugs, the lights are switched off, and the water is kept at the same temperature as your skin. The result is that all outside sensations are removed, and most people, even many who are highly stressed, relax deeply within minutes.

Flotation therapy may help stress-related problems, such as anxiety, migraines, and headaches. People with back pain and muscle fatigue may also benefit. The therapy tends to reduce pain because it stimulates the body to release its own natural painkillers, hormonelike substances called endorphins. Some people even experience euphoria.

HEALING ★

Healers usually talk about what they do in terms of energy—a vital life force, which everyone possesses. This force can become depleted when someone is ill, but healers believe that they can transfer their own vital energy to a sick person. There are many different types of healing, including faith healing, which is based on a religious faith shared by healer and patient, and spiritual healing, in which the healing energy is separate from the beliefs of the people taking part. Reiki (p. 65) is a form of healing therapy.

Some studies indicate that healing can be beneficial. It may help to relieve pain, or, by providing comfort, it may help the sufferer to cope with the illness more effectively, even though the actual disease remains.

Professional consultation

Healers work in a variety of ways. Some attempt to transfer their "healing energy" through their hands, touching you gently. Some hold their hands an inch or so away from your skin. Others channel healing energy by thinking or praying. You may feel

---

Therapeutic touch

Practitioners of therapeutic touch believe that every human being has an energy force that extends outside the body. When this force is blocked or out of balance, illness results. Practitioners try to correct these problems by passing their hands over the sick person (sometimes without touching). Many nursing schools teach this form of therapy.

---

a sensation of warmth as the practitioner places his or her hands on or near your body. A reputable healer may advise you to consult your doctor as well as undergoing healing. Beware of any healer who makes promises to cure or prevent disease, who charges an exorbitant fee, or who challenges your religious faith.

HELLERWORK ★★

Practitioners of Hellerwork believe that the bones and soft tissues of the body become misaligned from stress, illness, or bad posture. Hellerworkers aim to realign your body, banish tension, and correct the problems that originally caused the misalignment. They do this by manipulating the body and by teaching you how to move in a well-balanced way. People with a wide range of aches and pains, especially neck ache, back pain, and headaches, have responded well to this form of therapy. It may also help internal processes affected by muscle function, such as digestive problems.

Professional consultation

You normally attend a series of 11 weekly sessions, making up a complete Hellerwork course. After taking your medical history and assessing your needs, the practitioner will begin the first group of sessions, known as the superficial sessions. These concentrate on freeing tension in the chest, arms, and feet. Next come the core sessions, during which the therapist works on muscles that Hellerworkers believe to be at the core of the body—those of the pelvis, spine, head, and neck. A final group of sessions, known as the integrative sessions, draw together the work of the previous weeks.

HYPNOTHERAPY ★★★★

This therapy uses hypnosis, creating a state of mind in which normal thought processes are suspended for a short period of time. Hypnosis can be used to induce relaxation, to treat stress-related conditions, to help people overcome addictions, phobias, and eating disorders, and to treat lack of confidence and sexual problems. Some forms of hypnosis are also effective for pain relief, especially during labor and dental treatment.

Professional consultation

There are various ways of inducing a hypnotic trance, but the hypnotist will create a relaxing atmosphere, perhaps asking you to visualize a restful scene or repeat a phrase or sentence over and over. The therapist may suggest that your limbs are feeling heavy and that your eyelids are closing. When you go into a hypnotic trance, you will feel relaxed and you may be willing to accept the suggestions of the hypnotist. You may then go into a deeper trance, in which your heartbeat and breathing slow down and you enter a state that feels similar to that of meditation (see pp. 46–47). The hypnotist may make statements to address your problem—for example, ones that boost your self-esteem or tell you that you are going to stop a damaging form of behavior, such as smoking or drinking alcohol.

IRIDOLOGY ★

A technique said to help diagnose diseases, iridology is based on the idea that the iris of the eye contains a map of the body. Each part of the iris is believed to represent an organ. Iridologists believe that black marks on the irises indicate a disease and white marks signal some form of stress or inflammation. If an iridologist finds any problems, he or she will refer you to a doctor.

KINESIOLOGY ★

Like Chinese physicians, kinesiologists believe that an invisible form of vital energy circulates through the body. Treatment aims to restore imbalances in this energy flow. A kinesiologist tries to learn about your health by testing your muscles, and tries to correct imbalances of the muscles and other disorders by gentle massage, acupressure, and similar physical techniques.

Kinesiology can sometimes relieve muscular aches and pains. Practitioners also claim success in treating food allergies, although there is no evidence supporting these claims.

Professional consultation

The therapist will ask you about your medical history and health problems. He or she will then test your muscles by pressing them carefully, and will gently massage areas where the energy flow is thought to be blocked. The kinesiologist may touch acupressure points lightly or stimulate these points with an electrical device. He or she may also test your reactions to various foods and recommend dietary changes.

LAUGHTER THERAPY ★★

When you laugh, you feel good. The reason for this is partly that laughter boosts certain body chemicals, including endorphins, which are natural mood-enhancing and pain-relieving substances. There is also evidence that laughter has physical benefits—it relaxes tense muscles amd strengthens the immune system. A number of therapists run workshops in which you are encouraged to laugh—for example, by watching a clown, listening to a comedian, or being shown the funny side of problems. This can make your difficulties seem more manageable, so laughter therapy can also provide a way of managing stress.

LIGHT THERAPY ★★★

One form of this therapy involves sitting in front of a specially designed light box, which produces light at a higher intensity than ordinary bulbs. This helps many sufferers of seasonal affective disorder (SAD), or winter blues—people who get depressed during the winter months because of high levels of the hormone melatonin, which is produced by the pineal gland. The gland normally produces melatonin at night; the morning light makes it stop secreting the hormone. But during winter, when there is less daylight, the pineal gland may go on producing melatonin. About two hours of daily light therapy may alleviate the problem, but this should be done under a doctor's supervision.

MAGNET THERAPY ★

This therapy relies on the idea that the body responds to magnetism. The therapist applies magnets to your body, either in the form of a magnetic bracelet or as magnetic pads. Therapists claim success in treating the pain of rheumatism, but most research has shown that magnets have little or no therapeutic effect, and experts are therefore skeptical.

METAMORPHIC TECHNIQUE ★

This technique involves work on the feet and hands, using techniques similar to reflexology (see pp. 52–53). Just as reflexologists believe

that different zones on the feet affect different parts of the body, so practitioners of metamorphic technique believe that various areas on the feet affect the emotions.

NUTRITIONAL THERAPY ★★★

This form of therapy analyzes your diet and finds ways in which your body's strength and ability to heal itself can be improved by making changes in your eating habits. Besides dietitians and nutritional therapists, such practitioners as clinical ecologists and naturopaths often use nutritional therapy as part of their treatment.

When you first consult a nutritional therapist, you fill in a questionnaire about your health, illnesses, lifestyle, and diet. After the therapist has looked at your answers, he or she gives you dietary advice tailored to your particular situation. You should expect to make return visits so that the therapist can assess the diet's effectiveness and make any necessary adjustments. The practitioner may also advise you to consult your doctor if you have a condition that cannot be treated solely by dietary means.

OSTEOPATHY ★★★★

This system of medicine treats the mechanics of the human body—the bones, joints, muscles, ligaments, and other connective tissues. Osteopaths believe that many diseases are due to problems with the body's structure; therefore, fixing the structural problems helps the body heal itself. They use gentle, manipulative techniques to reduce tension and restore health. In most states, osteopaths have the same licenses as M.D.s.

Although osteopathy is especially effective in treating such problems as muscle and joint pains, an osteopath always tries to find out why these disorders occur, in case they are symptoms of some other disorder.

Professional consultation

A first visit usually lasts up to one hour. The osteopath asks about your lifestyle, work, and leisure activities, as well as your illness. He or she examines you standing, sitting, and lying on the treatment table. You may be asked to bend or stretch to see how your body responds in different positions.

Soft-tissue manipulation, with a range of massage-like techniques that help relax tight muscles and tighten loose ones, is often the first stage in treatment. The osteopath uses his or her fingertips to probe your muscles to seek out tension and other problems.

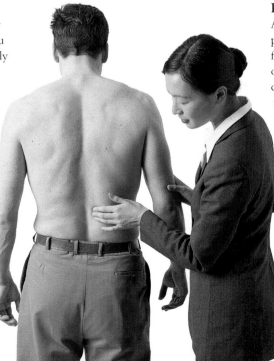

If you have joint problems, the osteopath may use gentle rhythmic strokes and stretches to ease them. He or she may also try a technique known as the high-velocity thrust. This is a rapid, painless movement, usually used on the spine. It makes the joint move and click and the muscles around the joint quickly relax. Pain around the joint can be relieved with this technique.

You may require several return visits, which usually last about half an hour each. The number needed will vary according to several factors—the condition itself, how long you have had the problem, and your age (younger people usually need fewer visits).

Besides joint and muscle problems, disorders that may respond well to osteopathy include sports injuries, migraine, premenstrual syndrome, constipation, and such respiratory problems as asthma.

POLARITY THERAPY ★

A mixture of Eastern and Western approaches, polarity therapy is based on the idea that a form of energy flows around the body from one pole to another, rather like a magnetic current. The energy, which may be positive, negative, or neutral, flows between energy centers known, as in yoga, as *chakras*. Polarity therapists use four techniques to balance energy and promote general health: bodywork (touch and massage), awareness skills (helping you talk through your problems), dietary recommendations, and stretching exercises (a series of yoga-like postures).

PSYCHOTHERAPY ★★★★

Trained to listen carefully and offer support in cases of distress, grief, stress,

and anxiety, psychotherapists treat many people with emotional and psychological problems. Therapists work by listening to you and talking with you about your experiences and relationships, so that you can gain insight into your problems. Gradually, you get closer to the roots of emotional difficulties that may be deep-seated.

Psychotherapists use a variety of different therapies, ranging from the warm and supportive to the more detached and analytical. When choosing a therapist, it is important to find out which technique he or she offers. Some of the most popular are behavioral therapy (which helps you "unlearn" problem behavior or habits), group therapy (in which you share your problems with a group of other patients), neurolinguistic programming (which works with the way personal experiences influence your perceptions), and gestalt therapy (which makes you more aware of such behavior as body language).

Depending on the type of therapy and the needs of the patient, psychotherapy may be short-term or may require a large number of sessions over months or even years. After a course of therapy, you should be able to confront and overcome your difficulties.

REIKI ★

The word *reiki* means "universal life energy," and this therapy offers a way of transferring healing energy from a giver to a receiver. Practitioners gain their ability to heal through reiki by studying with a reiki master teacher. The student practitioner undergoes "attunement," which is said to open up a channel through which healing energy can flow. Practitioners also learn specific hand positions for use during therapy sessions.

When you consult a reiki practitioner, the therapist lays his or her hands on your body, following intuition to adopt the positions that give the best flow of healing energy.

ROLFING ★★

The aim of rolfing is to improve the structural alignment of the body. Rolfers compare the human body to a tower of children's building blocks—if one block is pushed out of alignment, the structure of the entire tower is threatened. By manipulating the body's connective tissues and muscles—using the knuckles, fingers, palms, and elbows—the rolfer tries to realign your body, increasing range of movement, improving balance, and enhancing posture. Rolfing may be of benefit to people with poor posture and low vitality.

SOUND THERAPY ★★

Scientists now know that sound can alter our brainwaves. This therapy uses the power of sound to encourage healing. Treatment may be a simple matter of playing soothing sounds (such as chanting, the noise of waves, or the calls of dolphins) to induce relaxation. This type of sound therapy can be effective against stress, anxiety, and other emotional problems.

TAI CHI CHUAN ★★★

Performed as a series of graceful postures, one flowing into another, the Chinese "soft" martial art of tai chi chuan—or simply tai chi—works on both the body, by providing exercise, and the mind, by helping you concentrate. The movements relax the muscles, freeing the joints and easing tension. Tai chi provides gentle exercise suitable for most people.

Professional consultation
The best way to learn tai chi is to go to a class run by an experienced teacher. You will learn a sequence of movements known as a "form"—either a short form, lasting 5 to 10 minutes, or a full-length long form, which can take up to 40 minutes. Once you have learned a tai chi form, you will be able to practice it every day at home.

TIBETAN MEDICINE ★★★

The native medicine of Tibet is based on the theory that the body contains three substances called humors—vital energy, internal heat, and phlegm. In a healthy person, these substances are balanced, but when they are imbalanced, they turn into three poisons—desire, anger, and greed—and illness results.

When you consult a practitioner of Tibetan medicine, he or she will manipulate the artery in the wrist so as to feel the pulse in three different ways, examine a urine sample, ask you about your lifestyle and habits, and draw up your astrological chart. Treatment may involve advice about your lifestyle as well as recommendations of medicines made mainly of herbs.

TRAGERWORK ★★

This therapy uses gentle manipulation to help you relax. Practitioners claim that the movements used in Tragerwork can also benefit such ailments as high blood pressure, migraines, and asthma.

A Tragerwork practitioner uses his or her hands to find points of tension in your body. The Tragerworker then uses a range of movements—including rocking, gentle stretching, and cradling—to bring about a state of relaxation and a feeling of well-being.

65

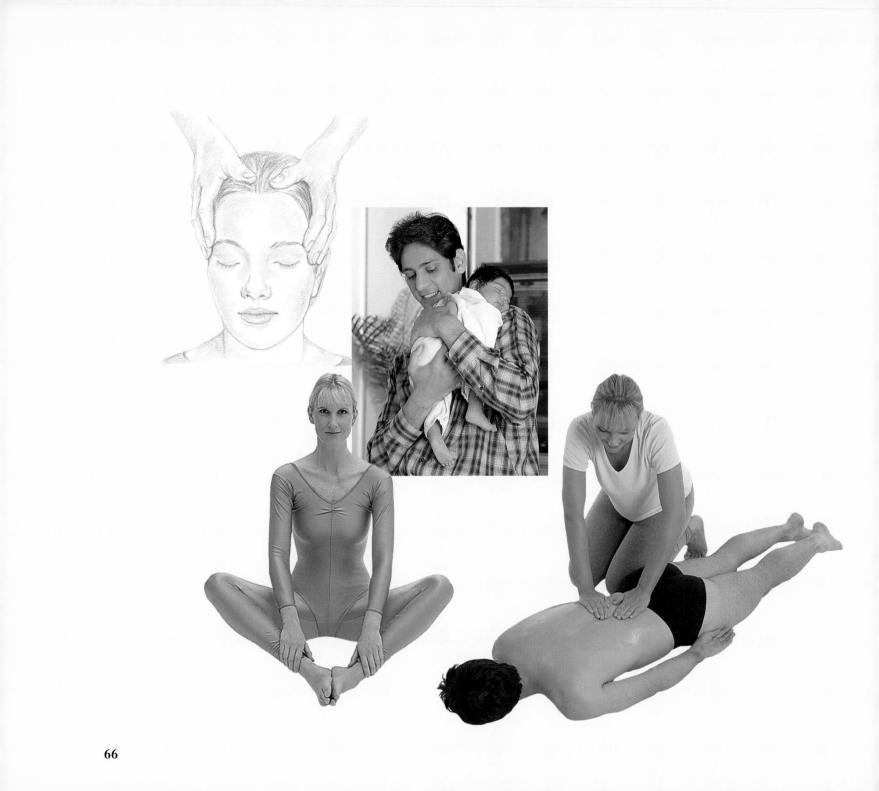

2 Symptoms & Ailments

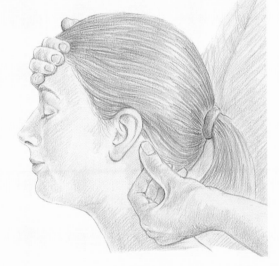

A range of ailments can cause us discomfort or even distress. When sickness strikes you or a family member, refer to this part of the book for advice on the natural remedies you can use to help alleviate the condition or symptom. Choose the treatments that fit your case best and that you feel most comfortable with. Also use this section to learn about steps you can take to prevent disease. Remember that while some minor problems can be treated at home, you should always seek your doctor's opinion for serious symptoms or when self-care isn't working.

Abdominal Pain

Most of us are familiar with a stomachache that results from anxiety or from eating too fast or too much. Natural remedies and lifestyle changes can ease discomfort in many such cases. More severe or persistent abdominal pain, however, requires medical attention, since it can be an indicator of a serious underlying condition.

Abdominal pain is frequently related to a problem in the digestive system. There may be infection (as with gastroenteritis or a peptic ulcer), inflammation (as with ulcerative colitis, diverticular disease, or appendicitis), or an obstruction (as with constipation or a stuck gallstone). An imbalance in the intestinal flora—the bacteria and other organisms normally present in the intestines—may occur, often as a result of treatment with antibiotics or steroids. In some cases pain may result from an oversensitivity to anxiety of the nerves supplying the intestines or from distension caused by gas (as with irritable bowel syndrome). Food allergies and other sensitivities can also involve irritation of the digestive tract.

PREVENTION

Once your physician has ruled out any serious underlying cause of your pain, you may be able to avoid a recurrence by making changes in your diet and lifestyle. To prevent digestive problems in particular, take the following steps:

- Eat a whole-food, high-fiber diet, avoiding rich, fatty, and spicy foods.
- Have regular meals, and take the time to eat in a relaxed way. If you are in the habit of eating too quickly, slow down, chew thoroughly, and avoid gulping air as you swallow. Also limit the amount that you drink while eating.
- Try to identify any food sensitivity, getting professional help, if necessary. Some people experience abdominal pain after eating certain foods or additives; the flavor enhancer monosodium glutamate (MSG) is a common cause of this problem.
- Drink enough water-based fluids to relieve thirst, prevent constipation, and produce pale-colored urine. This helps improve digestive efficiency. Too much alcohol, tea, coffee, and smoking can interfere with digestion and can make many types of abdominal pain worse.
- Do what you can to reduce unnecessary stress

Nondigestive causes

Abdominal pain can sometimes occur as a result of the following problems, which are unrelated to the digestive organs:

- Urinary-tract infection
- Strained muscles in the abdominal wall
- Kidney stones
- Hernia
- Gynecological disorders, such as dysmenorrhea (painful periods), pelvic inflammatory disease, fibroids, and endometriosis (in which cells of the type that line the uterus develop in the abdomen and cause painful cysts)
- Pressure or irritation from a disorder outside the digestive tract (as with certain tumors, pneumonia, and swollen lymph nodes surrounding the bowel)

in your life. Use effective stress-management strategies (see "Treatment"), and be sure to get enough sleep and exercise. Make mealtimes as leisurely as possible.

TREATMENT

Stress management: When you are stressed, blood levels of stimulating hormones, such as epinephrine, increase and make the muscles in your stomach and intestinal walls tense, leading to the sensation of "butterflies in the stomach"

or actual pain. Stress-relieving strategies include regular exercise, yoga, and relaxation classes and tapes. If these don't work, consider taking a stress-management course or seeing a therapist to help you work out better ways to cope with unavoidable stress.

Heat and cold: Abdominal cramps, indigestion, and painfully strained abdominal wall muscles may be eased with a well-wrapped hot-water bottle or a hot compress (see p. 295) over the

---

Relaxation through yoga

A daily half-hour yoga session is believed to balance the body's flow of energy, helping to reduce the harmful effects of feeling stressed, such as the muscle tension that is associated with many digestive disorders.

You can join a yoga class or buy a book or video that will teach you some simple yoga techniques. The yoga-based relaxation exercise described below can help dissipate tension and relieve related abdominal pain.

1 Lie on your back with back and shoulders relaxed, your legs comfortably apart and your arms away from your body and with the palms upward. If this is uncomfortable for your lower back, bend your knees.

2 Close your eyes and focus on your bodily sensations. Be aware of the contact your body makes with the ground and of your abdomen rising and falling as you breathe slowly and easily.

3 Try to allow extraneous or unwanted thoughts to pass through your mind quickly without attracting your attention, so your awareness is centered on the movement of air in and out of your body.

4 Count your breaths, noting the sensation as the air enters your lungs and as it leaves. When you inhale, think of the air as incoming energy, making you feel light. Then, when you exhale, feel your abdomen sink back down. Continue this exercise for five minutes.

69

sore area. You may want to put a thick, folded towel over the bottle or compress to hold the heat in longer.

Another method is to leave the bottle or compress in position for three minutes, then substitute a bottle filled with cool water, or a cold compress, for one minute. Continue alternating hot and cold applications in this way for about 20 minutes, ending with a hot one.

Aromatherapy: Add two drops of peppermint oil and two drops each of bitter orange and caraway oils to a teaspoon of sweet almond oil, olive oil, or other cold-pressed vegetable oil, and smoothe this gently over the painful area of your abdomen (see box, below). If you prefer, you can add two drops each of bitter orange and caraway

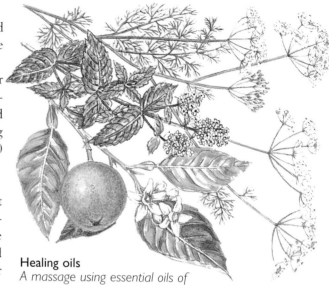

Healing oils
A massage using essential oils of bitter orange, peppermint, and caraway can soothe abdominal pain caused by indigestion or gas.

oils to a pint of hot water and inhale the fragrant vapor. Do not use caraway oil if you are or might be pregnant.

Herbal remedies: Herbs have been used for centuries to ease abdominal pain. It's worth trying several to discover which works best for you.

■ Chamomile is especially good for pain from tension or sluggish digestion, since it may relieve mental stress, help the intestinal muscles relax, and encourage food residues to pass through the intestines. It can also soothe inflammation and promote healing. Drink two or three cups of chamomile tea a day.

■ Parsley, eaten raw, may reduce pain from gas and indigestion. Parsley-seed tea relaxes the intestinal muscles and mitigates cramping.

■ Peppermint tea or capsules may alleviate

Abdominal massage

A circular abdominal massage can sometimes relieve pain. You can do it yourself, but it's easier for a partner or friend to do it for you. With this massage, try using some of the essential oils suggested under "Aromatherapy."

1 Lie on your back with your partner kneeling beside your hips.

2 Your partner should then put one hand gently on your abdomen and stroke firmly, smoothly, and slowly, with a clockwise circling movement, around your abdomen. The circle should begin just inside one hipbone, move up the side of your abdomen, go across the lower border of your rib cage, and then back down your other side to the other hipbone.

3 Continue the massage for several minutes or as long as is comfortable.

intestinal cramps; however, be careful not to take too much, as this herb can irritate the lining of the stomach.

Caution: For safety concerns, see pp. 34–37.

Homeopathy: Several homeopathic remedies may help abdominal pain caused by digestive problems. Depending on your symptoms, take:

- Nux vomica: if you have eaten or drunk too much and you feel queasy—especially if the meal was rich and you drank a lot of alcohol.
- Arsenicum: if you have a burning sensation in your stomach and you feel restless and chilly.
- Pulsatilla: if you've eaten too much rich food and it leaves an aftertaste, and you feel better in the fresh air.

- Carbo vegetabilis: if you are bloated but feel better after belching or passing gas, and you feel chilly but nevertheless prefer to be in the open air.

Acupressure

Apply thumb pressure on the point (St 36) four finger-widths down from the lower edge of the kneecap and one finger-width from the crest of your shinbone on the outside of your leg. Make firm, circling movements with the thumb for about two minutes on each leg. This point is said to regulate the functioning of the stomach and spleen.

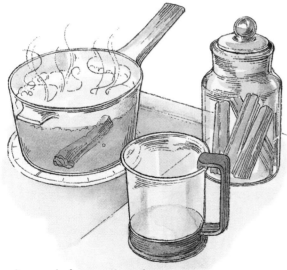

A remedy from ancient times
Cinnamon tea (made by simmering the bark in boiling water) has maintained its age-old reputation as an effective treatment for abdominal pain resulting from gas, diarrhea, or nausea.

When to get medical help

- Pain doesn't ease in two to three days.
- Pain recurs within a month.
- You have other symptoms, such as a fever, severe diarrhea, vomiting, menstrual or urinary problems, or general malaise.
- You have red or black blood in your stools.
- The usual frequency of your bowel movements changes with no obvious cause, such as a change in diet.
- You lose weight for no apparent reason.

Get help right away if:

- Pain is severe or continues to worsen.
- You vomit and see blood or what looks like coffee grounds in the vomit.

See also:
CONSTIPATION,
DIARRHEA,
DIVERTICULAR
DISEASE,
FLATULENCE,
GALLBLADDER
PROBLEMS,
INDIGESTION,
IRRITABLE BOWEL
SYNDROME, NAUSEA
AND VOMITING

71

Abscesses and Boils

Lumps containing pus, abscesses and boils are generally somewhat painful and tender. They are usually caused by bacterial infection. These disorders, especially if they occur repeatedly, may be a sign that your immune system is weak.

An abscess can develop in any organ and in soft tissue beneath the skin anywhere on the body. Common sites include the breasts, the gums, the armpits, and the groin. Boils develop in the skin, usually around a hair follicle, and common sites include the back of the neck, the armpits, and the groin. A carbuncle is a large boil or a cluster of boils. Carbuncles occur less frequently than regular boils, often on the neck or the buttocks.

Boils and carbuncles are readily visible, whereas an abscess is usually invisible or apparent only as a tender swelling. Most boils subside or come to a head and discharge through the skin. An abscess may subside, grow, burst inside, become a sac of uninfected pus, or discharge via a long track through the skin.

PREVENTION

Strengthen your body's resistance to infection by eating fewer foods containing sugar, white flour, and saturated fats, and more fresh vegetables and fruits. If you feel run-down, make sure that you are getting enough rest, fresh air, and exercise, and consider having a medical checkup.

TREATMENT

General measures

- Don't burst a boil yourself; there is a risk that this might spread the infection.
- For boils that have not burst, wring out a clean piece of cloth in warm water and place it over the affected area until the cloth cools. Do this every two hours to speed healing.
- For a boil on the torso or legs, add Epsom salts to your bathwater. Use two handfuls of salts, and soak for 15 minutes daily. (This treatment is unsuitable for the very young, the elderly, and those with high blood pressure.)
- If your boil, abscess, or carbuncle has burst, take a shower instead of a bath to reduce the risk of the infection spreading.

Herbal remedies: Hot herbal poultices encourage boils and superficial abscesses to come to a head. You can use various herbs, including marshmallow, slippery elm, and burdock (see box, facing page). Cabbage poultices also help draw pus from boils: Dip green cabbage leaves in boiling water for about a minute, until they have just

Natural antibiotic
Garlic, especially when raw, fights many types of bacteria.

wilted. Cool and wrap in gauze. Place this poultice over your boil as with an herbal poultice. Apply a fresh poultice each day.

Garlic and echinacea, taken orally, help strengthen the immune system and clear infection. Use several cloves of fresh garlic a day in your food, or take garlic capsules or tablets as recommended on the bottle. Take echinacea as a tincture or capsules, or as a tea made from two teaspoons of dried root added to one cup of water. Bring to a boil and simmer for 10 minutes; cool and strain. Drink three cups a day.
Caution: For safety concerns, see pp. 34–37.

Aromatherapy: Some essential oils have significant anti-infective properties.

- Add three drops of geranium oil or two drops of tea tree oil to a cup of warm water. Gently apply the mixture with a cotton ball. Use a new piece each time you wipe to avoid reinfection.
- When a boil ruptures, bathe the area in an antiseptic solution made with one tablespoon of tea tree oil or distilled witch hazel added to a pint of warm water. Apply and cover with a sterile bandage. Leave the bandage in place for two to three days, or until a scab forms and swelling and redness subside.

Homeopathy: Try the remedy given below that most closely matches your case. It can safely be used in addition to any treatment your doctor may recommend.

- Arsenicum: when a boil or abscess is very red and pain is eased by a hot compress.
- Belladonna: when a boil or abscess is red, hot, painful, and throbbing.

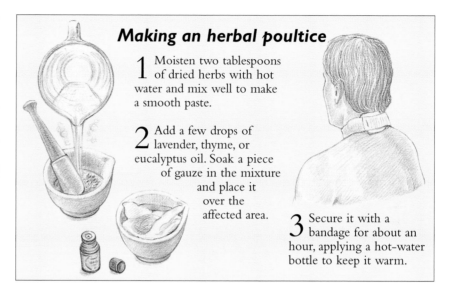

Making an herbal poultice

1 Moisten two tablespoons of dried herbs with hot water and mix well to make a smooth paste.

2 Add a few drops of lavender, thyme, or eucalyptus oil. Soak a piece of gauze in the mixture and place it over the affected area.

3 Secure it with a bandage for about an hour, applying a hot-water bottle to keep it warm.

- Hepar sulphuris: when pus has formed and the lump is very sensitive to touch.
- Tarentula cubensis: when a boil or abscess develops rapidly after a slow incubation, when it feels very hard and looks bluish, and when the pain is agonizing and burning.
- Silica: when a boil or abscess is slow to clear up.

When to get medical help
- A boil or abscess does not heal within a few days.
- You don't feel well.
- The skin is extremely tender.
- You have swollen or tender glands.
- You suffer from recurrent boils or abscesses.

Get help right away if:
- Inflammation or red streaks appear around a boil.
- You have a fever, chills, or night sweats.

See also:
ACNE, SKIN
PROBLEMS

Acne

Pimples on the face, neck, back, and/or shoulders characterize acne. The disorder often begins during adolescence, the very time when appearance becomes especially important. Although it can cause considerable distress, acne poses no risk to health. The malady is more prevalent in boys than girls and affects 80 percent of teenagers in Western countries.

The underlying cause of acne is an oversensitivity to normal levels of the sex hormone testosterone. This oversensitivity makes the sebaceous (oil-producing) glands in the skin produce an abnormally high level of sebum, the oily secretion that lubricates and protects the skin.

At the same time, an abnormal reaction of the lining of the sebaceous ducts makes the lining cells too sticky. Instead of being shed when they die, these cells build up and block the duct. The dammed-up sebum solidifies, forming a blackhead or whitehead. Bacteria that are normally present on the skin can then easily multiply in the trapped sebum, causing the typical redness and swelling of an acne pimple. In severe cases these pimples, or pustules, may develop into hard lumps (nodules) or fluid-filled cysts.

Certain medications—for example, some types of contraceptive pills, corticosteroids, and drugs for epilepsy—can make acne worse. In some women, acne is a symptom of polycystic ovary syndrome (see p. 274), a hormonal disorder that can also cause missed periods, infertility, excess body hair, and weight gain.

PREVENTION

The following general advice is helpful for anyone who tends to get acne, and it may be all you need to do to control mild acne. For more severe cases, try some of the treatments recommended on the next page.

- Wash your face with an oil-free soap that doesn't over-dry the skin.
- If you need a moisturizer, use a product that is light and nongreasy.
  - Ultraviolet rays can help relieve acne, so expose affected skin to daylight for a maximum of a half hour each day, but not when the sun is at its most intense (usually 10 A.M. to 3 P.M.).
    - Choose your sunscreen with care. Buy products that are PABA-free and oil-free or noncomedogenic (free of ingredients that clog pores).

Avoiding acne scars
Do not pick or squeeze pimples, as this can lead to scarring. Make sure your hands are clean before applying herbal teas or essential oil remedies with a fresh cotton ball.

- Avoid getting very sweaty or spending long periods in a humid environment. Many people find that this makes their skin condition worse.
- Iodine-containing food supplements and iodized salt may exacerbate acne, so avoid these.
- Apply tea tree oil to blemishes with a cotton swab or piece of gauze once or twice a day. If you prefer, dilute the oil with water.
- Keep your hair off your face, especially if it tends to be oily, and try to avoid touching your face too often.
- If you use hair gel or mousse and have acne on your forehead, do without these products for a couple of weeks to see if this helps.

TREATMENT

Aromatherapy: Some essential oils help regulate sebum production. These include juniper berry (avoid during pregnancy) and Atlas cedarwood (avoid during first 20 weeks of pregnancy). Lavender and geranium have antiseptic and healing properties, while Roman chamomile and petitgrain help reduce skin inflammation. Try the following treatments:

- Add two drops each of juniper berry and Atlas cedarwood oils to half a cup of water. Use a cotton ball to apply this solution to your skin every two hours during the day.
- Add two drops of juniper oil to a tablespoon of jojoba or sweet almond oil. Mix this and apply gently to the problem areas as above.
- Add two drops each of petitgrain and Atlas cedarwood oils to five teaspoons of jojoba oil. Also add these essential oils to five teaspoons of an unscented skin lotion. Use the oil each night, and the lotion each morning.

Acne and diet

Most surveys show that food has no effect on acne. However, it may be worth keeping a food diary— a record of what you have eaten each day—to see if any foods appear to cause breakouts. Some women find that chocolate is a problem just before menstruation.

Acne sufferers tend to have lower than normal levels of vitamin A in the blood, so make sure that you are getting enough of this vitamin. Vitamin A is present in milk, butter, eggs, and liver. Do not take supplements except on medical advice, because of the risk of overdose.

Herbal remedies

- Combine equal amounts of dried dandelion root, burdock, nettles, yarrow, cleavers, and echinacea, and make an infusion in the usual way. Drink a cup once or twice a day.
- Boil two to three teaspoons of dried basil in a cup of water. Cool and apply with a cotton ball to clean skin.
- Clean your skin once a day by steaming your face over a bowl of very hot water for 5 to 10 minutes with a towel over your head. Dry your skin, then apply rosewater, elderflower water, distilled witch hazel, or calendula tea. Alternatively, use warm water containing a few drops of calendula tincture.

Caution: For safety concerns, see pp. 34–37.

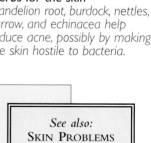

Herbs for the skin
Dandelion root, burdock, nettles, yarrow, and echinacea help reduce acne, possibly by making the skin hostile to bacteria.

When to get medical help

- Self-help treatments don't improve your acne.
- You suspect that your acne is a side effect of a prescribed medication.

See also:
SKIN PROBLEMS

Addictions

Compulsive behavior resulting from a physical or emotional dependence is commonly known as addiction. You may be dependent on a substance, such as drugs or tobacco, or an activity, such as overeating or gambling. Despite your cravings, simple treatments may help you break your habit. However, severe addictions often require professional help.

If you associate an activity with pleasure or with the relief of stress or uncomfortable feelings, you can fall into the habit of doing it whenever times are tough or when certain events in your everyday life easily lead to it. Some addictions, such as smoking and excessive drinking, are always physically damaging. However, any habit that becomes the dominant feature of your life can take a toll on your physical or emotional health and may even be dangerous to your family and others.

Such substances as narcotic drugs and the nicotine in tobacco are highly addictive; most of those who consume them become physically dependent on them. Research indicates that some people are genetically predisposed to addiction because they have a particular balance of chemicals in the brain. Depression or anxiety, for example, can be associated with an imbalance of neurotransmitters (such as serotonin) and hormones (such as epinephrine) that makes the cravings leading to addictive behavior more likely. Nevertheless, social, emotional, and behavioral influences are equally important. With determination, persistence, and support, patterns of addictive behavior can often be changed.

PREVENTION

If you have a tendency toward addictive behavior, try to recognize the warning signs that a new cycle is about to begin, and find alternative, less self-destructive ways of behaving. For example, if you react to depression or stress by reaching for a drink, a cigarette, or the cookie jar, you need to find a better way of meeting your underlying needs and managing stress (see p. 347).

TREATMENT

Support groups: Find out if there is a local support group for your type of addiction. The well-known 12-step Alcoholics Anonymous program, for example, is echoed by similar groups for people who have other addictions.

Increasing self-awareness

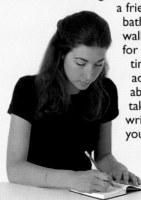

Buy a notebook and fill it with lists of alternative, life-enhancing behaviors—such as phoning a friend, having a scented bath, or going for a walk—you can substitute for your habit. Then any time you feel that your addictive behavior is about to break through, take out the notebook, write down exactly how you feel, and choose one of the alternative activities from your list.

Yoga and meditation: Studies show that yoga exercises, meditation, and visualization can help break addictions and enable you to attain a more positive attitude toward your health. A daily session of yoga postures, breathing exercises, and relaxation (see p. 69) may calm you down, reduce withdrawal symptoms, and increase willpower. Exercise of any type tends to lift mood and improve self-esteem, thereby providing a valuable weapon against addiction.

Diet: If you are a compulsive drinker, include in your diet foods rich in beta-carotene, magnesium, chromium, zinc, and vitamins B, C, and E, to help meet your body's increased need for vitamins, minerals, and essential fatty acids, and to reduce cravings. Addiction to alcohol or tobacco may be associated with low blood sugar. Maintain a steady blood-sugar level by eating regular, small meals and keeping sugar-containing foods to a minimum. Follow a diet high in protein and complex carbohydrates, such as whole-grain bread and pasta and brown rice. Drink plenty of nonalcoholic fluids; dehydration can be a trigger for addictive behavior.

Other therapies: Seek help from a counselor who uses cognitive techniques—ways of helping you understand what you are doing and why, and enabling you to discover other ways of achieving the same ends or meeting the same needs. Even when stress is not the trigger for addictive behavior, therapy can help. Acupuncture, hypnotherapy, and biofeedback can all be effective.

Replacing nutrients
Whole-grain cereals contain high levels of the vitamins and minerals that are often lacking in those addicted to alcohol.

Massage away cravings

Self-massage may help reduce some withdrawal symptoms and ease tension when you are trying to resist a substance or activity.

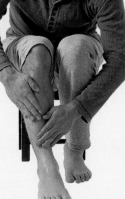

1 Sit somewhere comfortable and give each foot a firm massage, using a tablespoon of sweet almond oil mixed with two or three drops of lavender, geranium, neroli, or jasmine oil.

2 Using the same blend of oils, stroke your lower legs, working with long, slow sweeps from your ankles up to your knees.

3 Gently smooth moisturizing cream over your face and neck with your fingertips.

When to get medical help

- You realize that a habit is out of control.
- Addictive behavior causes emotional or physical problems.
- Addictive behavior starts to affect your relationships adversely.

Get help right away if:
- You have taken an overdose of an addictive substance.
- Addictive behavior makes you a danger to others or yourself.

See also:
ANXIETY, DEPRESSION, EATING DISORDERS, OVERWEIGHT, STRESS

Aging

There is as yet no wonder drug or other treatment to prevent all the physical symptoms of aging or to make us live longer. There are, however, many safe, natural methods of reducing some of the problems associated with aging and of helping ourselves to stay as fit and well as possible so that we can enjoy our natural life span to the fullest.

Aging is associated with increasingly slow cell division, mechanical wear and tear, the continued loss of brain cells, genetic damage from various environmental factors, and oxidative damage by free radicals. These unstable oxygen molecules are created through the normal process of generating energy within cells, but their levels are raised by smoking, an unhealthy diet, and anxiety. Their effects on the body as it ages include loss of elasticity in the skin, blood vessels, and tendons, as well as a progressive decline in organ and joint function. If you lay the foundations of good health in youth and middle age, however, you are much more likely to maintain it into old age.

PREVENTION

You may not be able to stop your hair from turning gray or your skin from losing the smoothness of youth, but you can do much to avoid a pot belly, mental confusion, dimming eyesight, stiff joints, and many of the other problems of aging. You can also keep your immune system working well and take steps to prevent age-associated diseases, such as Alzheimer's disease, arterial disease, arthritis, and osteoporosis.

It is important to stay active in mind and body. The principal ways of doing this are to maintain your interests and social activities, sustain close relationships, exercise regularly, eat a

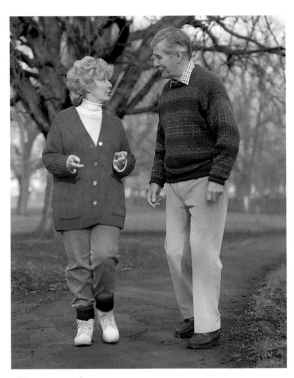

Always active
Keep physically and mentally lively in your later years. Those who enjoy friendships and explore interests tend to stay fitter.

healthy diet, and not smoke. You should also expose your skin to daylight so that you make enough vitamin D to keep your bones strong, but be careful to avoid ultraviolet rays at their most intense (10 A.M. to 3 P.M.).

Mental well-being: Such activities as engaging in stimulating discussion, reading a book or newspaper, doing a crossword puzzle, and playing chess or bridge help prevent the gradual loss of nerve connections in the brain.

Relationships: Fostering good relationships with family and friends is life-enhancing and life-lengthening, probably because it reduces stress, boosts the levels of natural body chemicals that foster a feeling of well-being, and provides another reason for living. Even having a pet can prolong life by reducing stress and lowering blood pressure.

Stress management: High levels of stress encourage more rapid aging. Stress can also lead to arterial disease and trigger such illnesses as infections, arthritis, and migraine. Minimize the pressures in your life and learn how to manage your reactions to those that remain (see p. 347).

Sex: Those who enjoy regular sex tend to live longer, perhaps because of the emotional intimacy and physical exercise of sex, the stress relief of cuddling, and the increased levels of hormones that are released during orgasm, which widen the blood vessels.

Exercise: At minimum, get a half hour of moderately vigorous exercise five days a week. This will make you feel happier, increase your mental powers, and improve the health of your heart, lungs, skin, eyes, and other tissues.

Consult your doctor if you are uncertain as to what type of exercise is suitable in your case,

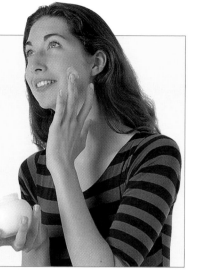

Youthful skin

Help slow the aging of skin by taking the following measures:
- Protect yourself from excessive sun exposure.
- Prevent skin dryness and wrinkles by applying a moisturizer with an SPF of at least 15 every day.
- Smooth on a little antioxidant oil each day. Make it by adding one drop of geranium or thyme oil to a teaspoon of sweet almond oil. (If you make this up fresh each time, no preservative is necessary.)

especially if you have a health problem. Popular forms of exercise for older people include swimming and low-impact aerobics. Weight-bearing forms of exercise, such as walking, tennis, and dancing, help ward off osteoporosis. Yoga and tai chi improve flexibility, and most types of exercise strengthen muscles to some extent. Regular yoga practice has been shown to reduce aches and pains in old age.

Diet: Well-nourished people who are not overweight tend to age more slowly and have fewer ailments. A poor diet—especially when combined with lack of exercise—can lead to the accumulation of fat around the abdomen. This form of weight gain carries an increased risk

Good fats
The omega-3 fatty acids in oily fish (such as sardines, mackerel, and tuna) can help keep your blood vessels in good condition. Try to have three three-ounce servings a week.

79

of diabetes and arterial disease, which may reduce quality of life and life expectancy.

As you grow older, your digestive system becomes less efficient, so you need a more nutritious diet, with fewer refined, fatty foods and more foods rich in antioxidant nutrients (beta-carotene, vitamins C and E, selenium, and zinc) and plant pigments (flavonoids). Avoid large amounts of alcohol. However, if you do drink, a daily glass of wine will stimulate appetite and may reduce your risk of heart disease.

Herbal remedies

■ Garlic: To help immunity and circulation, include a crushed raw clove in your food each day, or take garlic capsules.
■ Ginkgo biloba: For mental functioning (especially memory) and circulation, drink a daily cup of tea made from this herb.
■ Ginseng: To protect against loss of sex drive or general debility, take some ground ginseng root each day, either in tea or tablet form.
■ Green tea: For its antioxidant and blood-thinning effects, have at least a cup a day.
Caution: For safety concerns, see pp. 34–37.

From the drugstore: Consider taking supplements of the antioxidant nutrients beta-carotene, selenium, and vitamins B_{12}, C, and E.

Massage and aromatherapy

The overall benefits of massage, which include improved circulation and relaxed muscles, make it an excellent way to help maintain good health as well as to treat indigestion, arthritis, and aches and pains associated with aging. Ask a friend or partner to give you a massage from time to time. You can increase its therapeutic benefits by adding essential oils to your massage oil or lotion. Choose the oils according to the effect you want.

Massage oil for relaxation
Two drops of geranium oil, two of lavender, two of sandalwood, and one of ylang ylang added to two teaspoons of an unfragranced lotion or of sunflower or sweet almond oil.

Massage oil for revitalization
Two drops of clary sage oil, two of juniper berry, and two of rosemary in two teaspoons of lotion or oil as above. (Avoid this mix of oils during pregnancy.)

When to get medical help
● You feel depressed about growing older.
● You have symptoms of disease that aren't responding to natural treatments.

See also:
ARTERIAL DISEASE, ARTHRITIS,
DIABETES, EYESIGHT PROBLEMS,
HEARING LOSS, HIGH BLOOD
PRESSURE, MEMORY LOSS,
MENOPAUSAL PROBLEMS,
OSTEOPOROSIS

Allergic Rhinitis

*T*he runny nose, frequent sneezing, and watery, itchy eyes of allergic rhinitis are triggered by exposure to an allergen (allergy-causing substance), such as pollen or dust. You can take steps to avoid exposure, and natural remedies will provide some respite, but the best way to increase resistance is to strengthen your immune system.

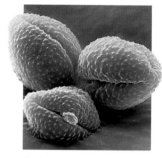

Airborne allergen
Pollen in the atmosphere is the most common cause of seasonal allergic rhinitis. Pictured above are pollen grains from the artemisia plant enlarged 1,500 times.

The symptoms of allergic rhinitis are similar to those of the common cold, but they are not caused by infection. Instead they represent an inappropriate response to a normally harmless substance. Your immune system reacts to the substance as if it were a dangerous invader, leading to inflammation and irritation.

The most familiar form is seasonal allergic rhinitis, also called hay fever or pollen allergy. Tree pollens are the main culprit in spring, grasses in summer, and weeds in autumn. If you are allergic to more than one kind of pollen, your symptoms may last for several months each year. The year-round symptoms of perennial allergic rhinitis result from such triggers as mold, animal dander, dust-mite droppings, certain foods, and environmental toxins.

PREVENTION

Bolster your immune system by eating a healthy diet, with plenty of foods rich in vitamins B and C as well as flavonoids (see p. 12). Vitamin C supplements may be helpful.

Seasonal allergic rhinitis: Pollen grains are so plentiful and minuscule that it is difficult to avoid them completely, but you can reduce the impact of exposure to them. Take the following measures in the three months before your hay fever usually begins:

- Eat a teaspoon of locally produced, non-heat-treated honey containing wax cappings from the honeycomb cells. This is thought to strengthen resistance to local plant pollens.
- Drink a daily cup of ginseng or echinacea tea to strengthen your immune system.

During hay fever season
- Stay indoors with the windows closed whenever feasible, especially in the early evening, when pollen levels often peak.
- Damp-dust regularly.
- Clear pollen from the air with an ionizer or a high-efficiency particulate air (HEPA) filter.
- Wear wraparound sunglasses and/or a cyclist's face mask when you go out.
- Trap pollen by applying petroleum jelly in and around your nostrils.
- Keep car windows and air intakes closed.
- Avoid city centers and smoky rooms, since polluted air traps pollen.
- Put on clean clothes when you come home, and launder clothes frequently.
- Stay indoors before a thunderstorm and for two to three hours after it's over. The high humidity that precedes a storm makes pollen grains swell and burst, releasing particles of pollen starch.
- Use a mask when cleaning dusty, moldy, or extremely dirty areas.

Other types of allergic rhinitis: If you are allergic to dust mites, see the tips on page 102. If you think you have a food sensitivity, see page 214 for advice on tracking down the source.

TREATMENT
General measures
- Splash or sponge your face frequently to remove pollen from your skin and eye area.
- Bathe itchy, runny eyes with a pint of cooled boiled water containing a pinch of salt or two teaspoons of witch hazel. Use the same solution to bathe inflamed nostrils.

Sore nostrils

Protect your nostrils from the moisture from a runny nose by smoothing on some petroleum jelly. Soothe already inflamed nostrils with a cotton handkerchief soaked in cooled chamomile tea.

Herbal remedies
- Inhale the steam from a pint of hot water to which you have added a tablespoon of dried chamomile or yarrow.
- For hay fever, drink two or three cups a day of tea made from eyebright, elderflower, lemon balm, echinacea, or chamomile.
- To help dry up a runny nose, drink a cup of nettle, elderflower, ginger, cinnamon, or clove tea up to three times a day.
- Reduce nasal congestion by adding garlic to food, or take garlic capsules or tablets each day.
- Have a daily cup of tea made from goldenseal, eyebright, elderflower, or chamomile.

Caution: For safety concerns, see pp. 34–37.

Homeopathy
- Allium: for the times when your symptoms are at their most severe.
- Euphrasia: when mainly the eyes are affected.
- Sabadilla: for persistent sneezing.
- Wyethia: for itching of the throat or mouth, or when the eustachian tube is affected.

Acupressure to ease congestion

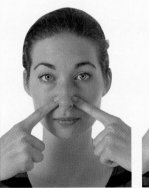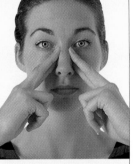

1 Press the tips of your forefingers firmly in the small depression (point LI 20) under the cheekbone to the side of each nostril for two minutes. Repeat every two hours.

2 Press the forefinger and middle finger of each hand firmly against each side of the bridge of your nose (*bitong* point) and hold for a few breaths. Repeat every two hours.

When to get medical help
- Your symptoms are new, severe, or persistent.

Get help right away if:
- You experience wheezing or difficulty breathing.

See also:
ASTHMA, COLDS, EYE IRRITATION AND DISCHARGE, HEADACHE

Anal Problems

With symptoms ranging from itching and soreness to bleeding and pain, anal problems are surprisingly common. The good news is that they are generally easy to treat or correct by using simple self-help measures. Bleeding, however, should always be checked out by your doctor to rule out any underlying disorder, such as cancer of the rectum or colon.

Anal fissure

This is a split in the lining of the anal canal that is usually caused by straining to pass a hard stool when constipated. Symptoms of a fissure are pain on defecation and bleeding, as the fissure is opened further. Treatment includes a high-fiber diet and plenty of fluids to soften the feces. A fissure usually heals after a few days, but persistent or recurrent splits may need medical treatment.

Most anal conditions are linked to intestinal problems, particularly those that cause constipation, diarrhea, or hemorrhoids. Poor hygiene, yeast (candida) infections, pinworm infestations, food sensitivities, and skin allergies may also contribute to such problems.

PREVENTION

You can avoid many of these conditions by eating ample amounts of fruits, vegetables, and whole-grain foods, and by drinking plenty of liquids. This provides fiber and fluid to help prevent constipation and supplies the nutrients needed to keep the intestines, the anus, and the skin of the anal area healthy. Avoid any foods that act as irritants, such as coffee and spicy foods.

Keep to the following guidelines to protect against anal problems:

- Clean the anal area gently but thoroughly after a bowel movement. (Women and girls should wipe from front to back to avoid bringing intestinal bacteria or pinworms near the vulva or the entrance to the vagina.)
- Wear cotton underwear, and change it daily.
- If you have sensitive skin or are prone to allergies that make your skin itchy and/or red, use nonbiological soap powder (available in health-food stores) to launder your clothes, and wash with unscented soap or a soap-free cleanser. Avoid fragranced bath products.

TREATMENT

Itching and soreness in the anal area can usually be soothed by the following simple measures:

- Keep the skin around the anus clean and dry.
- Don't scratch the anal area.
- Apply calendula (marigold) cream twice a day.
- Soak the area for 10 to 15 minutes at least once a day by sitting in a shallow bath or bidet of warm water containing a tablespoon of colloidal oatmeal or three drops of lavender oil.
- Take alternate hot and cold sitz baths (see p. 49) unless the skin is broken. Finish the sequence with cold water.
- Boost resistance to infection and inflammation by taking vitamins A and C with flavonoids, and zinc (with copper to aid absorption).
- If itching mainly occurs soon after going to bed at night, you may have pinworms and should treat this problem (see p. 314).

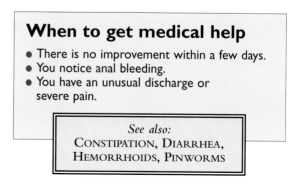

When to get medical help

- There is no improvement within a few days.
- You notice anal bleeding.
- You have an unusual discharge or severe pain.

See also:
CONSTIPATION, DIARRHEA, HEMORRHOIDS, PINWORMS

Anemia

Someone who is anemic has too little hemoglobin in their red blood cells. Hemoglobin is the iron-containing blood pigment that transports oxygen from the lungs to the cells and carbon dioxide from the cells to the lungs. You might think that someone who is anemic would look pale, but mild anemia doesn't cause a change in the skin color.

Anemia is the most common blood disorder, with the majority of cases caused by iron deficiency. Iron-deficiency anemia is usually triggered by the need for extra hemoglobin that comes about because of rapid growth or blood loss. Without sufficient iron, the body can't manufacture enough hemoglobin. In their fertile years, women lose iron during menstruation, so they need proportionately more iron-containing foods than men. It may be possible to cure iron-deficiency anemia by changing your diet.

SYMPTOMS

Any anemia that leads to a significant lack of hemoglobin can trigger fatigue, inertia, and headaches. If the anemia is very severe, physical activity provokes dizziness, breathlessness, chest pain (angina), and palpitations. Iron-deficiency anemia can make the tongue and corners of the mouth sore, the nails dry, thin, and brittle, and, in serious cases, the complexion pallid.

PREVENTION

Your risk of severe iron-deficiency anemia is relatively low if you are in good health and eat a healthy diet. However, if you have been losing blood—for example, from heavy periods over

Less frequent forms of anemia

Most cases of anemia are caused by a lack of sufficient iron in the diet and/or failure to absorb iron during digestion. However, there are a number of other causes of anemia.

- Megaloblastic anemia is caused by a lack of vitamin B_{12} or of folic acid. This form sometimes occurs during pregnancy.
- Pernicious anemia results from a lack of intrinsic factor, a substance necessary for vitamin B_{12} absorption. People with blood type A are the most susceptible.
- Aplastic anemia results from reduced or absent red cell production due to a damaged or inactive bone marrow.
- Inherited anemias have differing causes. Thalassemia, from faulty

hemoglobin production, occurs in people of Mediterranean, Middle Eastern, or Southeast Asian origin. Sickle cell anemia, from abnormally shaped red cells, is mainly found in people of African descent; it usually starts in childhood.
- Hemolytic anemia is caused by the premature breakdown of red blood cells, which may be brought on by drugs or infection.

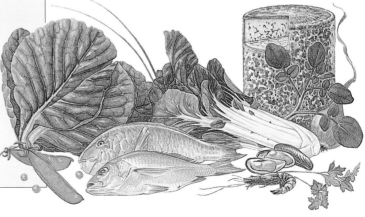

Anti-anemia diet
Eat plenty of foods that contain iron, copper, vitamin C, and/or folic acid. These include dark green vegetables, cheese, seafood, eggs, and fish.

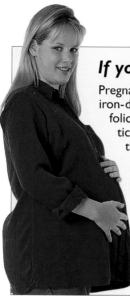

If you're pregnant

Pregnancy can bring about both iron-deficiency anemia and folic-acid-deficient megaloblastic anemia. Try to prevent these by eating foods rich in the following nutrients: vitamins A, B$_6$, C, and E, folic acid, pantothenic acid, flavonoids, iron, manganese, zinc, and essential fatty acids (see p. 12). Take any supplements your doctor recommends.

The role of stomach acid

Some anemic people make too little stomach acid and as a result don't absorb iron as well as they should. Carbohydrates may temporarily lower your stomach acid level. To improve iron absorption, therefore, avoid eating high-carbohydrate foods (such as bread, pasta, sugar, and rice) in the same meal as iron-rich, high-protein foods (such as meat, fish, and eggs). Protein requires the presence of adequate amounts of stomach acid for optimum digestion and iron absorption.

many months, untreated hemorrhoids, or bleeding in the digestive tract (due, perhaps, to ulcerative colitis or cancer of the stomach or colon)—you need an especially iron-rich diet.

- Enhance your meals with liver, lean red meat, fish, egg yolks, dried fruits, soy products, and blackstrap molasses.
- Eat plenty of onions, garlic, beans, peas, nuts, seeds, green leafy vegetables, and herbs (such as watercress, parsley, chives, nettles, cilantro, and dandelion leaves).
- Consume foods high in vitamin C, which boosts iron absorption. For example, have a glass of orange juice with your meals.
- Whole grains are a good source of iron, but they also contain phytates, which hinder iron absorption, so eat whole grains separately from other iron-rich foods.
- Limit consumption of spinach and rhubarb; their oxalic acid also reduces iron absorption.

- Eat foods that contain copper, which assists iron absorption. These include cheese, egg yolks, seafood, liver, whole grains, green vegetables, apricots, cherries, and dried figs.
- Avoid tea, coffee, cocoa, cola, and wine at mealtimes, since the tannins in these drinks block iron absorption from food.

TREATMENT

Your doctor may suggest an iron supplement, but it should only be taken under medical supervision; too much iron can be dangerous. The following measures, in addition to those described under "Prevention," may be helpful for iron-deficiency anemia:

- Consider kelp supplements, which are rich in minerals and may boost iron absorption.
- Take a daily dose of the homeopathic remedy Ferrum phosphoricum.
- Try teas or tinctures of yellow dock, which contains iron, and of dandelion or burdock, both of which may aid in absorbing iron.
- If you feel tired, drink teas or tinctures made from wild oats or licorice.

Caution: For safety concerns about the use of herbs, see pp. 34–37.

When to get medical help

- In all cases of suspected anemia.
- For regular checkups if you're under treatment.

Get help right away if:
- You are short of breath.

See also:
FATIGUE,
MENSTRUAL
PROBLEMS

Anxiety

Distress or tension is a normal response to an especially difficult situation, but the feeling should pass once your problem is resolved. During anxiety-producing times, use stress-management strategies and try natural remedies. If you're seeking an alternative or supplement to prescribed drugs, such as tranquilizers, check with your doctor first.

DID YOU KNOW?

Anxiety may underlie an obsessive-compulsive disorder, in which the person needs to keep doing something, such as washing hands, checking that lights are off, or repeating distressing thoughts. Seek professional help if this type of behavior is disrupting normal life.

Anxiety is the body's "alarm response" to a perceived physical or psychological threat. An acute anxiety state may occur before an important or difficult event, such as an exam or a job interview, and is usually short-lived. For some people, however, anxiety becomes an almost permanent state that seriously affects their ability to cope with everyday life. This condition is known as chronic anxiety.

SYMPTOMS

Acute anxiety can be either a vague or a focused feeling of foreboding. It may be accompanied by physical symptoms, such as stomach cramps, a dry mouth, a racing heartbeat, sweating, diarrhea, and insomnia. If you suffer from chronic anxiety, you may feel agitated without knowing why. Some people experience panic attacks, seemingly without warning. The symptoms, which may include a feeling of suffocation, chest pain, shaking, tingling in hands and feet, faintness, and terror, can be so extreme that sufferers —and onlookers—may believe they are having a heart attack.

Whatever form your anxiety takes, the symptoms can be distressing and disabling, and in the long run can damage your physical health. You need to find ways of dealing with the underlying cause. Consider seeking professional help from a therapist or support group.

PREVENTION

During periods of stress, the body uses up nutrients faster than normal, and unless these are replaced, the nervous system becomes progressively depleted, resulting in an anxious state. It is therefore important to eat a healthy diet—one high in complex carbohydrates, such as whole-wheat bread and brown rice, which may have a calming effect. Be sure to include essential fatty acids (for example, whole grains, nuts, seeds, and vegetables), vitamins (especially B complex), and minerals to nourish your nervous system. Eat

Restful foods

The amino acid tryptophan has a soothing effect on the brain. This is because tryptophan is converted in the brain to serotonin, a chemical messenger that exerts a calming action. Most protein-containing foods contain tryptophan. However, absorption of this substance is improved when it is taken with carbohydrates. Good sources include:
- Milk with cookies
- A turkey or cheese sandwich

small amounts often during the day to keep your blood-sugar level steady. A good balance of rest, exercise, and recreation will also help you feel better physically and thus more positive about life in general.

TREATMENT

If you are a very anxious person, you may need professional counseling, but there is also a lot you can do to help yourself.

Self-understanding: Many experts believe that some of us are naturally more fearful and fretful than others, but it may be that something in your past has triggered a tendency to become especially anxious. You might reflect on the possible origins of your anxiety as a first step to overcoming it. For example, overly protective parents, constantly warning you of risks and dangers inherent in normal life, may have passed along their own fears, or you may have had a traumatic experience that set off your anxiety. Anxious people often have a highly developed

imagination, too, so that they quickly foresee all the possible unpleasant or disastrous consequences of any action and can't help dwelling on them. If you have a phobia, such as an abnormal fear of flying, this may be a way of focusing your fear on something specific, even though that is no easier to handle than generalized anxiety. You

---

Hyperventilation

When you are anxious, and especially if you experience a panic attack, your breathing becomes fast and shallow. This disrupts the body's oxygen and carbon-dioxide levels. To correct this overbreathing, or hyperventilation, sit with one hand over the top of your abdomen and breathe in and out slowly so that your hand moves outward each time you inhale. This "abdominal breathing" helps slow and deepen your breathing.

Yoga breathing for calm

Yoga is excellent for people who often feel anxious, because it can relax both mind and body, encourage steady breathing, and help overcome negative emotions. This breathing exercise is designed to strengthen and relax the chest and abdominal muscles, and to harmonize the flow of life energy (prana). Take five breaths at each stage.

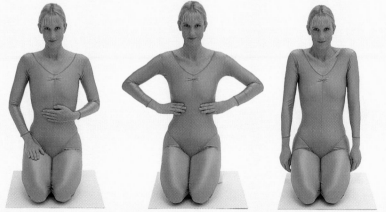

1 Kneel with one hand on your abdomen and the other palm placed downward on your thigh. Feel your abdomen expand as you inhale and retract as you slowly exhale.

2 Place your palms on either side of your rib cage. Lift and lower your rib cage as you breathe, pushing inward with your hands to help expel the last of the air as you exhale.

3 Tighten your abdomen. Lift your shoulders and upper chest as you inhale, and then let them drop as you exhale and release the muscles of your abdomen.

may find it easier to get to the root causes of your anxiety with the help of an understanding friend.

Relaxation: Evolution has programmed our bodies to react to dangerous situations with automatic physical changes that prepare the body for "fight or flight." Unfortunately, being ready to do battle or run away is of no use in many of the situations that frighten us today, so we are often left in a state of heightened tension with no physical outlet. You can help yourself disperse this tension by learning how to relax physically and mentally. This enables you to cope with difficult situations early, rather than keeping on the alert. There are several ways to do this:

■ Try an exercise class or other strenuous physical activity to release muscle tension and nervous energy.

■ Perform a quiet activity, such as gardening or listening to soft music.

■ Join a relaxation or meditation class, or use one of the many video- and audiotapes designed to teach you to relax.

■ Practice progressive muscular relaxation (see p. 245) twice a day or whenever you feel anxious, or try the yoga relaxation exercise described on page 69.

Affirmation: Practicing affirmations helps reprogram your thoughts to emphasize the positive aspects of your life and personality instead of the negative ones. Work out short phrases appropriate to your situation: for example, "I am qualified for this job," if you are facing an interview, or "I know and like everyone who will be at this party," if you are shy in large groups. It helps to repeat your phrase aloud (even if you feel silly) or to write it out several times.

This kind of mental exercise is part of cognitive therapy, which aims to change your natural or instinctive responses rather than understand the reasons for them. For example, a therapist might encourage you to think of more positive explanations for other people's behavior: the acquaintance who ignored you in the store did not do so because she dislikes you but because she didn't see you or had something on her mind. Once you get the idea, you can practice this for yourself, so that you learn to recognize automatically negative responses for what they are and to substitute more constructive, positive, and realistic ones.

Diet: Anxiety can depress or increase the appetite. (Follow the advice on diet under "Prevention.") Choose plenty of foods rich in the B vitamins, vitamin E, calcium, and magnesium, since a lack of these nutrients can contribute to anxiety. Cut down your sugar intake and eat fewer foods made with white flour. Avoid

Acupressure for relaxation

Pressing with your thumb on the point (LI 4) on the back of the hand where the base of the thumb and index finger meet may relax you and increase your sense of well-being; it helps trigger the release of endorphins, the brain's "feel-good" hormones. Do this three times for 10 to 15 seconds. Do not use this point during pregnancy.

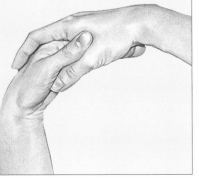

alcohol and caffeine-containing drinks. Choose spring water, fruit juices, or soothing herbal teas instead.

Aromatherapy: If you feel physically tense, give yourself a shoulder massage with essential oils or add them to your bath or your vaporizer.

- To make a massage oil, add two drops each of geranium, lavender, and sandalwood oils, and one of basil oil to two teaspoons of a cold-pressed vegetable oil, such as sweet-almond or olive oil. Omit basil oil if you are in the first 20 weeks of pregnancy.
- Put a few drops of geranium or lavender oil in your bath or into a bowl of very hot water, and inhale the scented vapor for five minutes.

Herbal remedies

- Have a cup of tea made from vervain, wild oats, or ginseng three times a day for two to three weeks. These herbs have a restorative effect on the nervous system.
- To ease tension in the day and aid sleep at night, add chamomile, kava, lime tree flower, valerian, hops, or passionflower to the above brew or take as tablets or tinctures.

Caution: For safety concerns, see pp. 34–37.

Flower essences: The following flower essences are all meant to treat negative feelings, and some are specifically for anxiety. You can use them individually or in combination, according to your personality type (see p. 33).

Tension-easing massage
Rest the palm of one hand on the opposite collarbone, and use your fingers to massage your shoulder muscle and the back of your neck.

- For generalized anxiety, take Aspen, Cherry Plum, Larch, Mimulus, Red Chestnut, Rock Rose, or White Chestnut four times a day.
- For a panic attack, take Rescue Remedy every few minutes until you feel better.

Homeopathy: The following remedies are useful, especially for short-term crises, and work well in conjunction with other therapies:

- Aconite: for anxiety before a stressful event.
- Arsenicum: for a constant need for reassurance.
- Gelsemium: for fatigue, weakness, and fear before an event.
- Phosphorus: for nervousness and sensitivity to loud noise.

Other therapies: Anxiety-related symptoms may also be helped by such therapies as psychotherapy and cranial osteopathy.

When to get medical help

- You are suffering from severe anxiety or panic attacks.
- You also feel depressed.
- You have insomnia or light-headedness.

Get help right away if:
- You have any of the physical symptoms described on page 86.

See also:
APPETITE LOSS, CHRONIC FATIGUE SYNDROME, DEPRESSION, EMOTIONAL PROBLEMS, GRIEF, IRRITABLE BOWEL SYNDROME, PALPITATIONS, SEX DRIVE LOSS, SHOCK, STRESS

Appetite Loss

Eating is one of life's necessities and also one of its greatest pleasures. Yet there are many reasons why you may not feel like eating from time to time. Most of these are minor and pose few problems. Natural remedies and changes in lifestyle often help. However, if you experience loss of appetite for a prolonged period, seek medical advice, especially if you have also lost weight.

Many people lose their appetite for a short period of time, for example, when suffering from indigestion or a fever. Anxiety or depression may also reduce the appetite (though some depressed people want to eat more). Once the underlying cause is over, the appetite usually returns to normal, with no harm done.

Drinking too much alcohol on a regular basis supplies so many calories that it usually removes the desire for proper nourishment. And anything that makes you nauseated—including motion sickness, gastroenteritis, early pregnancy, treatment with certain drugs, and exposure to pesticides, lead, and other poisons—will keep you from wanting to eat.

A continuously poor or nonexistent appetite can suggest a more serious disorder, such as infectious mononucleosis, rheumatoid arthritis, high blood pressure, stomach cancer, tuberculosis, hepatitis, or severe depression.

Surprisingly, perhaps, people who suffer from anorexia nervosa, which can involve life-threatening weight loss, don't often lose their appetite. While victims of this eating disorder consume only small amounts of food, most continue to feel very hungry.

PREVENTION

If your appetite loss is a symptom of illness, you need to treat the underlying cause. Otherwise, there are many ways in which you can encourage a good appetite.

- Eat small, regular meals, making them as nutritious and appealing as possible.
- Try a pre-meal appetizer containing a traditional, bitter-tasting appetite booster. Examples are olives, watercress, young dandelion leaves, rosemary, and chicory.
- Avoid excessive alcohol intake. However, if you drink, a bitter aperitif may whet your appetite before a meal. Having a small glass of wine with a meal may also encourage you to relax and you may therefore eat more.
- Take your time over meals and make them as stress-free as possible.
- Opt for meals composed of several smaller courses rather than one or two larger ones.

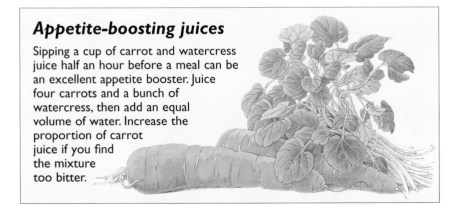

Appetite-boosting juices

Sipping a cup of carrot and watercress juice half an hour before a meal can be an excellent appetite booster. Juice four carrots and a bunch of watercress, then add an equal volume of water. Increase the proportion of carrot juice if you find the mixture too bitter.

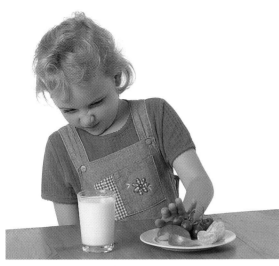

When a child doesn't eat
If your child's appetite is poor for no clear reason, find out whether there's a problem at home or at school. Refusal of school lunches, for example, may not be because of the food but instead for social reasons.

- Say no to foods containing white flour and added sugar, as these lack the nutrient quota of whole foods. If refined foods really are the only ones you feel like eating, take a daily multiple vitamin and mineral supplement.
- Drink coffee and tea that contain caffeine only after meals. Caffeine can suppress appetite. Excessive fluid intake during a meal can fill the stomach and hamper digestion.
- Exercise regularly to stimulate hunger.
- If you smoke cigarettes or use other tobacco products, get help to stop or at least cut down. Any tobacco use can inhibit appetite.
- Ask a friend to give you a relaxing massage, using five drops of lavender oil in two tablespoons of sweet almond oil, if stress is suppressing your interest in food.

TREATMENT

Your choice of treatment for appetite loss depends on the underlying cause. See, for example, advice on indigestion (p. 252), morning sickness (p. 318), and motion sickness (p. 282).

Nausea and tension at mealtime: Give yourself a soothing, gentle aromatherapy massage. Add two drops each of peppermint and black pepper oils, and one drop of rose otto oil, to five teaspoons of sweet almond oil. Use this mixture to massage your abdomen with slow, circular, clockwise strokes.

Anxiety or depression: Get expert assistance to address the source of the problem. In the meantime, care for yourself by preparing attractive, nutritious meals of foods that you normally like, and take a daily multiple vitamin and mineral supplement if you are still unable to eat much.

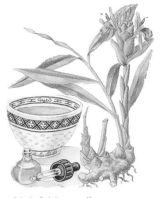

Helpful hors d'oeuvre
Chew a little fresh ginger or take it as a tea before meals. Or add a few drops of the essential oil to five teaspoons of olive oil for an appetite-stimulating abdominal massage.

When to get medical help

For children aged 1 to 3 years
- Reduced appetite lasts longer than a few days or is accompanied by other symptoms.

For older children and adults
- Appetite loss lasts longer than seven days, or there is also vomiting, diarrhea, a cough, abdominal pain, rapid weight loss, or other symptoms.

Get help right away for babies under 12 months if:
- Poor appetite is accompanied by fewer than five very wet diapers in a 24-hour period.
- Your baby refuses all feedings for longer than 24 hours.
- He or she vomits, cries uncontrollably, or shows other symptoms.

See also:
ANXIETY,
BREAST-
FEEDING
PROBLEMS,
DEPRESSION,
EATING
DISORDERS,
INDIGESTION,
NAUSEA AND
VOMITING,
PREGNANCY
PROBLEMS,
WEIGHT LOSS

Arterial Disease

Endemic in the Western world, arterial disease plagues the lives of many people and causes a high proportion of premature deaths. Cardiovascular disease claims the lives of nearly one million Americans each year. Lifestyle changes and other natural approaches can reduce—or even reverse—artery damage and make a significant difference to your well-being.

Diseased arteries can reduce the delivery of blood to the tissues and cause internal bleeding. They may also contribute to fluid retention. Arterial disease underlies most cardiovascular conditions, including the following: high blood pressure; angina and heart attacks; pain in the legs when walking; abnormally cold hands, feet, and nose; Raynaud's syndrome; migraine; and strokes and mini-strokes (transient ischemic attacks). The disorder can also cause dizziness, memory loss, and confusion. Less common manifestations include a group of inflammatory conditions known collectively as vasculitis or arteritis.

CAUSES

Many factors can lead to arterial disease. Often several factors are present, acting together to cause the disorder.

Irritation of the artery lining: This encourages the accumulation in the arteries of "bad" cholesterol (oxidized low-density lipoprotein, or LDL). The oxidized LDL collects as a layer of yellowish material, called atheroma, in the artery lining. This narrows the artery and encourages turbulence in the blood, leading to tiny tears in the artery lining that form scars as they heal. Scarred arteries can, at worst, tear through at their weakest points, resulting in hemorrhages that damage surrounding tissues. The roughened interior of a scarred artery promotes the formation of blood clots and further blockages.

Known irritants of the arterial lining include:
- A high level of oxidized blood fats
- A high blood-sugar level
- Smoking and passive smoking
- Autoimmune disorders (in which the damage is caused by a person's own immune system)

Possible irritants include:
- High blood levels of the amino acid homocysteine (the result of insufficient folic acid and vitamins B_6 and B_{12}, smoking, inactivity, and genetic flaws)
- Viral or bacterial infections, such as long-term lung or gum disease

Hardening of the arteries: This reduces the efficiency of the circulation. The artery walls may lose elasticity as a result of high blood pressure, smoking, inactivity, or atheroma.

Thickening of the blood: This encourages blood clots to form in arteries and can be caused by inactivity, infection of any kind, cold weather, and/or a diet that is low in nutrients and high in saturated fats.

Oversensitivity of the artery muscles: This leads to unexpected changes in artery diameter and blood flow. The condition can be caused by

low blood levels of magnesium and calcium, and also by stress, cold weather, smoking, changing hormone levels, insufficient intake of vitamin C, or a high fat intake.

PREVENTION

There are a number of established, preventable risk factors for arterial disease. By avoiding them, and by practicing other healthy habits, you can help keep your arteries strong.

Give up smoking: Smoking tends to narrow the arteries and to increase oxidation of fats in the blood. Stopping reduces your risk of serious arterial disease, and the longer you are a non-smoker, the lower your risk becomes. If you find quitting impossible, at least cut down, and eat plenty of foods rich in vitamins C and E. Each cigarette you smoke destroys about 25 milligrams of vitamin C, and you need both it and vitamin E to protect against heart disease.

Avoid inactivity: A half hour of exercise—strenuous enough to boost your circulation and make you feel warm (for example, a two-mile walk)—five or more days of the week is good for your heart and circulation. Exercise increases the ratio of protective HDL (high-density lipoprotein) cholesterol to the damaging LDL type, strengthens the heart, and promotes weight loss. Always warm up before exercise (see p. 13), especially after eating a fatty meal.

Ease tension: Make time each day to relax both mind and body. Good ways to do this include seeing friends, watching movies or TV, cooking

Reduce tension with yoga

By helping you deal with stress, yoga practice can make a significant contribution to the prevention of arterial disease. One relaxing yoga exercise is the standing forward bend: Stand with your feet together and your weight slightly forward. As you inhale deeply, raise your arms, stretching them above your head. Hold this position for 20 to 30 seconds. Then exhale while slowly bending from the waist and stretching your hands and arms down toward the floor. While breathing normally, hold the position for up to half a minute, then straighten slowly.

creatively, gardening, walking the dog, enjoying sex, and playing with your children. Or you can try progressive muscular relaxation (see p. 245), meditation, and yoga.

High stress levels trigger the release of epinephrine, cortisone, and other hormones. These raise blood pressure and increase oxidation of fat in the blood. Even slight depression raises stress hormone levels and makes the blood more sticky and prone to clot. Moreover, if you feel stressed or depressed, you are less likely to take care of yourself and more likely to indulge in such habits as smoking and compulsive eating—especially of sugary and fatty foods.

Stress and depression management skills include not only looking after your physical health, but also recognizing and dealing with your feelings—by, for example, learning safe

Risks dating from birth

Low birth weight and/or premature birth may make high blood pressure, heart attacks, and strokes more likely. If this applies to you, be especially careful to take steps to prevent arterial disease.

93

techniques for handling anger and other difficult emotions. This is especially important if you often find yourself hiding emotional distress, if you're argumentative, or if you've recently experienced the death of a loved one.

Choose a healthy diet: Avoid eating too much, and especially limit foods containing animal fats (as these are mainly saturated fats) and trans fats (present in many commercially hardened vegetable fats). A large, fatty meal creates a surge of fat in the blood, which encourages the formation of atheroma. Limit your intake of animal products—meat, eggs, butter, and other high-fat dairy products. Some people have an increased risk of arterial disease if they eat too much salt, because this can raise blood pressure.

Certain nutrients are good for the arteries and the heart. They include antioxidants, such as beta-carotene, the mineral selenium, and vitamins C and E, which reduce the oxidation of

LDL cholesterol. Omega-6 fatty acids (from vegetables, nuts, whole grains, seeds, and olive oil), omega-3 fatty acids (for example, from oily fish and pumpkin seeds), plant estrogens (for example, from soy products) and soluble fiber (in oats and apples, for example) help combat the effects of damaging fats in the blood.

These nutrients help maintain the health of the artery linings, strengthen the immune system, and counter danger from saturated fats and other artery irritants. Fruits and vegetables also contain natural salicylates, which help prevent blood from becoming too thick. Omega-3 fatty acids from fish also help prevent abnormal thickening of the blood.

An occasional glass of wine is safe for most people and may even be good for the arteries— partly because it dilates them, thereby increasing the blood supply to the heart muscle and other tissues, and partly because red wine (as well as some other alcoholic drinks) contains antioxidant plant pigments (flavonoids). Grape juice is an alternative source of flavonoids for those who need or prefer to avoid alcohol.

Manage your weight: Keep your weight down, especially if you are accumulating fat around your waist and abdomen and becoming "apple-shaped." Laying down fat in these areas makes a heart attack more likely.

Stay out of the cold: Living in a cold climate makes the blood thicker, increasing the possibility of clots. If you live somewhere cold, wet, and windy and also have additional risk factors, consider a move to somewhere warmer. If this isn't

Foods to counter artery damage
Consumption of onions, leeks, garlic, tomatoes, apples, oats, and oily fish is associated with a lower risk of heart disease because of their blood-thinning and/or antioxidant effects. Eating half a raw onion a day may help lower your blood level of damaging LDL cholesterol.

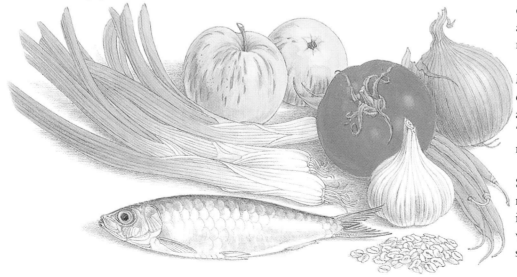

94

feasible, avoid the cold and cover up sufficiently when you must be outdoors.

Watch your breathing: Avoid overbreathing (hyperventilating) when stressed. Breathing too fast makes the blood relatively alkaline, which means that it is harder for red blood cells to supply enough oxygen to the cells of the artery walls. Try the breathing exercises on page 87.

Herbal remedies: Warming spices—such as ginger, cinnamon, cloves, and cayenne—added to recipes or used in a tea, aid arterial health by stimulating the circulation and dilating the blood vessels that supply the arms and legs.

■ Drink up to three cups a day of ginkgo biloba tea to help counter artery-wall inflammation and prevent the formation of damaging oxidized cholesterol.

■ Eat fresh garlic or take garlic tablets or capsules regularly. This can reduce high blood pressure and keep the blood flowing smoothly. Garlic lowers the level of cholesterol and reduces oxidation of LDL cholesterol.

Caution: For safety concerns, see pp. 34–37.

Supplements: There is evidence to suggest that certain food supplements, available at a drugstore or health-food store, can lower the risk of developing arterial disease.

■ The pectin in powdered grapefruit fiber may help reduce high blood cholesterol and open up blocked arteries.

■ The antioxidants beta-carotene, vitamins C and E, and selenium are thought to play an important part in protecting the circulatory system.

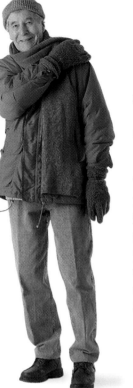

Dress warmly
Being cold causes the blood to thicken, thus becoming more likely to clot.

■ Bromelain, an enzyme derived from pineapple stalks, reduces blood stickiness.

■ The amino acid L-arginine helps form nitric oxide, which relaxes artery walls.

TREATMENT

If you develop arterial disease, remember that it is never too late to take steps to reduce or reverse the damage to your arteries. In consultation with your doctor, consider all of the preventive measures outlined above, as well as the following natural remedies:

■ Hawthorn, which is particularly valuable in treating high blood pressure caused by hardening of the arteries, angina, and arterial spasm. Use a teaspoon of the flowers or the crushed fruit to make one cup of tea, and sip at regular intervals throughout the day.

■ A daily dose (90–300 milligrams) of the antioxidant coenzyme Q_{10}, which may reduce the frequency of angina attacks.

When to get medical help

● You suffer pain when walking or unexplained dizziness or faintness.

Get help right away if:
● You experience pain in your chest, arms, or neck.
● You become unexpectedly short of breath, have sudden vision loss, or black out.
● Your arms or legs suddenly lose sensation or become very pale or bluish.

See also:
COLD HANDS AND FEET, DEPRESSION, DIABETES, DIZZINESS, HIGH BLOOD PRESSURE, MEMORY LOSS, MIGRAINE, OVERWEIGHT, PALPITATIONS, RAYNAUD'S SYNDROME, STRESS

Arthritis

More than 100 diseases fall under the heading of arthritis. The symptoms they have in common are joint stiffness and pain, which in some cases can severely limit movement. Arthritis is a chronic condition affecting about 43 million people in the United States. If you have arthritis, you may be able to relieve your symptoms by using a variety of natural methods.

Pain in a joint may be caused by an injury or a condition, such as rheumatoid arthritis, food sensitivity, or infection. Natural remedies can be used for pain that has not been directly caused by an injury. The main forms of arthritis are described in the box below.

PREVENTION

Although mainly associated with damaged cartilage in the joints from the wear and tear of aging, osteoarthritis may have a genetic component. To reduce your likelihood of suffering from joint damage, avoid becoming overweight, since this puts additional strain on the joints. Eat a healthy diet, containing plenty of fruits and vegetables, to provide the nutrients your body needs to repair damaged cartilage.

To help prevent rheumatoid arthritis, try to discover and avoid any trigger factors. Possibilities include stress and certain foods, such as (in order of likelihood) wheat and other cereal grains, red meat, sugar, animal fats, salt, coffee, dairy foods,

---

The main types of arthritis

Osteoarthritis occurs when the cartilage lining a joint—usually a weight-bearing joint, such as the knee or hip—wears away. Excess fluid can then accumulate in the joint, causing swelling, pain, and reduced mobility. Osteoarthritis is more common in people over 60. It affects almost three times as many women as men.

Rheumatoid arthritis results from inflammation of the membrane lining the joints and eventually the cartilage, too. The affected joints become swollen, stiff, and painful. In people with this arthritis, the normal immune response that is designed to protect against infection turns against the joint lining. The disorder usually begins in the fingers, wrists, and toes. You may inherit a tendency to rheumatoid arthritis, and one or more of several triggers may play a part. Some people with this condition have additional symptoms, such as fatigue, anemia, poor circulation, and trouble with the tendons, eyes, and thyroid gland. The disease generally begins in young or middle-aged adults and is two to three times more common in women. Women who have taken oral contraceptive pills seem to have a lower risk of developing rheumatoid arthritis.

Infective arthritis occurs when inflammation is caused by bacterial infection. This may be the result of germs entering a wound or may be linked to infection elsewhere in the body, as with, for example, tuberculosis, gonorrhea, or a urinary-tract infection.

Gout causes acute attacks of pain in the joints. It results from high levels of uric acid (a waste product) in the blood, which causes crystals of uric acid to form in a joint. High uric acid levels may be due to inefficient kidney function. Often only one joint is affected, frequently that of the big toe. In an attack the affected joint becomes red, hot, swollen, and extremely painful. Gout is 10 times more common in men. It is generally found in women only after they have gone through menopause.

and potatoes. Tomatoes, potatoes, peppers, and eggplants may promote arthritis in some people. Try excluding these foods to see if this eases your condition. It may be that pesticide poisoning and certain medications can also act as rheumatoid arthritis triggers.

You may be able to prevent attacks of gout by reducing alcohol consumption. Avoid eating liver and other organ meats, poultry, peas, and beans, since these are high in purines, substances that can raise the uric acid level in the blood.

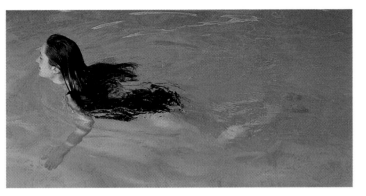

Stress-free exercise
Swimming is an ideal activity for those suffering from arthritis, because it helps strengthen affected joints without jarring them. Choose the stroke you find most comfortable.

TREATMENT

Most arthritis treatments aim to relax muscles and ease pain by reducing inflammation. Only a few try to correct the underlying causes.

Heat and cold: Heat can help relieve pain, aid circulation, and ease stiffness; cold is better for a hot and swollen joint. You may find relief by using one or more of the following:

- A compress made by dipping a small towel in hot or cold water and wringing it out. Place this over the affected joint(s).
- A pack of frozen peas wrapped in a towel and applied to the painful area.
- Gloves, socks, and other warm clothing.
- Warm (not hot) melted beeswax or paraffin. Immerse arthritic hands for 10 minutes. The wax peels off easily when cooled. It can be reused for further treatments.
- An Epsom salts bath for the discomfort of rheumatoid arthritis. Add two handfuls of

Epsom salts to a hot tub and soak for 15 to 20 minutes. (This treatment is unsuitable if you are very elderly or have high blood pressure.)

Rest and exercise: A joint that is very painful or inflamed should be rested. When it feels better, exercise daily for a half hour to warm the joint without stressing it. Do some muscle-strengthening exercises as well, to keep the muscles around the joint supple and to increase the production of joint-lubricating fluid.

Diet: Supply your joints and your immune system with the nutrients they need by eating a healthy diet, with five servings of vegetables and fruits daily. The essential fatty acids in oily fish (such as herring, sardines, and salmon), nuts, seeds (especially flaxseeds), and whole grains are particularly helpful for reducing inflammation. Some people find pineapple beneficial, possibly because it contains bromelain, an enzyme that aids digestion and increases the absorption of nutrients.

➤ continued, p. 99

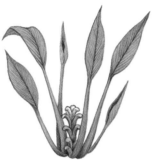

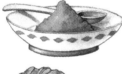

A spicy remedy
Turmeric contains powerful anti-inflammatory substances that ease sore joints. You can add the fresh or powdered root to curries and other dishes.

Relaxation with yoga

Ask your doctor if it would be appropriate for you to try yoga to ease your discomfort. Daily yoga exercises will not only help keep you and your muscles relaxed and your joints supple, but may also allow you to reduce your dosage of painkilling drugs. The gentle movements can, in addition, boost the immune system and stimulate the circulation of blood and lymph. If you think this form of exercise may suit you, try joining a yoga class. Some exercises for stiff joints are shown below. Do them slowly and carefully, without overstretching. Do not exercise joints that are red and painful.

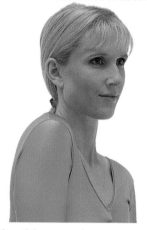

For knee pain
Sit comfortably with your legs stretched out in front. Bend one leg so that the heel is as close to your buttocks as you can manage. Flex the foot and then stretch out the leg without touching the floor. Repeat five times with each leg.

Shoulder rotation
Rotate arms one at a time, from the shoulder. Go forward a few times, then backward. Try it first with your arms straight, then bent.

Foot rotation
Use your hands to rotate the upper foot each way, then rotate the foot without using your hands. Wriggle your toes. Repeat with the other foot.

For hip pain
Lie on the floor with your lower back relaxed and feet together. Inhale slowly and bring one knee as close to your chest as is comfortable. As you slowly exhale, gently return your leg to the ground. Do this five times with each leg. Repeat the exercise, holding the bent knee and moving it in circles. Finally, repeat the exercise moving the bent knee from side to side.

Hand rotation
Slowly rotate each wrist a few times, first in a clockwise, then a counter-clockwise direction. Follow by wriggling your fingers.

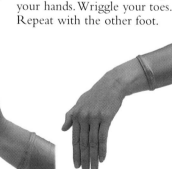

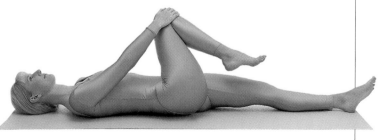

Bromelain can reduce inflammation in the body when taken between meals and is also available as an extract. Blueberries can also help combat arthritis. They are an excellent source of powerful antioxidants called proanthocyanidins, which can ease osteoarthritis.

Special advice for gout: In addition to the advice given above, try the following measures to relieve joint pain resulting from gout:
- Omega-3 fatty acids reduce inflammation, so take fish oil daily, which is a rich source of two such fatty acids: eicosapentaenoic acid (EPA) and docosahexanoic acid (DPA).
- Eat plenty of foods with high levels of beta-carotene (orange and yellow vegetables and fruits), vitamin C (citrus fruits), and vitamin E (vegetable oils, nuts, seeds, beans, and egg yolks—or from a vitamin E supplement), and selenium (whole grains, fish, and nuts).
- Eat cherries. They are an excellent source of proanthocyanidins, substances that are helpful for reducing the joint inflammation of gout. Cherry extract is an alternative when fresh cherries are unavailable.
- If you drink alcohol, reduce your intake.

Aromatherapy: German chamomile and lavender can ease inflammation. Juniper berry and cypress may reduce swelling. The warming properties of black pepper and sweet marjoram help relax muscles and relieve aching. Roman chamomile and cajuput may alleviate severe pain. Do not use cypress and cajuput oils in the first 20 weeks of pregnancy. Juniper berry oil should be avoided throughout pregnancy.
- Take a warm, scented bath: Sprinkle two drops of lavender oil into the water. Add two drops of either cajuput or Roman chamomile if you are suffering from severe pain.
- Make a warm compress by sprinkling two drops of lavender oil and two drops of juniper berry oil into a bowl of warm water. Place a piece of cloth over the surface of the water to pick up the oil film, then lay it over the affected joint. Cover with a towel, put a hot-water bottle on top, and leave for 30 minutes.
- Prepare some massage oil by mixing two drops each of juniper berry, black pepper, and Roman chamomile oils and five drops of lavender oil with 10 teaspoons of olive or jojoba oil. Smooth this scented oil over the affected joints each day.

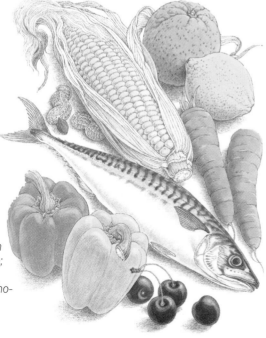

Anti-arthritis foods
To help alleviate symptoms, include in your diet foods containing beta-carotene, such as yellow and orange produce; omega-3 fatty acids, such as oily fish and nuts; and proantho-cyanidins, such as cherries.

Herbal remedies: Depending on your condition, choose from:

- Bogbean (buckbean) tea and celery-seed tea for rheumatoid arthritis. Drink one small cup three times a day. You can also add celery seeds to soups, casseroles, salad dressings, and pizzas.
- Devil's claw tea for rheumatoid arthritis. Add one teaspoon of the herb to a cup of water; simmer for 15 minutes. Drink a cup three times a day. Or buy devil's claw tablets from a health-food store or drugstore. Devil's claw can cause indigestion; stop taking it if you experience this problem.
- Wild thyme tea if stress is making your arthritis worse. Have one small cup three times a day.
- Nettle or coriander tea for gout. These herbs help the kidneys get rid of uric acid.
- Two or three dandelion roots, boiled in two pints of water in a covered pan for one hour. Drink this tea three times a day before meals.

Caution: For safety concerns, see pp. 34–37.

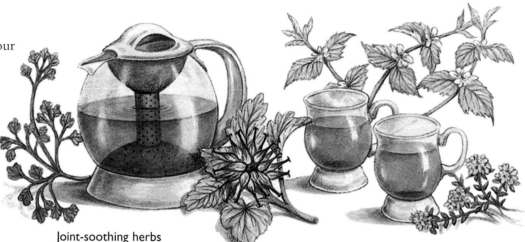

Joint-soothing herbs
Teas made from wild thyme, devil's claw, nettles, or coriander contain natural anti-inflammatory substances.

- A mixture of four parts olive oil, eight parts spirit of camphor, and one part cayenne pepper, used to massage the joints.
- Two large teaspoons of apple-cider vinegar in a glass of hot water flavored with a teaspoon of honey, taken twice a day.
- Tea made by adding boiling water to two teaspoons of powdered ginger.

Breathing: Some people find that their joint pain is worse if they breathe too fast or deeply. Exhaling too much carbon dioxide makes the blood more alkaline and prevents red blood cells from releasing oxygen. The lack of oxygen results in a need to breathe even more deeply or quickly. Practice breathing more slowly. Consult your doctor before trying breathing exercises if you have a disorder of the heart or lungs.

Kitchen cabinet remedies: Some people find the following traditional treatments effective:

When to get medical help

- Pain is severe.
- You also have a fever or don't feel well.
- Self-help treatments don't improve your symptoms.
- Your arthritis is getting worse, or discomfort impairs sleep or everyday functioning.

Get help right away if:
- The joint swells suddenly or severely.

See also:
BACK PAIN, PAIN

Asthma

Recurrent attacks of wheezing and breathlessness—known as asthma—can develop at any age, but they usually begin early in life and sometimes lessen or clear up completely by adulthood. Asthma is becoming more common; according to estimates, it now affects 12 to 15 million North Americans, including 5 million children.

Asthma occurs when the small airways in the lungs become overly sensitive, reacting to one or more substances that have no effect on non-asthmatic people. This reaction makes the lining of the airways swell and produce mucus, reducing the space available for incoming air. Principal symptoms include breathlessness (with particular difficulty in exhaling), wheezing, coughing, and tightness in the chest. Attacks vary in severity, from mild breathlessness to life-threatening respiratory failure. Frequent asthma attacks can interfere with everyday life.

Some people have an inherited tendency to get asthma, while many develop it for no known reason. Asthma is caused by an allergic reaction in 1 in 20 children and in 1 in 30 adults who are over 30 years old. A wide variety of things can trigger the oversensitivity of the airways that underlies the condition (see box below).

There are several possible reasons for the increase in asthma. The improved living conditions of people in developed countries mean that they have fewer early childhood infections and parasitic infestations. Because their immune systems don't have the early stimulation derived from exposure to foreign organisms, they may overreact not only to these organisms, but also to certain other substances later. The widespread

---

Asthma triggers

Allergens (inhaled or eaten), activities, or conditions may set off an asthma attack. They include:

- Dust-mite or roach droppings
- Pollen
- Dander (hair and skin scales) shed by pets
- Certain drugs (including aspirin)
- Certain foods (such as peanuts, shellfish, and eggs)
- Mites in food (cereals, flour, and other dried foods) well past the expiration date
- Mold spores
- Respiratory infection
- Cigarette smoke
- Vehicle exhaust fumes
- Vapor from air fresheners, perfumes, finishing chemicals in new clothes, dry-cleaning solvents, paints, glues, shoe-waterproofing sprays, and pesticides
- Nitrogen dioxide in burnt gas fumes from gas appliances
- Industrial chemicals and other substances (for example, dusts from paper, wood, and flour; fumes from welding and soldering; vapor from hardening agents and isocyanates)
- Cold air or a sudden temperature change
- Exercise
- Strong emotion

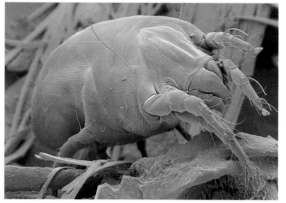

Tiny troublemaker
The dust mite, shown above at 245 times life-size, thrives in the modern super-insulated, heated home. Soft furnishings and wall-to-wall carpets provide its ideal environment. Dust-mite droppings are one of the most common asthma triggers.

use of antibiotics to treat relatively minor childhood infections also makes asthma more likely. This may be because antibiotics disturb the development of normal immunity by altering the population of bacteria in the intestine. As children grow older, they are more likely to overreact to viral infections and to substances in the environment. Environmental pollutants—from, for example, nitrogen dioxide, sulfur dioxide, ozone, and airborne particles in vehicle exhaust emissions—are also to blame.

PREVENTION

Try to identify your asthma trigger and take steps to avoid it. In cold weather, wind a scarf loosely around your nose and mouth so that you breathe warmer air. Air pollution is often at its worst when it's hot and humid, so you may want to stay inside on those days. Don't use spray products, and make your home a no-smoking zone.

If allergy tests reveal a sensitivity to dust mites, consider replacing wall-to-wall carpets or rugs with hard flooring, such as tiles or wood. Vacuum upholstery and drapes frequently, and clean them regularly. Wash bedclothes often, at as high a temperature as the fabric can withstand. Put your pillow and mattress in allergen-proof covers. Buy a vacuum cleaner or air purifier with a high-efficiency particulate air (HEPA) filter, or install such a filter in your heating system. Dust mites thrive in moist conditions, so purchase a dehumidifier if indoor humidity is high.

Once a week, kill dust mites in soft toys by laundering washable ones and putting others in the freezer overnight. If a pet causes asthma, you may have to give it away, though bathing it weekly may help.

Diet and supplements: A healthy diet (see p. 9) reduces the risk of wheezing. A magnesium supplement may help, and vitamins C and E may lessen the frequency of asthma triggered by smoke or air pollution. Garlic tablets may reduce production of mucus, which can contribute to narrowing of the airways. Take measures to identify and exclude any foods to which you might be allergic (see p. 214).

Exercise: Improving your general fitness with a daily half hour of strenuous exercise will boost your sense of well-being and your lung fitness.

Breathing and yoga: Regular breathing exercises, such as those taught by Buteyko instructors (see p. 60) or yoga practitioners, can increase your ability to relax your chest muscles. They may also improve your control over anxiety and

---

Spotting danger signs early

You may want to buy a peak flow meter and use it each morning and evening to measure how fast you can expel air. If your performance decreases, you can step up preventive actions.

other stress responses that can narrow the airways. Together these skills will make you less susceptible to frequent or severe asthma attacks.

Frequent episodes of feeling overstressed can readily instill the habit of rapid breathing. This eliminates too much carbon dioxide from the body, reducing the blood's acidity and thus diminishing the oxygen available to cells. All this leads to "air-hunger," a desire to get more oxygen by breathing even more rapidly.

Herbal remedies: Certain herbs may help relax airways and expel mucus, including echinacea, coltsfoot, elecampane, licorice, hyssop, and

---

Better breathing

When resting, always breathe deeply enough to expand both the lower and upper parts of your lungs. As your diaphragm descends, it presses against the abdominal organs, causing your abdomen to expand visibly. The exercises described below may reduce the severity and frequency of asthma attacks by helping to improve your breathing.

Rapid abdominal breathing
This relaxes the chest wall and helps reduce the severity of attacks.

1 With the neck, shoulder, and facial muscles relaxed, exhale strongly by contracting your abdominal muscles, then relax your abdomen as you inhale. Continue to breathe in this way, moving your abdomen with a slow rhythm, taking one breath every two seconds.

2 Gradually increase the speed until you are taking two breaths a second. Start with three sequences of 10 breaths each, then each week add another 10 until you do 30 in each sequence. Take a 20-second break between each sequence.

Breath-holding after exhaling
If you can hold your breath for no more than 30 seconds after exhaling, you may be in the habit of hyperventilating. This exercise allows you to measure and increase your breath-holding ability. Set aside a half hour each day to practice. Aim to increase the length of time you can comfortably hold your breath to 40 to 60 seconds. This may take several months of regular practice. To help you achieve this goal, be sure to get some form of aerobic exercise daily (see p. 13) and take steps to manage the unavoidable stress in your life effectively (see p. 347).

1 Use a stopwatch or a clock with a second hand. Sit in a relaxed manner but with your back straight, and keep your mouth closed throughout the exercise.

2 Exhale normally, then hold your nose and count how many seconds you can hold your breath. Then inhale slowly and smoothly. Reduce your breath-holding time if you feel faint or dizzy or get "pins and needles" in your fingers.

thyme. Vervain and chamomile are especially good if you feel tense. Drink one to two cups of one of these teas daily.
Caution: For safety concerns, see pp. 34–37.

TREATMENT

As soon as you feel an attack coming on, remove yourself, if possible, from any trigger, stay in a warm room, and summon help.

Breathing exercise during an attack: Sit comfortably upright, put one hand on your chest and the other on your stomach, and concentrate on relaxing, taking slow, easy breaths through your nose and filling your chest by using your abdominal muscles. The hand on your stomach should move farther up and down with each breath than the one on your chest.

Homeopathy: The following remedies may relieve a mild attack of asthma. Choose the one that most closely matches your symptoms.
- Arsenicum: if attacks often occur at night and make you feel restless and anxious.
- Ipecacuanha: if you feel that your lungs are congested with mucus and you have coughing along with nausea.
- Natrum sulphuricum: if attacks are brought on by damp conditions.
- Pulsatilla: if you feel better in the fresh air.

Other therapies: Acupuncture can help some asthma sufferers.

Massage to avert an attack

If you are feeling stressed and sense that you may be on the verge of an asthma attack, ask a friend to perform the back massage described below to relieve chest tension. You should lie on your front with your head to one side, while your friend does the following:

1 Kneel at a right angle to the person's back and place the heels of your hands on the far side of the upper back, avoiding the spine.

2 Leaning forward and pressing firmly, slide your hands over the ridge of muscle running alongside the spine from top to bottom.

3 Repeat this action, moving the starting point slightly down the spine toward the waist each time, until reaching the bottom rib. Do the same on the other side.

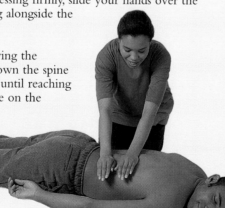

When to get medical help
- You need to find the cause of your asthma.
- Preventive measures don't stop attacks.
- You have an attack along with a worsening upper respiratory infection.

Get help right away if:
- You feel very breathless or dizzy, turn pale or bluish, or have chest pain during an attack.

See also:
ANXIETY, FOOD
SENSITIVITY

Back Pain

The health of your back is affected mainly by how you carry and use your body, but also by diet, digestion, and the way you cope with stress. Back pain affects most people at some time in their lives and is the leading cause of disability in the United States. Many natural therapies can be used to provide relief from back pain, even when orthodox therapies fail to help.

Back pain may be a slight problem lasting only a few days or a serious, long-lasting disability. Pain can result from any weakness in the back or from injury. Carrying heavy objects, exercising without due care, using a poor lifting technique, twisting or turning awkwardly—all these can cause damage. Bad posture, lack of exercise, sitting in one position for long periods, pregnancy, and being overweight make back pain more likely and may worsen existing pain. Stress is another major cause of back pain. Less commonly, backache results from a condition unrelated to the back, such as a urinary-tract infection.

CAUSES

Pain can result from problems with any part of the complex structure of the back (see illustration, below). Often it is caused by a combination of factors, such as:

- Strained muscles or ligaments.
- Damage to a facet joint in the spine.
- Muscle spasm, which occurs as a protective measure to immobilize the spine following injury, strain, or stress. The muscles surrounding the damaged area become tense and painfully stiff, often preventing all movement.
- Herniation of an intervertebral disk ("slipped disk"). This is a less frequent cause of back pain than was once thought. The pain results from the soft center of a disk bulging out and pressing on a nerve or irritating nearby tissues. Disks tend to dry out in later life, making them more vulnerable to injury. Inactivity also increases the risk of disk problems.
- Sciatica, a sharp, severe pain in the buttock that shoots down the back of the leg. The most common causes of this are a herniated disk pressing on the sciatic nerve and osteoarthritis.
- Osteoarthritis, which is one of the most common causes of back pain among those over 50.
- Osteoporosis, which can weaken the vertebrae so that they are easily crushed or fractured.
- Spinal stenosis, which is the narrowing of the spinal canal, causing pressure on the spinal cord or the nerves joining it.

➤ *continued, p. 106*

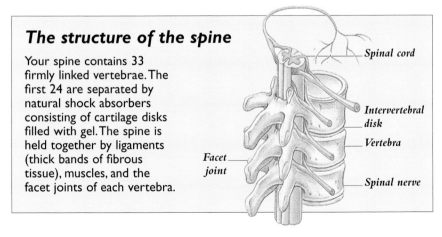

The structure of the spine

Your spine contains 33 firmly linked vertebrae. The first 24 are separated by natural shock absorbers consisting of cartilage disks filled with gel. The spine is held together by ligaments (thick bands of fibrous tissue), muscles, and the facet joints of each vertebra.

Spinal cord

Intervertebral disk

Vertebra

Facet joint

Spinal nerve

PREVENTION

The most important way to prevent back pain is to maintain your back's strength and flexibility with daily exercise. It is also essential to avoid excessive or awkward movements that can cause stress and strain. Take the following precautions to protect your back:

■ Never carry a heavy bag in one hand or on one shoulder. Instead, divide the contents between two bags, held one on each side. Better still, carry a backpack (use both straps), or sling a long-handled bag over the opposite shoulder.

■ To lift a heavy object, get as close to the object as possible, bend your knees, then lift by straightening your knees while keeping your back as straight as you can.

■ Don't twist your back while holding something heavy; move your feet to turn your whole body instead.

■ Sit with your back straight, making sure that your lower back is well supported. When driving, recline the seat to increase the thigh-to-trunk angle.

■ Wear comfortable shoes with good support that will not cause an abnormal gait. Placing orthotics prescribed by a podiatrist in the shoes can often reduce back strain.

■ If you work for long hours at a computer, make certain that you sit correctly (see photograph, left). Use a footrest if you can't place your feet flat on the floor.

■ Never stoop to do a ground-level job, such as weeding in the garden. Kneel instead.

■ Check that your mattress is firm enough to support your back, but not overly hard. If it is too soft, you can make it firmer by placing a board between the mattress and base.

TREATMENT

If stress is a contributing factor, try to reduce the sources of stress in your life, and use stress-management techniques (see p. 347).

Heat and cold: This form of hydrotherapy improves circulation and promotes healing.

■ To ease the pain of strained muscles or sciatica, apply a towel that has been dipped in hot water and wrung out.

■ Apply a hot towel (see above) for two minutes and then a towel wrung out in cold water for one minute. Alternate the two for about 15

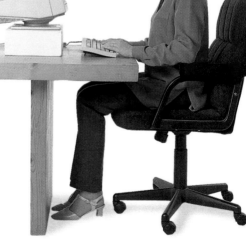

Avoiding strain
When working at a computer for any length of time, be sure that your knees are bent at a 90-degree angle and that your lower back is well supported by a correctly adjusted chair.

The supine twist

This gentle exercise can ease back stiffness. (Stop if it causes pain.)

Lie on your back. Place your right foot on your left knee, and lower your right knee to the left, twisting from the waist. Rest your left hand on your right thigh. Raise your right arm upward to the right, palm up, and look toward it. Relax in this position for one minute and then repeat on the other side.

Exercises for your back

Prolonged bed rest is no longer recommended for back pain. Instead, get up and about as soon as possible and, after checking with your doctor, begin to do a few minutes of gentle exercise each day. Build up a regular exercise routine to strengthen your back and abdominal muscles and to increase your flexibility. The following exercises help relieve strained muscles or ligaments, irritated facet joints, and sometimes sciatica. As with any exercise, stop immediately if you feel pain.

1 Lie on your back on the floor, with a small cushion or rolled towel under your neck. Bend your knees, then press the small of your back to the floor, tilting your pelvis slightly upward. Placing both hands around one knee, gently pull your thigh toward your chest for 10 seconds, then lower your foot to its original position. Do the same with the other leg, and repeat the sequence 10 times.

2 Lie on your back on the floor, with legs straight and feet flexed. Rest your linked hands on your lower abdomen. Breathe slowly and deeply, and as you inhale, slowly raise your straight arms—keeping your hands linked—until they are vertically above your face. Without stopping the movement, start exhaling, moving your arms down behind your head to rest on the floor. Reverse this procedure, inhaling as you raise your arms, and exhaling as you lower them to rest your linked hands on your lower abdomen. Press down firmly with your hands. Repeat the whole exercise five or six times.

3 Lie on your back with your knees bent to your abdomen and your hands holding your lower thighs. Curl your back slightly, with your weight on your lower back, then rock from side to side several times.

4 Lie face down with your palms on the ground just below shoulder level.

5 Raise your head and shoulders as far as is comfortable for you, using the muscles of your back and without pushing with your arms. Do this 10 times.

107

minutes. This is especially helpful if your pain results from muscle strain. Use just the cold towel for pain resulting from inflammation.

Herbal remedies: These can help relieve pain and stiffness, as well as stimulate circulation.
- Rub equal amounts of glycerin and tincture of cayenne into the skin over the painful area.
- Apply frequent hot compresses of cramp bark, valerian, chamomile, or ginger to the back.
- For sciatica, rub the skin with St. John's wort oil (see p. 192).
Caution: For safety concerns, see pp. 34–37.

Homeopathy
- Arnica: if back pain has followed an injury, take orally twice a day.

- Hypericum: to relieve back pain resulting from nerve irritation, take orally twice a day.

Other therapies: Chiropractic and osteopathy may help relieve persistent back trouble.

When to get medical help

- The pain does not improve after a few days or worsens at any time.

Get help right away if:
- The pain is sudden and severe.
- You lose sensation or strength in a limb.

See also:
ARTHRITIS, NECK AND SHOULDER PAIN, OSTEOPOROSIS

Massage for back pain

Gentle massage of the muscles on either side of the spine can often ease pain. Try these special massages to alleviate sciatica (below left) and stretch the spine (below right). Stretching the spine can help some back pain by relaxing tense bands of muscle on either side of the spine. Lie on a mat or on folded blankets or towels.

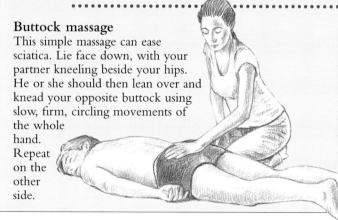

Buttock massage
This simple massage can ease sciatica. Lie face down, with your partner kneeling beside your hips. He or she should then lean over and knead your opposite buttock using slow, firm, circling movements of the whole hand. Repeat on the other side.

Spinal stretch
Kneel on the floor with your forehead touching the ground, your arms pointing back, and your hands near your feet. You may need a cushion between your calves and buttocks for comfort. Have your partner kneel beside you with one hand at the top of your spine and one at the base. He or she should then push down with each hand pressing slightly away from the other, so as to stretch out your spine.

Bad Breath

Unpleasant breath, or halitosis, usually results from eating strongly flavored foods, such as garlic or onions, smoking cigarettes, or drinking alcohol. Your breath may also be affected by disorders involving the mouth, lungs, or digestive tract. Sweeten your breath by using herbs, spices, and other kitchen-cabinet items. Paying attention to oral hygiene is also vital.

Mouth freshener
Add two drops of peppermint oil to a cup of warm water and gargle.

Persistent bad breath is frequently caused by poor oral hygiene, tooth decay, or gum disease. Fasting or eating too much food of animal origin may also be to blame. Occasionally, bad breath is a symptom of sinusitis, a respiratory disorder, anemia, diabetes, or a fever. In addition, if you produce insufficient stomach acid and eat fruit after a protein meal, the fruit may ferment in the stomach, producing gases that cause bad breath.

PREVENTION

Eat plenty of green leafy vegetables, because these contain the plant pigment chlorophyll, a natural breath freshener. Limit your intake of refined carbohydrates, coffee, alcohol, and dairy products, since they encourage bad breath.

If you also suffer from poor digestion or flatulence, you may be producing insufficient stomach acid. To boost your digestion, add vinegar to meals of meat, fish, or eggs. Apple-cider vinegar provides acetic acid in roughly the same strength as that of normal gastric acid. Some people benefit from gargling (do not swallow) with a solution of two teaspoons of this vinegar in half a pint of warm water each day. Brush your teeth meticulously twice daily, then use

dental floss or tape. If you are not sure how to do this correctly, consult your dentist. Brushing the tongue also helps prevent bad breath.

TREATMENT
Herbal remedies

- Chew parsley leaves to counteract the scent of garlic on the breath.
- Chew aniseed or fennel, dill, cardamom, or caraway seeds to prevent bad breath at any time.
- Drink fenugreek or peppermint tea to sweeten breath after a meal.
- A daily mouthwash of echinacea tea helps treat gum infections that cause bad breath. Add two teaspoons of echinacea root to one cup of water. Simmer, covered, for 10 minutes, then cool before using.

When to get medical help

- Your gums bleed or you have mouth ulcers.
- Bad breath persists despite self-help treatment.
- Bad breath is a new problem and does not stop within a week.

See also:
CANDIDA INFECTIONS, COLDS,
GUM PROBLEMS, INDIGESTION

Bloating

*D*istension of the stomach and intestines is a very common problem. It often results in discomfort, especially if the swollen abdomen makes clothes too tight. Bloating has a variety of possible causes, including fluid retention and excess gas, most of which can successfully be treated with a range of natural remedies and lifestyle changes.

The most likely cause of abdominal distension is an overfull stomach and intestines. Overeating—especially of foods high in refined carbohydrates and fats, such as cookies, cakes, and pies—may result in excess gas production, leading to bloating. Other causes include fluid retention, gastroenteritis, food sensitivity, constipation, irritable bowel syndrome, celiac disease (intolerance to gluten, a cereal protein), lactose intolerance (inability to digest lactose, the sugar in milk), inflammation or ulceration of the stomach or intestinal lining, and candida infection. Bloating may also result from a disruption in the population of bacteria in the intestines, leading to an insufficient number of "friendly" bacteria, such as *Lactobacillus acidophilus*.

Many women experience bloating just before their period, when hormonal changes lead to fluid retention. Occasionally, heart, kidney, or liver disease, an ovarian cyst, or another condition or complication causes distension.

PREVENTION

Bloating from fluid retention: Fluid retention can be associated with a salty diet. Many commercially processed foods contain high levels of salt and other sources of sodium (including baking soda and monosodium glutamate, or MSG), so always read labels. Minimize your sodium intake in the following ways:

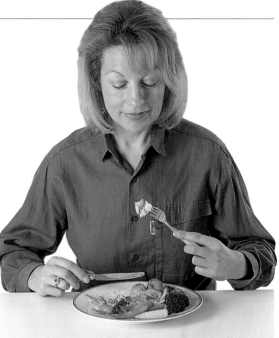

How you eat and what you eat
Choose your foods carefully, and take your time during meals to relax and chew well.

- Avoid processed meats (such as bacon, ham, sausage, and corned beef), stock cubes, yeast extract, and salted snacks.
- Buy low-salt foods. Look for low-salt bread, cereals, canned and frozen vegetables, butter and spreads, sauces, pickles, and soup.
- Don't cook vegetables in salted water.
- Don't add salt or sodium products to home-cooked recipes or to the food on your plate.

Bloating from digestive problems

- Eat small, frequent meals.
- Chew each mouthful well and avoid talking while eating. Powerful enzymes in the mouth aid digestion.
- Avoid carbonated beverages.
- Don't drink during meals. Fluid dilutes stomach acid and digestive enzymes, which may slow the passage of food through your stomach. In particular, any fruit eaten is then more likely to ferment and produce gas.
- Avoid eating starchy foods, such as pasta and potatoes, in the same meal as protein or fruit.
- Avoid excessive quantities of legumes, fatty foods, and raw fruits and vegetables, as these can increase the volume of gas in the intestines.
- Curtail a high fiber intake, especially of insoluble fiber, such as wheat bran.
- Take some papain, an enzyme preparation made from papaya, with each meal.
- If you suspect a food sensitivity, follow an exclusion diet to identify the cause (see p. 214).
- Try for one day eating only finely grated or puréed apples and drinking only mineral water or peppermint tea. On the next day, add some vegetable soup or steamed vegetables to the midday and evening meals, and then expand your diet over the next two days to include savory rice and yogurt with live cultures. After that, continue with a normal healthy diet.

Bloating from abnormal intestinal flora

- Eat foods, such as yogurt, containing *Lactobacillus acidophilus*. If you're milk-sensitive, take an acidophilus supplement, widely available in health-food stores.

Premenstrual bloating: Try the following for the three days before bloating usually begins:

- Eat more foods rich in vitamins B_6 and E, magnesium, and essential fatty acids (see p. 12).
- Cut out caffeine and added sugar and salt.
- Mix three drops of juniper berry oil and two drops each of rosemary and lavender oils with five teaspoons of grapeseed or wheat-germ oil. Omit juniper berry and rosemary oils if you are trying to conceive. Ask a friend to use this mixture to massage the backs of your legs (with upward strokes), lower back, and abdomen (with clockwise circular movements).
- Take 500 to 1,500 milligrams of evening primrose oil capsules twice a day, in this case starting one week before your period.

TREATMENT
Herbal remedies

- For bloating that occurs with indigestion or gas, pour a pint of boiling water over an ounce of cut angelica root, cover, and steep for 10 minutes. Take two tablespoons of this tea three times a day before meals. Or, chew some raw angelica leaves or root.

➤ *continued, p. 112*

A fragrant compress
To prevent premenstrual bloating, use a compress. Place a towel in a bowl of warm water to which you've added three drops each of rosemary and juniper berry oils and two drops each of lavender and cypress oils. Wring out and apply to the abdomen and chest for as long as is comfortable. Do not use this treatment if you are trying to conceive.

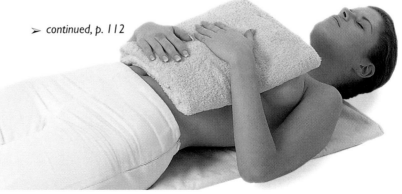

■ Have tea made from wild yam, peppermint, ginger, cinnamon, fennel, lemon balm, or chamomile after a meal to prevent gas-related bloating. If preferred, drink half a cup of warm water containing a few drops of a tincture made from one of these herbs.

■ Prevent gas by adding warming spices—such as cayenne, ginger, and cardamom and caraway seeds—to your meals.

■ For bloating resulting from premenstrual fluid retention, drink a cup of celery seed or horse-tail tea twice daily.

Caution: For safety concerns, see pp. 34–37.

Aromatherapy: For bloating with indigestion, gas, or fluid retention, try the following treatments with essential oils (but not if you are or might be pregnant):

■ Add three drops of black pepper oil to three tablespoons of sunflower oil. After a meal, smooth gently onto your abdomen, using clockwise movements.

■ Add four drops of peppermint oil and two drops each of juniper berry and black pepper oils to half a teaspoon of

Plant remedies for fluid retention
Cucumber, parsley, nettles, yarrow, elderflower, and meadowsweet have all been used to remove excess fluid. Include them in your diet or make herbal teas.

Abdominal massage
Clockwise massage of the abdomen using appropriate essential oils (see "Aromatherapy") can help shift excess gas or fluid.

unscented skin lotion. Apply to your abdomen with slow, clockwise movements.

■ Soak in a bathtub of warm water to which you have added three drops of black pepper oil and three drops of fennel oil.

■ Massage your abdomen with two teaspoons of grapeseed or wheat-germ oil to which you have added two or three drops of cinnamon, ginger, clove, or peppermint oil.

When to get medical help

● You have persistent or worsening pain.
● You have vomited or you have a fever.
● Your ankles are swollen.
● You have a chronic condition, especially if it suddenly worsens.

See also
CANDIDA INFECTIONS, CONSTIPATION, DIARRHEA, FLATULENCE, FOOD SENSITIVITY, INDIGESTION, IRRITABLE BOWEL SYNDROME, PREMENSTRUAL SYNDROME

Breast-feeding Problems

Your milk is the best food for your baby. It provides all the nutrients he or she needs as well as protection against infection and allergy. Nursing also gives you and your baby a special sense of closeness, and it has health benefits for you. Any difficulties can usually be overcome with proper information and the support of family, friends, and health-care professionals.

Breast milk is nutritionally perfect for babies and contains enzymes that make it easy to digest, as well as substances that boost immunity and enhance growth. Nourishing your baby with breast milk alone for the first six months and continuing to breast-feed for at least another six months protects against many infections. Breast-fed babies rarely develop gastroenteritis and are less likely to suffer from lung, ear, and urinary-tract infections or to develop such allergic conditions as asthma and eczema. Breast-feeding may also reduce the risk of sudden infant death syndrome (SIDS), or crib death.

Almost every woman is able to breast-feed, although some, especially first-time mothers, experience problems. Common difficulties include sore or cracked nipples, engorged breasts, blocked ducts, and a poor milk supply.

PREVENTION

Diet: To maintain your energy level and ensure an adequate milk supply, increase your calorie intake by 400 to 600 calories a day, concentrating on nutritious foods. You will need to maintain a calcium intake of about 1,200 milligrams a day (see "Calcium-rich Foods," p. 298). Eat small amounts often, with a meal or snack between each feeding. Drink at least eight glasses of caffeine-free fluids a day. Be aware that most substances you consume will be present in

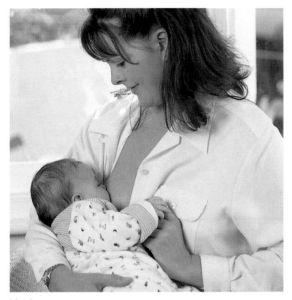

Vital protection
In the first few days after giving birth, your breasts produce a special milk called colostrum. This contains antibodies to help protect against infection.

your breast milk. Therefore avoid hard liquor and ask your doctor before taking any medications. Don't have beer or wine for at least two hours before nursing.

Everyday routine: Your baby will feed frequently at first, so delegate other tasks whenever possible. Get as much rest as you need, especially in the first few weeks following the birth,

when your milk supply is becoming established. Breast-feeding triggers the release of hormone-like substances called endorphins, as well as prolactin (a hormone that causes milk glands to produce milk), all of which can induce a feeling of calm and well-being.

Relaxation: Try to be relaxed when you feed your baby. If you feel tense or anxious, you may fail to release enough oxytocin, the hormone that triggers the initial flow of milk. Your hungry baby will then become frustrated, making you more tense. Simple measures, such as sitting quietly with a warm drink or watching TV, may be enough to make you feel relaxed. If this does not work, try using the relaxation techniques, such as deep breathing exercises, that you learned in prenatal classes.

TREATMENT

It is important to know how to tackle the common breast-feeding problems that can beset any mother. If you can't solve a problem yourself, get advice from a trained breast-feeding counselor or other health-care professional.

Engorged breasts: When the mature milk comes in a few days after the birth, your breasts may feel tight, swollen, and painful. This makes it difficult for your baby to "latch on"—to take hold of the nipple and areola properly—and this in turn can make the nipples sore.

- Nurse frequently, day and night, to prevent too much milk from accumulating in your breasts.
- To relieve some of the engorgement and allow your baby to take the breast more easily,

Breast milk by bottle

There is no reason why breast-feeding your baby should restrict your independence. Invest in a breast pump that allows you to express your milk into a bottle. This can then be given to your baby by your partner or a babysitter. If you will be expressing milk only at home, a full-size electric pump may be appropriate. These can often be rented. If you need to use a pump outside the home, choose a smaller type—either manual or electric. Remember to follow the instructions on sterilizing the breast pump and to use sterilized bottles or milk-collection bags (for freezing).

express a little milk before a feeding, either by hand or with a breast pump (see box, above).
- If your breasts are so full that expressing is impossible, bathe them in hot water for several minutes or place a hot compress on each breast before a feeding to help the milk flow. Place a cold compress on each breast between feedings to reduce discomfort.

Sore or cracked nipples: If your nipples hurt when your baby suckles, try the following:
- Place your baby so that he or she takes the whole areola into the mouth. Change the position in which you hold your baby at each feeding to ensure that no one part of the nipple takes too much of the force of your baby's sucking action. Your counselor can advise you.
- Treat any engorgement as soon as possible (see previous section).

- Encourage your milk to flow—before you put your baby to the breast—by relaxing and making yourself comfortable.
- Feed your baby frequently, but if your nipples are very sore or cracked, limit the length of each feeding for a day or two, and express any remaining milk.
- Offer the less sore nipple first.
- Don't use soap on your nipples.
- After a feeding, dry nipples, then apply some breast milk or calendula (marigold) ointment.
- Allow your nipples to air-dry as much as you can. If possible, expose your nipples to sunlight for just a few minutes each day.
- If leakage is a problem, keep your nipples dry by wearing breast pads (not plastic-lined), changing them frequently.

Blocked ducts: A tender, red lump in your breast may be a sign of a clogged milk duct. Try to clear the duct as soon as possible to avoid infection. The following measures will help:

- Empty your breasts thoroughly each time your baby feeds. Feed your baby from the affected breast first.
- Feed your baby more often, and express between or after sessions, if necessary.
- Gently but firmly massage the lump toward the nipple during a feeding.
- In the bath or shower, soap the area of the affected duct and then gently run a wide-tooth comb over it to stimulate milk flow and help clear the blockage.
- Do some arm-swinging exercises (see right).
- Ensure that your bra fits well and isn't pressing too hard and causing the blockage.

Boosting circulation
Prevent and treat blocked milk ducts by swinging your arms in big circles— forward and backward— for five minutes every hour or two.

- Vary your feeding position at each nursing.
- To relieve pain, place a hot, wet compress or a covered hot-water bottle on the breast every hour. Before a feeding, splash the breast or immerse it in hot water for 5 to 10 minutes.
- Increase your intake of vegetables, whole grains, oily fish, and vegetable oils. A supplement of vegetable lecithin may also help.

Poor milk supply: Only rarely is a woman unable to produce a sufficient amount. Nurse frequently and for as long as your baby wants, since sucking stimulates the milk to flow.

- To try to increase your milk supply, drink a cup of tea once or twice daily of chasteberry, nettle, fennel, vervain, raspberry leaf, cinnamon, blessed thistle, or marshmallow. Caraway, coriander, cumin, sunflower, sesame, celery, and fenugreek seeds are also said to help.

Caution: For safety concerns about herbs, see pp. 34–37.

Homeopathy: Calcarea carbonica, Pulsatilla, and Urtica are believed to promote milk flow. Silica may help cracked nipples.

When to get medical help

- A breast-feeding problem worries you or doesn't clear up in a few days.
- A lump or a red area persists or worsens.

Get help right away if:
- Your baby has not been feeding for 24 hours.

Bruises

Most bruises are the result of minor bumps or falls and disappear after only a few days. Even so, they may cause pain, especially if the site of the bruise is pressed or knocked. You may be able to keep a bruise from developing, or at least reduce its severity, if you carry out self-help treatment of the affected area as soon as possible after the injury.

A bruise is a discolored area of skin that forms usually after a blow damages underlying small blood vessels (capillaries). At first the blood leaking from the capillaries makes a bruise appear black and blue. Then, as the blood breaks down, the bruise turns yellow, green, or purple.

TREATMENT

Immediate action: Apply a cold compress as soon as possible after the injury. Soak a cloth in ice-cold water and place over the area for 10 minutes, or use a pack of frozen peas wrapped in a towel. Take one or two pilules (tiny tablets) of the homeopathic remedy Arnica 30c as soon as possible to minimize bruising. Repeat the dose every 15 to 60 minutes, depending on the severity of your injury, and continue for several doses. Also apply herbal arnica ointment or cream if the skin is not broken.

Herbal remedies: A number of herbs are effective in reducing the severity of bruising.
- If the skin is not broken or scraped, make a compress of comfrey (also known as bruisewort) by soaking some gauze in comfrey tea and placing over the injured area for an hour. Make the tea by pouring a pint of boiling water over one ounce of dried—or two ounces of fresh—leaves, infuse for 10 minutes, then strain. (Do not drink the tea.)

- A cabbage-leaf poultice is also soothing. Take the greenest leaves of a cabbage and discard the ribs. Warm the leaves in hot water, then drain them and flatten with a rolling pin. Place several leaves over the bruise, and secure them with a bandage or taped plastic wrap. Change the poultice every few hours.
- Calendula ointment and witch hazel solution are time-honored remedies for bruising, as both help stop bleeding under the skin.
Caution: For safety concerns, see pp. 34–37.

Aromatherapy: Mix five drops of sweet marjoram oil and two drops each of myrrh (omit during the first 20 weeks of pregnancy) and German chamomile oils with five teaspoons of calendula (marigold) oil or lotion. Apply to unbroken skin as soon as possible after the injury and repeat hourly until the pain subsides.

When to get medical help
- Bruises appear for no apparent reason.
- Skin discoloration is accompanied by severe pain and swelling.
- A bruise does not fade after a week.

See also:
STRAINS AND SPRAINS

Burns

Heat, friction, and chemicals can all burn or scald the skin. Many burns result from accidents at home, and prompt first aid can mean the difference between rapid recovery without scarring or further damage to the skin. After applying standard first aid, try natural treatments to soothe discomfort and promote healing.

Fast action is essential for both major and minor burns. You can safely self-treat small burns that affect only the top layer of skin. Carry out first aid as described in the box below. Deeper or more extensive burns and those caused by electricity need emergency medical attention.

TREATMENT

After first-aid treatment, you can let minor burns heal by themselves, but the following may help.

Aromatherapy: Apply lavender oil to the burn and cover it with gauze, secured at the edges with tape. Reapply the oil every two hours for 24 hours, without removing the gauze. If the burn has not then healed, apply six drops of lavender oil and two of geranium oil mixed with one teaspoon of grapeseed or sweet almond oil. Repeat four times daily until healed.

Herbal remedies: Apply one of the following:
- Aloe vera gel
- St. John's wort oil
- Calendula (marigold) ointment
- A compress soaked in diluted witch hazel or cooled tea made from chamomile, marigold, elderflower, or chickweed (or use a washcloth soaked in whole milk)
- Elderflower lotion or ointment
- Crushed yellow dock leaves

Homeopathy
- Apply Urtica or Hypercal (ointment or tincture) to burns that do not blister.
- Take Cantharis by mouth every hour for burns that blister.

Flower essences: Take Rescue Remedy to counter the emotional shock of the burn.

First aid for minor burns

- As soon as possible, immerse the area in cold water for at least 10 minutes. This cools the skin, stops burning, and relieves pain. If water is unavailable, use any cold, non-irritating liquid, such as milk or iced tea.
- Remove jewelry or clothing that may constrict the area should swelling occur.
- Cover the burn with a sterile dressing. If unavailable, use any clean, dry, absorbent cloth.
- Don't break blisters.
- Seek medical help as necessary (see box, right).

When to get medical help

Get help right away if:
- A burn covers more than two inches.
- A burn is deeper than the top layer of skin.
- A severe burn affects the mouth or throat.
- There is pus or increasing swelling or redness.
- The burn was caused by an electric shock or by chemicals.

Candida Infections

A yeastlike fungus, Candida albicans usually lives in the intestines, along with many other varieties of microorganisms. These organisms are known collectively as intestinal flora. The balance among them normally prevents overgrowth of any one type. However, sometimes the balance is upset, allowing candida to multiply unchecked, causing infection.

Also called thrush or a yeast infection, a candida infection can affect any area of mucous membrane or moist skin. In the vagina it causes a thick, whitish, curdlike discharge and, frequently, itching and soreness. A candida infection of the mouth—oral thrush—causes sore, raised, creamy-yellow patches in the mouth and on the tongue. Candida can also affect the nipples and the folds of skin at the sides of the nails. Some babies develop a diaper rash infected with candida; this is typically bright red with white patches. Generalized infection of the body with candida is a rare but serious condition.

Some alternative therapists believe that an overgrowth of candida in the intestines can cause a variety of symptoms, including poor digestion, gas, bloating, and even such problems as fatigue, headaches, and other aches and pains.

Candida infection can be triggered by anything that upsets the balance among microorganisms in the body—for example, poor general health, pregnancy, stress, and taking antibiotics, oral steroids, or contraceptive pills. Other possible causes include uncontrolled diabetes, reduced stomach-acid production, and a diet high in yeast-containing foods, alcohol, and refined carbohydrates, such as sugar and white flour.

PREVENTION

Diet: If you are vulnerable to candida infections, there are a number of adjustments you can make to your diet to boost your resistance.

- Cut out, or at least limit, foods containing added sugar and refined carbohydrates.
- Reduce your intake of foods containing natural sugars, such as milk, fruit, and wine.
- Drink no more than three cups of caffeine-containing tea or coffee a day.
- Eat two crushed or finely chopped cloves of raw garlic three times a day, perhaps in a salad dressing or added to soup at the last minute. Alternatively, take garlic capsules or tablets.
- Choose more foods containing B vitamins, particularly biotin and vitamins B_6 and B_{12}.
- Eat some yogurt with live *Lactobacillus acidophilus* cultures each day. These bacteria help

Anti-candida foods
Base meals around foods that discourage candida, such as yogurt with live cultures, leafy green vegetables, garlic, and olive oil.

118

maintain a beneficial balance of microorganisms in the intestines. You can also take acidophilus in tablet, capsule, or powder form.

■ Eat a healthy diet containing plenty of iron, magnesium, selenium, zinc, flavonoids, and vitamins A, C, and E (see p. 12).

Preventing vaginal yeast infections: If you are prone to vaginal candida, try the following:

■ Wear cotton rather than nylon underwear, and stockings rather than pantyhose. Avoid tightly fitting pants. Good circulation of air in the genital area discourages infection.

■ Make the water in your bath or shower as cool as is comfortable for you.

■ Change your towel frequently. Don't dry your genital area too roughly; sore skin is more prone to infections.

■ Avoid perfumed soaps, bubble baths, and other bath additives. Do not use fragranced vaginal deodorants, which may irritate the skin, making it more vulnerable to infection.

■ Use a lubricant during sexual intercourse if you feel dry, since too much friction can cause soreness, which promotes candida infection.

■ When using the toilet, wipe from front to back to prevent intestinal microorganisms from entering your vagina.

TREATMENT
From the drugstore

■ For vaginal yeast infections, douche gently with a boric acid solution: dilute one teaspoon of boric acid in a quart of tepid water.

■ For intestinal candida, take caprylic acid in tablet or capsule form.

Herbal remedies: The following are known to inhibit the growth of intestinal candida: black walnut seed hull, goldenseal, and oregano oil. These can be taken as capsules or tinctures.
Caution: For safety concerns, see pp. 34–37.

Aromatherapy: The antifungal action of lavender, sweet thyme, and tea tree oils may help clear up vaginal yeast infections.

■ Kneel in bathwater to which you have added essential oils (see illustration, right) and splash the water around the external genital area several times before sitting down. Remain in the tub for at least 10 minutes.

■ Mix two drops of sweet thyme oil and four of lavender oil with two and a half teaspoons of a cold-pressed oil, such as sweet-almond or olive oil. Smooth over your vulva to soothe soreness.

■ Apply two drops of tea tree oil to the top of a slightly dampened tampon and insert into your vagina. Leave there for three to four hours.

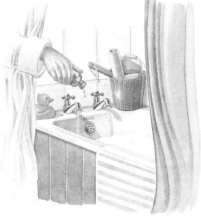

A healthy soak
To treat a yeast infection, sprinkle six drops of tea tree oil and two of sweet thyme oil into your bathwater, or add a few dandelion leaves.

When to get medical help

● A candida infection does not clear up after a few days of self-treatment.
● A baby or young child is affected.
● You develop a mouth infection.
● You suspect you may have a candida infection of the nipples.

See also:
DIABETES,
DIAPER RASH,
VAGINAL PROBLEMS

Cellulite

Up to four out of five Western women have lumpy, dimpled, fatty areas known as cellulite. Occasionally men are affected, too. The belief that the fat in cellulite is fundamentally different from fat elsewhere is popular among non-scientists, but incorrect. There is no special health risk associated with cellulite, unless you are also significantly overweight.

Certain parts of the body, such as the thighs and buttocks, are especially prone to developing dimpled fat. This cellulite can be hard to shift and usually appears when the reproductive hormones are in a state of flux—for example, at puberty, during pregnancy, around menopause, and when contraceptive pills are being taken.

HOW CELLULITE FORMS

The fat of cellulite is separated by inelastic bands of connective tissue. These bands run between the skin and the deeper tissues, where they are firmly secured. Many people with cellulite are overweight. As a person gains weight, the fat cells swell but the connective bands stay the same length. The fat then bulges the only way possible—toward the skin—and as this happens, the bands pull at the skin, creating the characteristic dimpled appearance of cellulite. The problem often becomes more apparent with age.

Poor circulation of lymph may contribute to cellulite formation. Lymph is a milky liquid that carries excess fluid, waste products, and toxins from the tissues to the bloodstream via the lymphatic vessels. Poor circulation of lymph—because of excess fat, lack of exercise, or fluid retention—may allow these wastes to build up in the tissues. This may be one reason that some women who are not overweight have cellulite.

PREVENTION

Try to keep your weight at a normal level and avoid rapid increases in weight. Exercise regularly to improve your body tone, reduce fat, build muscle, and boost the circulation of lymph and blood. Avoid sitting or standing for long periods. Eat five servings of vegetables and fruits each day. Limit your intake of alcohol and caffeine. Drink enough water-based fluids each day to relieve thirst and produce pale-colored urine.

TREATMENTS

A number of natural therapies can help improve the appearance of the affected areas temporarily.

Massage and skin brushing: A firm massage improves the circulation, and massaging with a blend of essential oils may be especially helpful. Stimulation of the skin surface contributes to an improvement in the appearance of the skin.
- Mix four drops each of cedarwood and rosemary essential oils, and three drops each of cypress and patchouli oils, into five teaspoons

Exercise for cellulite control
Working out tightens the muscles and improves the appearance of areas of cellulite. Ask a fitness trainer about exercises for the parts of the body that are affected by cellulite in your case.

of cold-pressed vegetable oil, such as olive or sweet almond oil. Avoid cedarwood, cypress, and rosemary oils in the first 20 weeks of pregnancy. Massage the cellulite areas twice a day.

- Gently brush the affected parts with a soft, dry bristle brush. Start at the feet and work toward the heart. This boosts the circulation, removes dead skin cells, and may improve the appearance of the skin.

Herbal remedies: Dandelion contains substances that enhance the liver's ability to break down waste products and toxins. It also aids elimination from the blood of water and waste by the kidneys.

- Add dandelion leaves to salads, or cook them as you would spinach.
- Drink a cup of dandelion tea each day, using two ounces of fresh leaves to a pint of water.

Caution: For safety concerns, see pp. 34–37.

Detoxifying diet: This type of diet may help clear excess fluid, waste products, and toxins from the body. However, seek advice from your doctor or a nutritional therapist before embarking on such a program.

- Eat a high percentage of your food in the form of fresh, raw fruits and vegetables, as well as brown rice, seeds, and bean sprouts.
- Drink plenty of fluids, especially spring water. Fruit and vegetable juices and herbal teas are

Firming foods
Fresh fruits and vegetables are the mainstay of a detoxifying diet, since they are rich in nutrients, are easily digested, and contain a lot of fiber.

also helpful. Eliminate alcohol and caffeine-containing beverages.

- Avoid refined, processed foods, and limit your intake of animal products, such as meat and dairy products.

When to get medical help

Although you may not find cellulite attractive, there is little treatment other than a healthy diet and exercise that your physician can suggest. If you are considering cosmetic surgery to remove excess fat, ask your doctor to recommend a reputable surgeon and take the opportunity to discuss the risks inherent in such a procedure.

See also:
BLOATING, OVERWEIGHT

Chapped Lips

The lips may easily become chapped and sore, especially after exposure to hot, cold, or windy weather—for example, when taking part in outdoor sports. They are particularly vulnerable to chapping because, unlike skin elsewhere, they have no sebaceous (oil-producing) glands and therefore lack a protective oily barrier.

Lip care
Apply lip balm at frequent intervals when chapping occurs.

Hot or windy weather dries out the skin, while cold weather reduces the circulation in exposed areas. These adverse weather conditions can lead to sore, cracked, rough skin on the lips. Constantly wetting the lips is also likely to cause chapping. It is often tempting to lick sore lips to soothe them, but this will give only short-term relief. Not only is the prolonged wetting of the skin likely to dry it out and worsen the chapping, but as saliva dries, it can irritate the lips and increase soreness.

PREVENTION

Always protect your lips against the elements, especially if they are already dry. This means applying a barrier, such as lip balm or salve, every time you go outdoors. Reapply frequently, especially after eating, drinking, brushing your teeth, or washing your face.

On sunny days, especially during the summer, use a sunscreen or sun block formulated for use on the lips. Lipstick can act as a barrier, but some types, especially those designed to last all day, can be drying, so buy only those containing moisturizers. In winter, use a humidifier or place bowls of water on or near radiators to counteract the drying effect of central heating on the skin and the lips.

TREATMENTS

- Massage dry lips with a generous dab of petroleum jelly. Then leave it on for two minutes to soften the skin. To remove the petroleum jelly together with any loose flakes of dry skin, rub your lips with a warm, damp washcloth or gently brush them with a soft toothbrush (kept for the purpose) dipped in warm water.
- Apply a little olive oil, which has soothing properties and makes the skin more supple.
- Combine rosewater with the same quantity of glycerin, which also has soothing properties and can reduce irritation and inflammation. Apply two or three times a day to chapped lips. Or mix two drops of rose oil with a teaspoon of cold-pressed vegetable oil, such as olive or sweet almond oil, and smoothe a little of this mixture onto your lips several times a day.
- Puncture a vitamin E capsule and apply the oil directly to the skin.

When to get medical help

- A sore on or near your lips fails to heal within a week.
- The sore area is encrusted or oozes.

See also:
COLD SORES, DRY SKIN

Childbirth

A woman about to give birth needs not only good obstetric care but also practical and emotional support. There are many ways in which you and your partner can prepare for the event and a wide variety of natural techniques you can use during labor to promote a trouble-free delivery and a positive start to your new relationship with your baby.

DID YOU KNOW?

Many women in labor prefer quiet, dimly lit surroundings, and some experts believe that it is also better for the baby to be born into a gently lit room. Ask your attendants to shade the windows, if necessary, and to turn off any lights they don't need.

Childbirth in the United States generally takes place in the hospital under close medical supervision, often with the assistance of a battery of equipment. However, even in this high-tech environment it is possible, in consultation with your birth attendants, to use natural therapies to relieve discomfort and promote a healthy labor.

Many women and their partners choose to attend childbirth classes to learn how to use Lamaze and similar techniques for breathing and relaxation to ease childbirth. Most experts agree that preparation for the birth helps reduce anxiety. The presence of a supportive, encouraging midwife and a trained birth companion (called a doula) can also ease childbirth.

POSITIONS FOR LABOR

Until relatively recently, American women could expect to give birth lying on their backs, often with their feet up in stirrups. Today, however, many professional birth attendants encourage women to adopt the position they find the most comfortable, and one in which the contractions can be aided by the force of gravity. Upright and semi-upright positions have the advantage of widening the pelvic outlet.

In the early stages, walking around the room can relieve discomfort and promote a speedier labor. When you feel the need to rest, try the positions suggested in the box on page 124. You

The three stages of labor

1 Intense and regular contractions of the uterus begin, and the cervix starts to dilate. The cervix opens wider with each contraction, until it is fully dilated. A transitional stage occurs at this time.

2 The second stage lasts from the end of stage one, when the mother feels the urge to push, until the delivery of the baby is complete.

3 Some minutes after the birth of the baby, the placenta is expelled, along with the amniotic membrane that enclosed and protected the baby in the uterus.

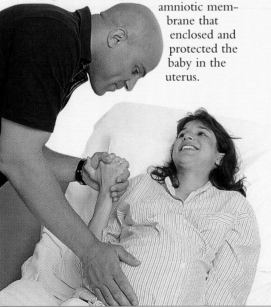

123

Has labor started?

In the following circumstances, labor may have started or be about to start. Call your doctor or midwife if:

- Your water sac breaks.
- A plug of mucus (possibly bloodstained) is expelled from the vagina.
- You are having contractions in the abdomen, back, or thighs at least every 10 minutes.

may find it easier to go through labor on a sheet on the floor rather than on a bed, because it is easier to move and change position. Even when you need to be on a bed—for example, if your attendants wish to monitor the baby—you can return to a more comfortable position later.

FLUID AND ENERGY LEVELS

Delivery rooms are often very warm, and you will lose fluids through sweating during labor. You will need to drink to avoid dehydration and thus help maintain your strength and energy.

- Take frequent sips of water or fruit juice (if allowed) throughout labor.
- You may prefer to suck on a washcloth dipped in ice water or to suck crushed ice.
- Add Rescue Remedy, a standard blend of flower essences, to your drinking water to help you remain calm and in control.
- Homeopathic Arnica is said to help control

Positions for labor

Some popular and effective positions are shown here. Practice them during pregnancy, and during labor alternate among those that help you feel most comfortable.

- Kneeling with the support of a bed or chair relieves pressure on the lower back between contractions.

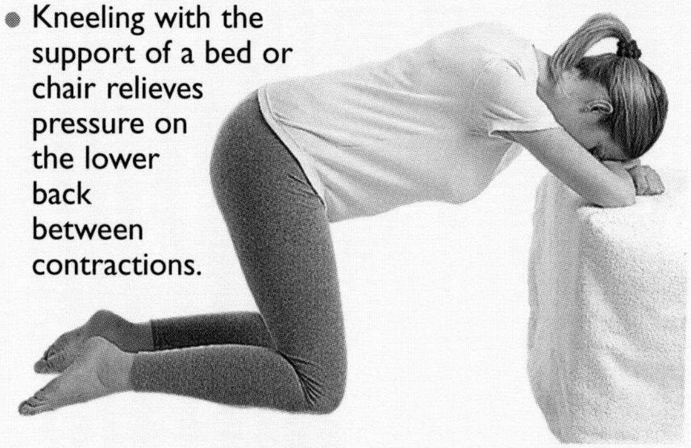

- Kneeling on all fours with your buttocks raised and legs wide apart can be restful in early labor.

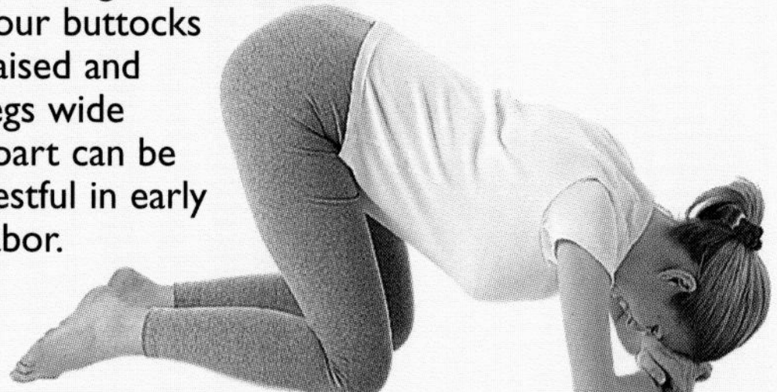

- Practicing squatting during pregnancy may encourage opening of the pelvic outlet. In the second stage of labor, adopt a semi-squatting position (p. 319) while supported by a partner; full squatting may speed delivery too much.

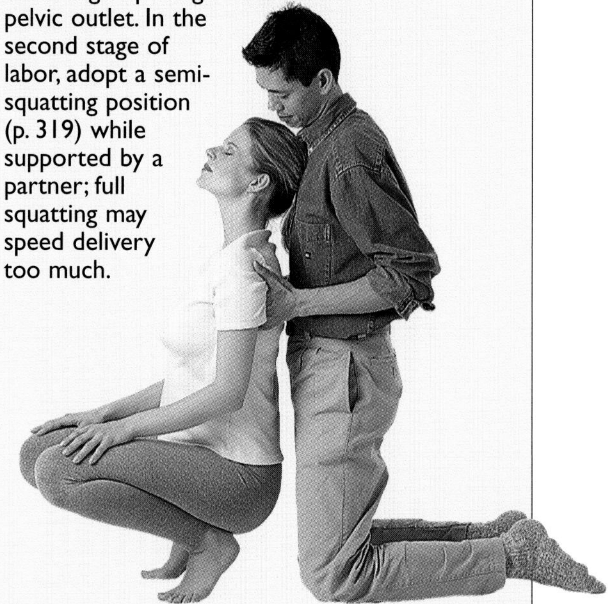

pain. Take three drops or one tablet every two hours, if your doctor agrees.

■ In the early stages of labor, eat one or two small snacks to maintain your energy level—as long as your medical attendants agree that you are not expected to need an anesthetic. Suitable foods include cereal bars and bananas and other fruits. Vegetable broth, honey, and even glucose tablets also provide energy.

■ You will almost certainly feel hungry once your baby is born, so ask your partner to bring a picnic in a cooler or hot soup in a thermos.

COPING WITH CONTRACTIONS

Breathing and relaxation: Instead of tensing and holding your breath as you feel the pain of a contraction begin, concentrate on exhaling slowly through your mouth while keeping your face, neck, and shoulder muscles relaxed. Once your lungs have emptied, you automatically inhale—do so deeply, lowering your diaphragm toward your abdomen and breathing through your nose. This slow abdominal breathing will help you through the first stage of labor and ensure that you and your baby receive plenty of oxygen. When your baby is about to be born, resist the urge to hold your breath. Instead, breathe quickly and lightly, inhaling and exhaling from your chest rather than your abdomen. Your birth partner can help by reminding you of the breathing techniques you have learned.

Lamaze teachers encourage focusing on a particular point, sound, or sensation to help their clients relax through the contractions. Some

Massage strokes for your partner

Lie against a large pillow or on your side, whichever is more comfortable, while your partner tries these massage techniques to help you while you're in labor. These strokes can be learned and practiced during the term of pregnancy.

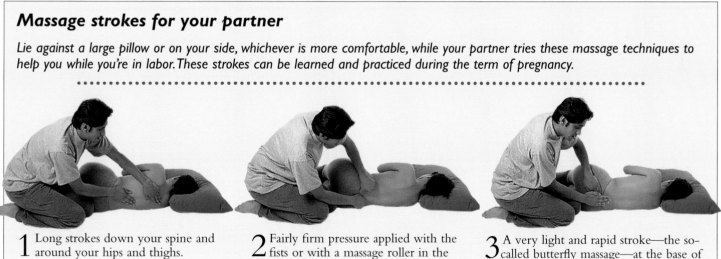

1 Long strokes down your spine and around your hips and thighs.

2 Fairly firm pressure applied with the fists or with a massage roller in the small of the back or the buttocks. This may be especially useful for backache.

3 A very light and rapid stroke—the so-called butterfly massage—at the base of your spine, just above the crease between the buttocks.

women like to have a photograph or illustration to focus on. Many other relaxation techniques can assist you through labor. For example, you may want to try a type of meditation or visualization that you have practiced during your pregnancy (see pp. 46–47). Soft music can also be calming during labor, although some women prefer the room to be quiet.

Massage: Besides being emotionally soothing, massage can relieve backache or abdominal pain during labor. Your partner should be well-practiced in the techniques involved, which can be learned at Lamaze classes. He can use either his hands or, since massaging for long periods can be tiring, a wooden massage roller. Apply talcum powder, oil, or cream to lubricate the skin,

Acupressure for easing labor

If you would like your partner to use acupressure during labor and delivery, identify the points beforehand, so that he can work quickly and easily when labor begins. However, none of the points below should be pressed before labor has started. The pressure exerted on these points during labor should be only as firm as is comfortable.

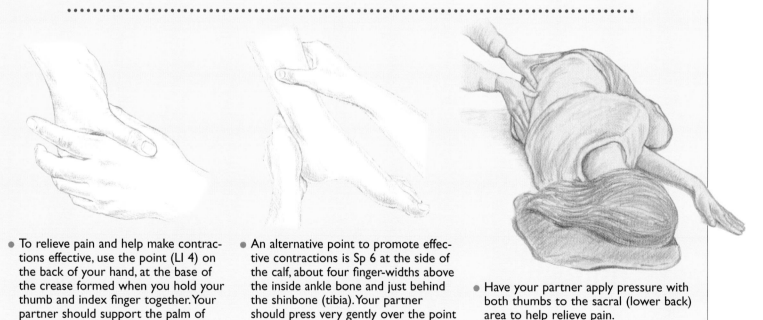

- To relieve pain and help make contractions effective, use the point (LI 4) on the back of your hand, at the base of the crease formed when you hold your thumb and index finger together. Your partner should support the palm of your left hand in his or her right, and then use the right thumb to apply pressure toward your wrist.

- An alternative point to promote effective contractions is Sp 6 at the side of the calf, about four finger-widths above the inside ankle bone and just behind the shinbone (tibia). Your partner should press very gently over the point or slightly up toward your knee.

- Have your partner apply pressure with both thumbs to the sacral (lower back) area to help relieve pain.

choosing one that is not strongly scented; you may be extra-sensitive to smells while in labor. Experiment with the massages shown on page 125. Some strokes may not be soothing for you; tell your partner which help most. You may no longer want to be touched during the "transition" stage of labor—the stage just before your cervix dilates fully.

Hot and cold therapy: A well-covered hot-water bottle or a hot pack can help ease the discomfort of contractions early in labor and can be especially useful if backache is predominant. Or try rubbing an ice pack or a bag of ice cubes quickly over your back. Refresh yourself during labor by spraying mineral water on your face or wiping it with a cool, damp sponge or cloth.

Aromatherapy: Many essential oils can have a calming effect during labor. They're best used in a vaporizer. Experiment with different mixtures in advance to discover which you prefer. For example, try mixing four drops each of lavender and sandalwood oils with two drops of geranium oil and sprinkling eight drops of this mixture into the vaporizer bowl. This scents the air in a gentle, rather than overpowering, way.

Homeopathy: These remedies should present no risk to you or your baby, but consult your doctor before taking them at this time.
- Arnica: to reduce bruising and soreness after the birth. It is especially effective if you start

taking it as soon as you go into labor and then for several days after the birth.
- Caulophyllum: to help promote effective contractions, especially when they are short or stop altogether. Take a daily dose if your baby is overdue.
- Coffea: to reduce pain.
- Kali carbonicum: for backache.
- Pulsatilla: for weak or ineffective contractions, or for when you feel very discouraged or especially emotional.

Flower essences: The following relate especially to the difficulties of childbirth:
- Olive: if you are exhausted during or after childbirth.
- Walnut: if you need help adjusting to the changes in your body afterward.

Traditional tonic
Some herbalists recommend raspberry leaf during pregnancy and childbirth for its alleged strengthening and toning effects on the uterus. Check with your doctor before taking.

See also:
PREGNANCY
PROBLEMS

Childhood Viral Infections

Chicken pox, measles, mumps, and rubella (German measles) are viral illnesses that can occur in childhood. Immunization has made most of these diseases much less common than in the past. Symptoms may include a fever, a rash, and swollen lymph nodes ("glands"). Natural therapies provide a range of treatment options that can alleviate symptoms.

The symptoms of the childhood viral infectious diseases are distinct, but treatment of these conditions at home is similar. If you suspect such an infection, seek medical diagnosis to exclude the possibility of a more serious disorder and to prevent complications, as with measles.

Chicken pox: Most nonimmunized children catch chicken pox, the most common of the childhood viral infections. Two to three weeks after exposure to infection, an itchy rash appears, first on the torso and then on the rest of the body. The rash consists of crops of pink spots that quickly become fluid-filled blisters. After about five days, they form crusty scabs, which gradually disappear within about 14 days. There is also usually a fever for the first few days.

Measles: This disease is now rare in the United States. It starts with a fever, runny nose, cough, and inflamed eyes. After three or four days, a rash

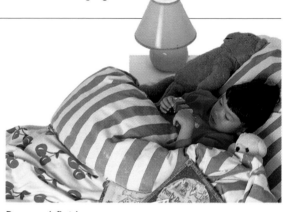

Rest and fluids
A few days in bed are usually all that's required to recover from a childhood viral infectious illness. Your child may not feel like eating much, but be sure to provide plenty of drinks.

of brownish-pink spots begins behind the ears. This spreads to the rest of the body, usually lasting five to seven days. The child may feel ill and have small white spots inside the cheeks. When the rash stops spreading, the temperature falls, and the child begins to feel better. Possible complications of measles include ear and chest infections and, more seriously, encephalitis (inflammation of the brain).

Mumps: This illness produces swelling and tenderness of one or both of the salivary glands below each ear. There is often fever as well as earaches and headaches. Chewing may be painful. The illness usually lasts about a week.

When infections strike adults

These illnesses are rare in adults, but when they do occur, they often produce more severe symptoms than in children. Even if she has had the infection, a pregnant women should avoid contact with chicken pox, measles, and, in early pregnancy, rubella, since any of these diseases may harm the baby. Mumps is more likely to cause inflammation of the testes and ovaries when it occurs in adulthood.

Adolescent boys and men may develop painfully swollen testes, and girls and women may have abdominal pain from swollen ovaries. Mumps occasionally leads to fertility problems.

Rubella: Also known as German measles, this is usually a mild disease that causes a light red rash, sometimes accompanied by slight fever and swollen lymph nodes. The rash lasts between one and five days, and joint pain may occur after the rash has faded and continue up to 14 days. Rubella may make your child headachy and fussy.

PREVENTION

These viruses are spread by airborne droplets. Sufferers are highly infectious during the incubation period (usually two to three weeks, depending on the infection), which means that they can pass on the disease before symptoms appear. Immunization is the preferred way of preventing these diseases (see p. 130), since it also limits the spread of the infection in the community, but an attack of any of these infections usually provides natural immunity for life.

TREATMENT

General measures: Treatment of all these diseases includes rest, reducing any fever, and general nursing care. Keep an infected child, or one who may be incubating an infection, away from young babies and others who are at particular risk, such as pregnant women, the elderly, and the chronically sick.

Chicken pox: Discourage your child from scratching the spots, which could damage the

Recognizing symptoms

Chicken pox: The blistery rash normally first appears on the torso and later spreads to other parts of the body. The photograph below shows a typical blister.

Measles: The dark, brownish-red rash, shown below, typically starts behind the ears and then spreads to the torso and abdomen.

Mumps: The hallmark of this infection is swelling of the parotid glands, the salivary glands located below each ear.

Rubella: The light red rash is usually first seen on the face and chest. It may later affect the limbs, as in this photograph.

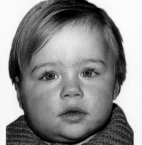

Immunization

Infants in the United States are routinely immunized against measles, mumps, and rubella. Infants who are thought to be at particular risk from chicken pox may also be immunized against that disease. According to medical experts, the scientific evidence suggests that the risk of side effects from immunization is much smaller for the average child than that of developing complications from these diseases.

---

skin and lead to bacterial infection and scarring. Keep the fingernails short and smooth, and, if feasible, have your child wear cotton gloves at night to reduce damage from scratching while asleep. Give the child frequent cool showers or baths, if this seems comforting. Colloidal oatmeal added to a bath can counteract itching. Gently pat the skin dry with a clean towel. Apply calamine lotion or aloe vera gel to soothe itching.

Measles: Your child may be more comfortable resting in bed in a darkened room, though a

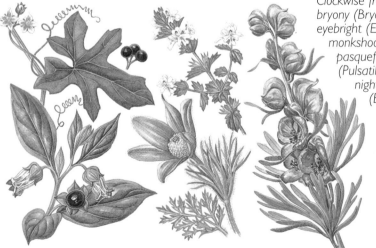

Homeopathic helpers
Remedies derived from the following plants may ease symptoms of childhood viral infections. Clockwise from top left: bryony (Bryonia), eyebright (Euphrasia), monkshood (Aconite), pasqueflower (Pulsatilla), deadly nightshade (Belladonna).

young child will probably not wish to be left alone. Be sure he or she drinks plenty of fluids.

Mumps: If chewing causes pain, offer bland soups and other soft foods, and avoid highly flavored or acidic foods, such as orange juice, pineapple, and tomato.

Rubella: Your child may want a little extra company, entertainment, or rest, but otherwise will probably feel well enough to carry on with everyday activities at home.

Homeopathy

- Aconite: for the early stages of measles, when the child is restless, or when measles or mumps appears very suddenly.
- Apis: for measles, when the child has red, puffy eyes, swollen lymph nodes ("glands"), and restlessness; or when he or she has a fever but does not want to be covered, and is drowsy but finds it hard to fall asleep.
- Belladonna: for measles, mumps, or chicken pox in the early stages, when the child has a high fever and very red complexion but no thirst; and for mumps, when there is a lot of swelling and pain in the lymph nodes, especially on the right side.
- Bryonia: when a measles rash or a mumps swelling develops slowly, the child is very thirsty, and movement is painful and makes him or her want to stay still.
- Euphrasia: for sore, streaming eyes and sensitivity to light with measles.
- Mercurius solubilis: for a child with mumps who alternates between feeling hot and cold

Aromatherapy tips

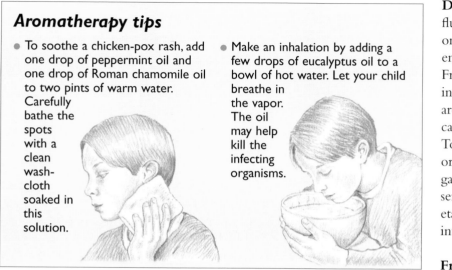

- To soothe a chicken-pox rash, add one drop of peppermint oil and one drop of Roman chamomile oil to two pints of warm water. Carefully bathe the spots with a clean wash-cloth soaked in this solution.

- Make an inhalation by adding a few drops of eucalyptus oil to a bowl of hot water. Let your child breathe in the vapor. The oil may help kill the infecting organisms.

and has bad breath, thirst, profuse saliva, sweating, and swollen lymph nodes.

- Pulsatilla: for a child with mumps, measles, or chicken pox who is clingy or weepy, has a slight fever and a cough, and feels better when cool; and when mumps swells the testes or makes them sore.

- Rhus toxicodendron: for mumps, measles, or chicken pox, when there is extreme restlessness, and when the child is better in a warm room. Also for itchy chicken pox.

Herbal remedies: Reduce the itching from chicken-pox spots by bathing them with tea made from elderflowers or from lavender flowers and leaves, or with a solution made from a teaspoon of distilled witch hazel in half a pint of warm water.

Caution: For safety concerns, see pp. 34–37.

Diet: If your child has a fever, give plenty of fluids to prevent dehydration. Give solid foods only as tolerated in the first few days. Try chicken soup and carbohydrates, such as potatoes. Fruit and vegetable juices provide fluid and infection-fighting nutrients. Good combinations are orange juice with a little lemon juice, and carrot or beet juice with a little watercress juice. To boost the immune system, give garlic tablets or capsules or, if your child will eat it, add raw garlic to food. If your child has diarrhea, avoid serving dairy products and sugary foods. Vegetable soup or plain rice is less likely to cause an intestinal problem.

From the drugstore: Give the recommended daily dose of vitamin C with flavonoids to combat infection and help skin heal. Topical applications of vitamin E may also help.

When to get medical help

- Your child won't eat for longer than a day or cannot swallow.
- Chicken-pox spots are very inflamed.
- You suspect measles.
- Your child coughs repeatedly or vomits more than once.
- There is severe joint pain.
- Your child has swollen or sore testes.
- Your child has rubella and you are or might be pregnant and have not had rubella or been immunized.

Get help right away if:
- Your child has a high fever, a severe headache, sensitivity to light, a stiff neck, or is excessively drowsy.
- A baby under 12 months is affected.

See also:
DIARRHEA,
FEVER

Chronic Fatigue Syndrome

*T*his disorder is characterized by attacks of unexplained and disabling tiredness over a period of more than six months. The condition has been previously known as myalgic encephalomyelitis (ME), chronic fatigue and immune dysfunction syndrome, post-viral fatigue syndrome, Epstein-Barr virus syndrome, persistent virus disease, neurasthenia, and "yuppie flu."

About four out of five people with chronic fatigue syndrome are women, and the condition most often strikes people in their 20s and 30s. Diagnosis is made by excluding other disorders, such as infectious mononucleosis, that could account for the symptoms. Chronic fatigue syndrome can be disabling as well as lengthy, lasting months or even years, with symptoms varying in severity. Relapse is common, but many sufferers retain only minimal symptoms within five years, and others make a complete recovery.

The cause of chronic fatigue syndrome is unknown. Sometimes it follows a viral infection (with the flu virus or with the Epstein-Barr virus, which causes infectious mononucleosis); however, some experts think such infections are coincidental or the result of lowered immunity in the early stages of the syndrome. Recent research has found that people with the condition have higher than normal levels of melatonin, a hormone produced by the pineal gland and thought to influence daily body rhythms. Other suggested causes include pesticide or lead poisoning, and a low estrogen level.

Psychological factors are often significant. One in two sufferers feels depressed, and one in four has some other mental health problem, but it is unclear whether this is a cause or an effect of the disorder. While studies show that the strongest risk factors for the condition are

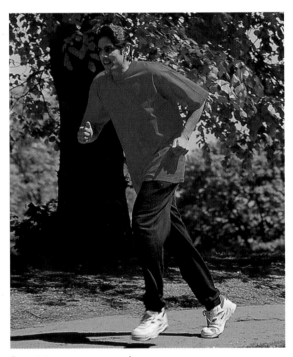

Regaining your strength
Exercise is a vital part of any treatment program for this condition, but build up your fitness gradually.

depression, anxiety, and stress, these are also an understandable result of the experience of having the illness, especially if it lasts for months or years. Mind and body are intimately linked by hormones, neurotransmitters, and other body chemicals whose levels can be altered by both "physical" and "mental" illness.

SYMPTOMS

Besides overwhelming weariness, chronic fatigue syndrome can cause headaches, nausea, sleep problems, and weak, aching, or twitchy muscles. Some sufferers have poor concentration and memory, difficulty keeping warm, or swollen lymph nodes ("glands"). Other possible symptoms include dizziness, slurred speech, sore throat, fainting, breathlessness, and an abnormal sensitivity to sound, light, touch, and smells.

PREVENTION

Improve your lifestyle with a good diet and regular exercise. Try to reduce sources of stress in your life, and learn and practice more effective stress-management strategies (see p. 347), especially if you've already had one or more episodes of chronic fatigue syndrome.

TREATMENT

Experts recommend a graduated program of physical exercise. People who are depressed as well may benefit from cognitive-behavioral therapy. This attempts to help you change the way you think about your illness and deal with your symptoms.

Rest and exercise: When your symptoms are at their worst, a daily rest is essential, perhaps in the form of an afternoon nap. However, since too much rest can lead to loss of muscle bulk and therefore increased weakness, step up your physical activity gradually when you feel well

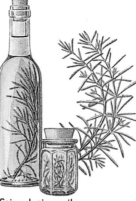

Stimulating oil
Add one tablespoon of fresh rosemary, which can relieve fatigue, to a bottle of olive oil. Use this fragrant oil for cooking or for salads.

Instant relaxation
Sit comfortably with your eyes closed. Take slow, regular breaths and focus your mind on a peaceful scene. Let any intrusive thoughts pass through your mind.

enough. Start with gentle exercise, such as walking or swimming. As you get better, increase the intensity and duration of exercise, but stop before you feel tired. If your symptoms come and go, take particular care to rest as soon as you feel them coming on. With luck, this will shorten the duration of an attack.

Stress management: Reduce stress by asking others to limit the demands they make on you, and learn to say no when necessary. Listening to relaxation tapes or practicing gentle yoga postures and breathing techniques on a regular basis can have a calming effect.

Diet: A healthy diet can boost your immunity and enhance your ability to manage stress well. Avoid eating too many foods containing added sugar, especially if your appetite is poor. A reliance on sugary foods can cause a succession of rapid peaks in your blood glucose level, with each peak being followed by a dip below normal that can make you feel tired. Cut down on caffeine and alcohol, and drink plenty of fluids.

Sensitivity to one or more foods may coexist with chronic fatigue syndrome and make the symptoms worse. If you suspect a food sensitivity, take steps to discover any foods (see p. 214) that may provoke symptoms, and then avoid them. Common trigger foods include milk, wheat, and fermented foods, such as vinegar, cheese, pickles, and soy sauce.

➤ continued, p. 134

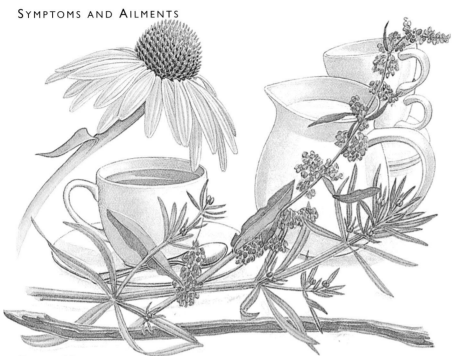

Botanical boosters
Many herbs enhance the immune system and increase resistance to stress. Among the best for those suffering from chronic fatigue syndrome are echinacea, cleavers, yellow dock, and licorice.

Supplements: Some people believe that vitamin supplements have a positive effect on this disorder, though there is little scientific evidence to support this. If you want to try bolstering your immune system and energy in this way, take an antioxidant supplement containing vitamins A, C, and E, as well as selenium, coenzyme Q_{10}, vitamin B complex, magnesium, potassium, and zinc. Or choose a multiple vitamin and mineral supplement. Fish oils may help some sufferers.

Herbal remedies
- Drink teas made from a combination of echinacea, yellow dock, cleavers, and wild indigo. Take a cup daily for at least six weeks. It may be necessary to continue the treatment for several months.
- Licorice has an antiviral action and can increase the body's level of cortisol, a natural hormone that helps us deal with stress. Take 2,000 to 3,000 milligrams of licorice root twice a day. If you feel better after six to eight weeks, gradually reduce the amount of licorice and start taking a daily small dose of ginseng for its antidepressant and restorative capacities for up to three months. Astragalus is an alternative.
- St. John's wort is often helpful because of its antidepressant properties.
- Evening primrose oil may be of benefit.

Caution: For safety concerns, see pp. 34–37.

Aromatherapy
- Inhale the scent from a handkerchief sprinkled with a few drops of lavender oil when you need to relax and recover from stress.
- Take a relaxing warm bath to which you have added two drops each of geranium, lavender, and sandalwood oils, and one of ylang ylang oil.

Portable pick-me-up
Inhale the scent of a handkerchief sprinkled with a few drops of rosemary oil when you feel mentally and physically exhausted (but not in the first 20 weeks of pregnancy).

■ To help lift your spirits when depressed, each morning and evening inhale the vapors from a handkerchief sprinkled with a few drops taken from a mixture of 20 drops of clary sage and 10 drops each of rose otto and basil oils. Avoid clary sage and basil oils in the first 20 weeks of pregnancy.

Flower essences: These are specifically intended to alleviate the mental and emotional problems that accompany conditions affecting both mind and body, such as chronic fatigue syndrome. They are especially useful if you feel depressed or find it difficult to take an interest in anything. One reason for their effectiveness may be the need to identify specific emotional concerns before choosing a remedy. Identifying a problem is always the first step toward finding a solution, yet many people in distress—and perhaps particularly those most likely to suffer from chronic fatigue syndrome—bury, ignore, or otherwise avoid their difficult emotions, which can prolong the healing process. Choose one or more of the following remedies.

■ Clematis: to increase alertness.
■ Olive: for all kinds of stress.
■ Rescue Remedy: to counter the aftereffects of sudden stress, especially if you are feeling faint and shaky.
■ Wild Rose: for apathy.
■ Willow: for resentment at the limitations imposed by this illness.

Homeopathy: The following remedies are often used to treat fatigue and exhaustion.

■ Arnica: for when you're feeling stressed by

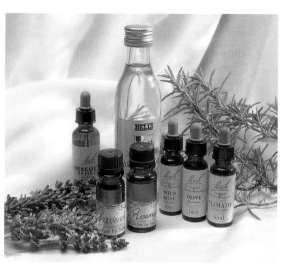

Countering negative emotions
In chronic fatigue syndrome both physical and psychological symptoms are generally present. Flower essences are said to help you overcome emotional difficulties that obstruct physical recovery.

overworking or being too busy in other ways.
■ Eupatorium: for aching muscles and other flu-like symptoms.
■ Ignatia: for stress leading to depression, and disturbed sleep.
■ Rhus toxicodendron: for aching muscles and flulike symptoms, especially if they are worse at night and you tend to feel chilly.
■ Sepia: for tiredness accompanied by depression, tearfulness, and the inability to cope.

When to get medical help

● Exhaustion and other symptoms don't improve with home remedies.
● Symptoms interfere with work, sleep, relationships, and other important aspects of life.
● You suffer a significant relapse after a long period of doing better.

See also:
DEPRESSION,
FATIGUE, INFLUENZA,
MUSCLE ACHES
AND STIFFNESS

Cold Hands and Feet

Hands and feet feel cold when they don't receive an ample supply of warm blood containing oxygen and nutrients. The most common reason for this problem is exposure to cold air, especially from a draft or the wind. An underlying health problem may be responsible, but whatever the cause of the condition, there is much you can do to relieve symptoms.

Although cold extremities can be uncomfortable or even painful, the problem is usually relatively minor. When you are inadequately protected from the cold—especially if you also smoke or feel tired, faint, or anxious—your peripheral arteries become narrower. This restricts the circulation of warm blood to your hands and feet with the purpose of keeping the rest of your body warm. Cold extremities can also result from hormone fluctuations before menstruation or a lack of circulating nutrients, as when a person is on a very strict diet or is suffering from an eating disorder. In addition, they may occur during the incubation period before an infection.

Other causes of cold hands and feet include Raynaud's syndrome and circulatory problems associated with such conditions as chronic bronchitis and arterial disease. Prolonged restriction of the blood supply may lead to chilblains— shiny red or purple lumps on the fingers or toes that can be painful and itchy.

PREVENTION

Prevent cold hands and feet and the development of chilblains in four simple ways:
- Dress warmly in cold weather.
- Stop or reduce smoking.
- Get exercise that raises your pulse rate for about 20 minutes every day.
- Eat regular, nutritious meals to fuel your body so that it raises metabolism and creates heat. Small, frequent meals are better than one or two large meals a day.

TREATMENT
Keeping warm

Protect yourself from the cold with several layers of thin fabric, since this traps heat more effectively than wearing a single thick layer. Close any gaps in clothing where cold air can enter, especially around the neck, wrists, and ankles. Wear shoes with thick soles, and insert insulating boot liners.

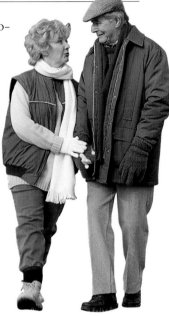

Winter clothing
Keep warm by wearing a hat (a large proportion of body heat is lost from the head), scarf (to close gaps), wind-proof warm coat, gloves or mittens, sturdy shoes, and thick socks.

Diet: Avoid heavy, fatty meals, which divert blood from the extremities to the stomach and intestines for several hours afterward. Eat three servings of oily fish each week to encourage the production of prostaglandins (hormonelike

substances that help keep the blood flowing smoothly through the veins and arteries).

Herbal remedies: To improve your circulation and keep the blood from becoming too thick and slow-moving:

- Add warming spices, such as ginger, mustard, and cayenne, to food and drinks.
- Eat three cloves of fresh garlic, or take garlic tablets or capsules, each day.
- Take a daily dose of ginkgo biloba, a traditional remedy for boosting the circulation.
- Drink a cup of hawthorn tea either alone or with ginger, cinnamon, prickly ash, or dong quai twice a day.
- Soothe chilblains with ointment containing calendula (marigold) or cayenne. (Do not use cayenne on broken skin.)
- Soak your feet until they feel warm. Add to a basin of hot water one tablespoon of dried—or two of fresh—thyme, marjoram, or rosemary; two teaspoons of powdered ginger or crushed black pepper; or one tablespoon of mustard powder.

Caution: For safety concerns, see pp. 34–37.

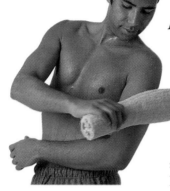

A stimulating massage
In the bath or shower, rub your arms and legs with a loofah or bath brush. Cover up well afterward. This may warm your hands and feet for several hours.

A circulation-booster
Hawthorn (Crataegus oxyacantha) has the ability to dilate blood vessels, thus making the blood flow more quickly.

Aromatherapy: Massage with stimulating essential oils can boost the circulation in the hands and feet.

- Mix three drops each of rosemary and black pepper oils into a tablespoon of warm almond or olive oil, and massage your hands, arms, feet, and calves with the mixture. Use a firm stroke as you sweep your hand up your leg or arm, and a lighter one as you sweep down toward your hand or foot. (Avoid rosemary oil in the first 20 weeks of pregnancy.)

Hydrotherapy: To help the circulation before you go outdoors:

- Place a hot compress on your feet or hands for three minutes, then a cold compress for one minute. Repeat several times, ending with a cold compress. Dry yourself briskly.

Homeopathy: To relieve chilblains, apply a thin layer of Calendula or Hypercal ointment. The following remedies, taken by mouth, may be useful for chilblains:

- Agaricus: if chilblains are worse when cold.
- Pulsatilla: if they are worse when hot.

When to get medical help

- The condition occurs often or suddenly.
- Self-help remedies have no effect.

See also:
ANXIETY, ARTERIAL DISEASE, EATING DISORDERS, RAYNAUD'S SYNDROME

Cold Sores

A cold sore not only looks unsightly and feels unpleasant, but the condition is also highly contagious. You therefore need to be careful to avoid passing on the infection to others. If you act as soon as you feel the tingling or hot sensation that heralds the advent of a sore, you can sometimes prevent a fresh outbreak.

Don't spread infection

Cold sores are contagious, so take care to avoid passing them on. Don't kiss anyone when you have a cold sore. Change your towel, washcloth, and pillowcase daily, and don't share them. Try not to touch a sore, but if you do, wash your hands as soon as possible. Avoid touching your eyes, since this could lead to a potentially serious eye infection.

Cold sores are small blisters that occur on or near the lips or around the nose. There are usually some warning signs that a sore is about to erupt. The area may suddenly itch and tingle or feel hot, sore, and irritated. A day or two later, a blister appears. It enlarges and bursts to form an open sore that gradually crusts over and dries up. Most cold sores disappear in about a week with or without treatment.

Cold sores are usually caused by Herpes simplex type I viruses. You can become infected by direct contact with a sore, the fluid from a sore, or the saliva of someone with a sore. There are usually no outward signs of the first infection, but children occasionally become very ill. Newborn babies are particularly at risk.

Once infected, you either develop immunity to further infection or the virus lies dormant in the skin until something reactivates it. The most common triggers of a new outbreak are:

- Exposure to very hot or cold temperatures
- Strong sunlight
- A cold (which is why they're called cold sores)
- Stress
- Fatigue and exhaustion
- Menstruation
- Deficient nutrition

PREVENTION

You may be able to prevent further cold sores from forming by boosting your immunity. Eat a vitamin-rich diet (see p. 9), get enough sleep, and get some exercise each day. Herbal remedies containing echinacea root are a traditional immune system tonic. You can take echinacea in tablet or tincture form or use the roots to brew a tea. Garlic, licorice, and ginseng are believed to strengthen the immune system, but avoid licorice root if you have high blood pressure.

The amino acid lysine can be a deterrent, although its effect is not immediate. Take 500 milligrams twice a day for several weeks. You can also boost your lysine intake by eating more lysine-rich foods (meat, potatoes, milk, yogurt, fish, beans, and eggs), while avoiding foods rich in another amino acid, arginine (chocolate, peanuts, nuts, seeds, and cereal grains).

TREATMENT

Start treatment as soon as possible.

Kitchen cabinet remedies: These traditional treatments are all reported to help cold sores heal. As soon as you feel the initial symptoms, apply a wet tea bag or, with a cotton swab, cooled black coffee or an alcoholic spirit (such as gin, vodka, or whiskey). An ice cube applied to the affected area may also be effective.

Aromatherapy: Geranium, bergamot, eucalyptus, and lavender oils are all astringent and antiseptic, and geranium contains substances that are thought to help fight viral infections.

■ Add four drops each of bergamot, eucalyptus, and geranium oils to two and a half teaspoons of calendula (marigold) oil or lotion. Protect this mixture from bright light by keeping it in a brown glass bottle, and apply a little to the affected area several times a day with a cotton swab. Because this mixture may increase sensitivity to light, avoid exposure to bright sunlight for at least 30 minutes after use.

■ Combine 10 drops of thyme or tea tree oil with two teaspoons of lavender tincture and four teaspoons of water. Apply with a cotton swab two or three times a day.

Marigold power
Remedies containing marigold (calendula) are antiseptic, helping prevent the broken skin of a cold sore from becoming infected with bacteria. The yellow pigments are also thought to promote the healing effect of light.

Genital herpes

Infection with another strain of the herpes virus, Herpes simplex type II, leads to blisters and sores in the genital area. This type of infection can be sexually transmitted and can also be passed from mother to baby during childbirth. Do not rely on self-treatment for this condition; see a doctor.

Herbal remedies

■ Dab a little diluted marigold tincture or cooled tea onto the area with a cotton swab.

■ Crush some marigold flowers and apply the liquid that oozes out directly onto your cold sore with a cotton swab.

■ Apply lemon balm (melissa) cream to the affected area.

Caution: For safety concerns, see pp. 34–37.

Homeopathy: Natrum muriaticum or Rhus toxicodendron can sometimes help speed healing of cold sores.

Other remedies: Some people find that covering a cold sore with a greasy substance speeds healing. Apply vitamin E oil to your cold sore, or dab on some petroleum jelly or zinc cream.

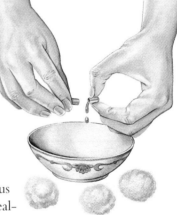

Healing vitamin
Break open or puncture a capsule of vitamin E oil and apply a little of the oil to your cold sore.

When to get medical help

● Your cold sore doesn't heal within a week.
● You have frequent or severe sores.
● You develop eye pain or light sensitivity.

See also:
MOUTH ULCERS,
SKIN PROBLEMS

Colds

Most of us are familiar with the classic symptoms of the common cold: a sore throat followed by sneezing and a runny, stuffy nose. Fatigue, headache, and a slight fever may also occur. In some cases, the lymph nodes in the neck become swollen. Although there is no cure, natural remedies can offer plenty of help to reduce discomfort and speed recovery.

More than 200 viruses can cause the annoying common cold. These are generally kept at bay by our immune systems, but when our resistance is lowered, colds may develop. Most adults catch a cold once or twice a year, usually in winter. Young children may get colds more frequently, as they have not yet built up sufficient resistance to the many strains of cold viruses.

PREVENTION

The key to preventing colds is to build up and maintain a healthy resistance to infection. To do this, you need a well-balanced diet that is high in vitamin C and flavonoids and low in sugar (see p. 12). You should also avoid factors that reduce immune function, such as stress, lack of sleep, and excessive consumption of caffeine and alcohol. Wash your hands frequently, since cold viruses are often spread by hand-to-hand contact.

TREATMENT

At the first sign of a cold: If you think you may be developing a cold—for example, if you notice a dry tickle in the back of the throat—you can stave off or lessen the severity of the infection by taking one or more of the following:

- Twenty drops of echinacea tincture in water every two hours (for up to two weeks)
- Tea from an appropriate herb (see facing page) every two hours
- The homeopathic remedy Arsenicum
- 250 milligrams of vitamin C with added flavonoids every two hours, but limited to 2,000 milligrams a day
- 25 milligrams of zinc, in the form of lozenges, four times a day (for one week maximum)
- Half a clove of garlic or two garlic tablets or capsules every two hours

General cold relief: Make yourself more comfortable by taking the following steps.

- Stay in a warm but well-ventilated environment. Keep the air from becoming too dry by

Acupressure to prevent colds

1 Place both hands over the point (GB 20) behind the ears at the top of your neck and rub your palms back and forth about 30 times.

2 Then apply pressure to the point (LI 4) on the hands in the fleshy web between the thumb and index finger. Press toward the bone at the base of the index finger for several seconds, until it aches. Repeat on each hand several times. Do not use this point if you are or might be pregnant.

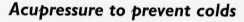

placing bowls of water near heat sources, such as radiators, or by using a humidifier.

- Eat light, vitamin-rich foods—vegetable and chicken soups are ideal.
- Drink plenty of fluids, excluding drinks containing sugar, caffeine, or alcohol.

Herbal remedies

- Take elderberry extract according to the instructions on the package.
- Drink tea made from fresh or dried ginger, sweetened with a little honey, if preferred.
- Steep one teaspoon of dried oregano or thyme

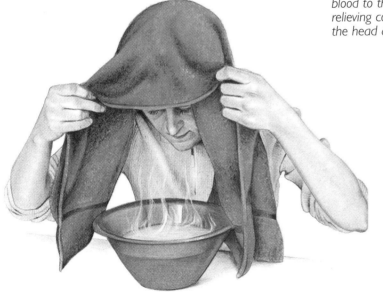

Winter foot-warmer
A mustard footbath, prepared by adding two teaspoons of mustard powder to two pints of hot water, is said to draw blood to the feet, thereby relieving congestion in the head and lungs.

in a cup of hot water. Drink this brew three times a day while symptoms persist.
Caution: For safety concerns, see pp. 34–37.

Aromatherapy: Clear congestion with a steam inhalation to which you have added eucalyptus, lemon thyme, clove, and/or tea tree oils (see illustration, below left), or add up to 10 drops to your bathwater. Do not use clove oil at any time during pregnancy.

Homeopathy

- Aconite: if symptoms strike after a chill.
- Allium: if you have a very runny nose that leads to soreness of the nostrils and upper lip.
- Ferrum phosphoricum: if you feel generally run-down. Repeat the remedy daily for a week or more, if necessary.

Clearing congestion
Add a few drops of essential oils (see "Aromatherapy," above right) to a bowl of hot (but not boiling) water to make an inhalation. Position your face over the bowl and drape a towel over your head to capture the rising vapor. Inhale through your nose.

When to get medical help

- You have facial pain, an earache, or a significant fever that lasts for more than two days.
- You have severe coughing with phlegm and tightness in the chest.
- You have yellow-green phlegm along with a feeling of pressure in the head or chest lasting more than two days.
- You have a severe sore throat, and other cold symptoms do not develop within a day or so.

See also:
ALLERGIC RHINITIS, COUGHS, EARACHE, FEVER, HEADACHE, INFLUENZA, SORE THROAT

Colic

Some 25 percent of newborns suffer from unexplained bouts of inconsolable crying—often called colic. This disorder begins in the first few weeks of life and is often at its worst at about six weeks. Nearly all colicky babies grow out of the problem within three months. In the meantime, various treatments may mitigate your child's discomfort.

Living with colic

If nothing seems to help your baby's colic, you will have to resign yourself to a challenging few weeks until the problem resolves itself. In the meantime, minimize other stresses in your life, and try to rest whenever your baby sleeps.

A baby with colic may cry for several hours a day, often mainly in the early evening. The infant's knees may be drawn up to the chest, and the abdomen may feel hard and look distended. When the baby does eventually fall asleep, he or she may wake up screaming in an hour or so.

Most babies with colic are otherwise healthy. Babies cry for many reasons, but the crying of colic is distinctive, and the infant is obviously in pain, rather than simply tired or hungry. The pain is believed to arise from tense muscles in the intestinal wall, but the underlying cause is unknown. Possible explanations include:

- Trapped gas
- A feeding problem
- A reaction to breathing tobacco smoke or drinking nicotine-tainted breast milk
- A sensitivity to formula or to something in a breast-feeding mother's diet
- Immaturity of the nerves in the digestive tract
- Having solids before the age of three months

TREATMENT

Diet: If you are breast-feeding, give your baby plenty of time to drink the hind-milk—the milk released (let down) from the breast only after the first few minutes of a feeding. If you switch to the second breast too soon and then take your infant off that breast before he or she has been able to drink the hind-milk, the baby may seem

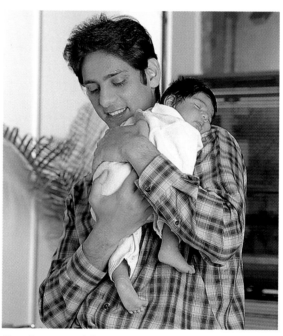

Comforting cuddles
When your baby is colicky, walk around with the infant held securely against your chest. The warmth of your body is calming and makes your baby feel safe.

satisfied but may actually be filled only with fore-milk—the lower-fat milk released from the breast first. Without the presence of hind-milk, fore-milk quickly passes from the stomach into the intestine. Its lactose (milk sugar) may then ferment in the intestine, producing gas. If you

have a large amount of milk, breast-feed your baby from only one breast at each feeding.

Adjust your own diet, if necessary, to exclude possible irritants that may enter your milk. Dairy foods can cause problems for some breast-fed babies, and others are sensitive to substances in eggs, bananas, apples, oranges, strawberries, tomatoes, chocolate, coffee, cola, or alcohol.

Traces of foods that produce gas in the intestines may also enter breast milk. Possible culprits include cauliflower, broccoli, Brussels sprouts, peppers, onions, garlic, beans, rhubarb, and cucumber. If you eat any of these and your baby cries after the next feeding or two, try excluding the suspected food. Add soothing herbs and spices to your meals, such as ginger, caraway, dill, thyme, fennel, and cinnamon.

If your baby is formula-fed, don't change to a different formula unless advised to do so by a health professional.

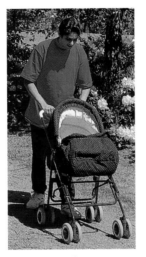

Rocking to sleep
Many colicky babies are soothed by the gentle motion of a stroller or by a car ride.

Herbal remedies: Ask your pediatrician if it would be appropriate to try herbal treatments. If so, give your baby small sips of warm herbal tea from a cup or spoon before each feeding. Fennel, chamomile, ginger, lemon balm (melissa), or peppermint will help relax the stomach and intestines and prevent the painful spasms that are probably the cause of colic. Give no more than a quarter of a cup of herbal tea daily.
Caution: For safety concerns, see pp. 34–37.

Homeopathy: Magnesia phosphorica is an effective all-round remedy if your baby draws the knees up to the chest and is generally better with warmth and gentle massage. If your baby appears to be extremely upset, try Chamomilla or Colocynthis.

Other therapies: Cranial osteopathy seems to provide relief for some babies.

Massage for baby

Each day, when your baby is calm, lay him or her on your lap or on a towel on the floor or bed. Gently massage the abdomen with a slow, clockwise movement. As you do the massage, lubricate the skin with a teaspoon of warmed olive or jojoba oil combined with a drop of sweet marjoram, Roman chamomile, or mandarin oil. All of these oils—when their vapor is inhaled—encourage is inhaled—encourage the baby's tense stomach and intestines to relax.

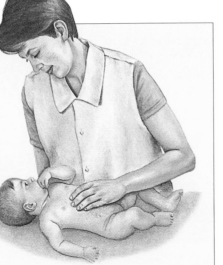

When to get medical help

- You find it hard to cope or find yourself becoming angry with your baby.
- Your baby continues to cry for long periods after four months of age.

Get help right away if:
- Your baby vomits, passes unusual stools or blood, or has a fever, a rash, or a rigid abdomen.
- Your baby feeds less or is unresponsive.

See also:
BREAST-FEEDING PROBLEMS

Constipation

This increasingly common disorder among people living in the Western world involves infrequent bowel movements, with stools that are difficult or painful to pass. Constipation may make you feel generally out of sorts, and it can lead to other problems, such as hemorrhoids. It may be a symptom of an underlying intestinal disease.

Working out
Inactive people who have sedentary jobs are especially susceptible to constipation. Make sure you build plenty of exercise into your daily routine.

The last stage in the digestive process occurs in the colon, the major part of the large intestine. The colon is five feet long and populated by billions of bacteria, yeasts, and other microorganisms, collectively known as intestinal flora. Some of these help detoxify waste and guard against infection. A good balance of the microorganisms helps prevent constipation as well as diarrhea.

Food residues and other waste material move through the bowel by peristalsis—involuntary rhythmic movements. The healthy transit time from eating to having a bowel movement is 12 to 48 hours, though up to 72 hours is acceptable if bowel movements are regular. People with healthy intestines generally have at least one movement a day, and their stools are smooth, soft, and easily passed. As we get older, the intestines may become more sluggish.

The usual cause of constipation is a poor diet. Highly refined, low-fiber foods and insufficient fluids almost inevitably slow down the digestive system. Other possible factors include too little exercise, long-term stress, pregnancy, and, very occasionally, a more serious underlying disorder, such as an underactive thyroid gland or colon cancer. Certain medications—including some painkillers, antidepressants, antibiotics, and contraceptive pills—

may produce constipation. Paradoxically, regular use of laxatives can cause constipation by making the intestines weak and sluggish.

PREVENTION

Most of us can easily avoid constipation if we eat a high-fiber diet and avoid too many refined, processed, and fatty foods. However, adding fiber in the form of extra wheat bran to your food is not recommended; it can be irritating to the intestines. Oat or rice bran is a gentle alternative.

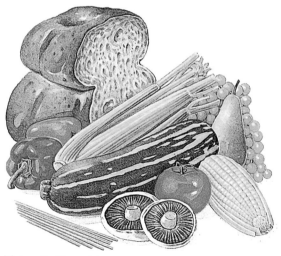

Naturally fiber-rich
Fruits, vegetables, and whole-grain foods (such as whole-wheat bread and brown rice) help waste matter move quickly through the digestive tract.

Check that you eat plenty of foods rich in magnesium (shrimp, nuts, seeds, beans, whole grains). If this is a problem, consult your doctor about taking a magnesium supplement.

Drink at least six glasses of water-based fluids every day to make your stools softer, bulkier, and easier to pass. Increase your intake if you are large or active or if the weather is hot. Fruit and vegetable juices can actively stimulate the intestines. You can buy many juices in the super-market, but it's better to make your own juice and drink it right away (see box, right).

TREATMENT

Compresses: Putting alternately hot and cold compresses on the abdomen can stimulate the intestines. Start with a hot one. Wring out a small towel in very hot water, fold it over the abdomen, and leave for three minutes. Remove

---

Juices for regularity

These recipes, which are especially recommended for alleviating constipa-tion, each make one large glass of juice. Drink up to three glasses a day.

Spinach juice
Juice a handful of fresh spinach leaves, a third of a cucumber, and two toma-toes. Dilute with the equivalent volume of uncarbonated bottled or filtered water. You can substitute watercress for the spinach if you prefer.

Apple and grape juice
Juice two apples and six ounces of grapes. You can substitute pears, papaya, or pineapple for the apples for variety.

---

and replace with a towel wrung out in very cold water and leave in place for one minute. Continue to alternate the hot and cold com-presses for 10 to 20 minutes.

Psychological factors: Just as some people react to stress by getting a migraine or eczema,

---

Massage for constipation

With a partner
A friend can give you the following gentle abdominal massage, but ask to stop if you feel any discomfort: Rest both hands on the right side of the lower abdomen, then make big, slow, circling movements, moving the hands slowly upward, beneath the lower left ribs, then down to the inside of the left hipbone. Slide the hands across to the starting point and repeat, moving in rhythmic circles for up to 10 minutes.

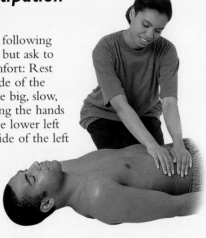

Self-massage
Make massage oil by adding two drops each of rosemary and sweet marjoram oils plus two drops of Roman chamomile oil to five teaspoons of sweet-almond or a cold-pressed vegetable oil. (Omit rosemary oil in the first 20 weeks of pregnancy.) Massage the oil into your lower abdomen and then the small of your back—using firm, gentle, clockwise strokes—for several minutes every day.

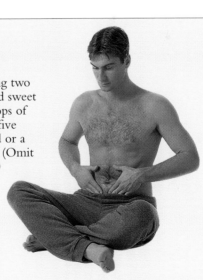

others develop diarrhea or constipation. If you feel pressured, try to find healthy ways of managing your reaction to stress (see p. 347).

Diet: Try the following measures in addition to those outlined under "Prevention":

■ Drink the juice from five or six stewed prunes each morning, and eat the prunes themselves late at night. Figs are good alternatives.

■ Eat yogurt with live cultures, which help re-establish the balance of intestinal flora if this has been upset by antibiotics or gastroenteritis.

■ Take one teaspoon of molasses daily.

■ Soak one to two teaspoons of flaxseeds or psyllium seeds in a cup of hot water for two hours. Add lemon and honey to taste and drink the

Acupressure for constipation

Apply thumb pressure to the point (TH 6) four finger-widths above the wrist on the back of the forearm. Do this for two minutes each day while the problem persists.

liquid and seeds at bedtime. While using this remedy, make sure you drink extra fluids.

Herbal remedies

■ Make a tea of licorice, ginger, dandelion root, yellow dock root, and burdock. Drink a cup of this mixture three times a day.

■ Take three garlic capsules each night for up to one week to help rebalance intestinal flora.

Caution: For safety concerns, see pp. 34–37.

Yoga to start the day

Try this exercise if you tend to be constipated in the morning. (Do not attempt it, however, if you have high blood pressure.) Ask a yoga teacher to check that you are doing it safely.

1 Start by drinking two glasses of tepid water. Lie on your back and raise your legs as you inhale, bending your knees, if necessary.

2 Exhale, lifting your legs higher, so that your hips come off the floor and are supported with your hands. Your torso should remain at an angle of 45 degrees and your legs should be as vertical as possible.

3 Exhale forcibly from your abdomen, then inhale and relax. Continue breathing like this for 40 breaths, then put your legs down and rest. Do this 40-breath sequence twice more. Then sit on the toilet with your feet raised to encourage the bowels to open.

When to get medical help

● Onset is sudden and self-care measures do not work within three days.
● Your feces are black or blood-stained.
● You have abdominal pain or a fever.
● You suffer from long-term constipation.
● New medication may be the cause.

See also:
ABDOMINAL PAIN, ANAL PROBLEMS, DIARRHEA, DIVERTICULAR DISEASE, HEMORRHOIDS, IRRITABLE BOWEL SYNDROME

Convulsions

A sudden episode of violent involuntary contractions of the muscles, often with loss of consciousness, is known as a convulsion, or seizure. It results from chaotic electrical activity in the brain. Recurrent attacks can be caused by a form of epilepsy. An isolated convulsion may be provoked by a very high fever or a reaction to a medication.

One person in about 200 has recurrent convulsions—known as epilepsy—but one in three affected people eventually grows out of the condition. The two main types of epilepsy are grand mal and petit mal seizures. A person having a grand mal convulsion may become unconscious for a few minutes, falling to the ground. The muscles may twitch and jerk in an uncontrolled way. Petit mal epilepsy results in momentary loss of consciousness but no convulsions. It mainly affects children.

Causes of epilepsy include head injury, birth trauma, brain infection or tumor, withdrawal from alcohol or drugs, stroke, and metabolic disturbance. Often there is no apparent cause.

PREVENTION

In a minority of people with epilepsy, convulsions are triggered by flashing or flickering lights, as from a television or computer screen, a failing fluorescent tube, or strobe lighting in a disco.

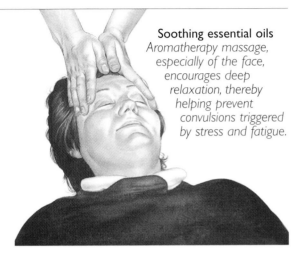

Soothing essential oils
Aromatherapy massage, especially of the face, encourages deep relaxation, thereby helping prevent convulsions triggered by stress and fatigue.

Some individuals appear to be sensitive to certain wavelengths of light.

- Stay away from risky environments. When you watch TV, sit several feet away from the screen in a well-lit room. If a fluorescent tube flickers, get it fixed or replaced. And don't go to places with strobe lighting.
- Ask your doctor or optometrist about the possibility of obtaining eyeglasses with specially colored lenses, tailored for the individual. There is some evidence that this might help reduce the frequency of convulsions.

Diet: Some people experience convulsions due to a food sensitivity that affects their brain chemistry. Use an elimination diet to check for foods

Trigger factors

If you are prone to convulsions, try to identify and avoid anything that may bring them on. Common triggers include:
- Flashing or flickering lights
- Stress or fatigue
- Changing hormone levels before a period or during pregnancy
- Food sensitivity
- High fever—especially in babies and young children (see box, p. 148)

147

that may provoke attacks (see p. 214). Keep a diary of what you eat, so that you can look back to see whether eating any particular food always precedes your convulsions. A lack of certain nutrients can make convulsions more likely. Increase your intake of foods containing:

- Vitamin B$_6$ (lean cuts of meat, fish, whole grains, nuts, seeds, egg yolks, bananas, green leafy vegetables)
- Calcium (milk and yogurt, the soft bones of sardines or canned salmon, beans, peas, green leafy vegetables, nuts, seeds)
- Magnesium (shellfish, beans, whole grains, green leafy vegetables, nuts, seeds)

Stress: Avoid becoming fatigued, and use stress-management strategies (see p. 347) if you think convulsions occur when you are under pressure.

- When you feel tense, ask a friend to give you a massage (or massage your own feet, hands,

abdomen, or face) using four drops of lavender oil in two teaspoons of sweet almond oil.

- To relieve tiredness, use four drops of lemon oil instead of lavender in the recipe above.

TREATMENT

Most convulsions are not serious, and recovery is usually rapid. Knowing what to do for a victim is important (see box, left). If you suffer from recurrent convulsions, make sure your family and colleagues know how to look after you if you have a convulsion. Wear an ID bracelet that gives details of your condition, so that you can be given suitable treatment, should the need arise.

Fever and convulsions in children

Some children are especially susceptible to convulsions caused by excessively high body temperature. This can occur if the child has a feverish illness, is too warmly wrapped, or is in a room that is hot. If your child has a fever, take appropriate action (see p. 207). If a convulsion occurs, seek immediate medical help.

What to do

If someone has a convulsion, take the following steps to keep the person safe:

- Remain calm, and protect the victim from injury by moving hard or sharp objects—such as furniture— out of the way.
- Place the victim on his or her side, loosen tight clothing, and keep onlookers away.
- Don't restrain the victim or put anything in the mouth (the possibility of biting the tongue is slim, and you might break the person's teeth).
- When the attack has ended, place the victim in the recovery position (see p. 195) and stay nearby until he or she regains consciousness.

When to get medical help

- Convulsions recur or increase in frequency despite treatment with anticonvulsant drugs.
- Symptoms are new or different from usual.

Get help right away if:
- You have never had a convulsion before.
- A person not known to have epilepsy has a convulsion.

See also:
FAINTING, FATIGUE, FEVER, STRESS

Coughs

A reflex action, coughing serves to clear the breathing passages of irritants and excess mucus. Dry or smoky air, vehicle exhaust fumes, chemical vapors, mucus from the nasal passages trickling down your throat, or an allergy or respiratory infection can provoke coughing. A cough may bring up mucus (phlegm), or it may be dry.

The most common cause of a cough is an upper respiratory infection, such as a cold, the flu, or bronchitis. The resulting inflammation produces irritation and swelling of the lining of the upper airways—and sometimes mucus, which you cough up as phlegm. A dry cough may be caused by asthma, which narrows the bronchioles (small airways in the lungs), often as a result of an allergic reaction to a substance in the air, such as pollen or dust. Coughs are more common in winter and in areas with significant air pollution.

PREVENTION

The most important way to reduce your risk of developing a cough is not to smoke. Avoid smoky atmospheres and insist on a smoke-free working environment. When possible, stay out of crowded public spaces during severe cold or flu outbreaks in your community.

You can also help prevent coughs by boosting your immune system. This means eating a healthy diet with plenty of vitamin C–rich foods, such as citrus fruits, getting regular brisk exercise, and learning to manage stress (see p. 347).

TREATMENT

If you are bringing up phlegm, don't take any over-the-counter cough medicines designed to suppress coughs. Also avoid decongestants, meant to dry up mucus. Instead, you may want to try an expectorant, a remedy that helps loosen phlegm, and there are many natural types available from the drugstore. If your cough is dry, try a home remedy that can relieve irritation.

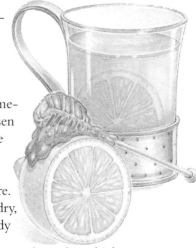

A soothing drink
Lemon juice and honey blended with hot water is a tried-and-true cough remedy.

➤ continued, p. 150

Special causes of coughing

- Coughing in babies and toddlers may be caused by bronchiolitis (a viral infection of the small airways in the lung).
- Acute bronchitis (inflammation of the bronchi, the large airways in the lungs) results from a viral or bacterial infection. Viral bronchitis generally produces a mild cough, with minimal or clear phlegm. Bacterial bronchitis, which

requires antibiotics, may cause a more severe cough with thick green or yellow phlegm.
- Chronic bronchitis, which involves a persistent phlegm-producing cough, is nearly always associated with smoking.
- Viral or bacterial infections of the lung, such as pneumonia or tuberculosis, may cause a painful, phlegm-producing cough.

149

Fluids: For all types of coughs, drink plenty of fluids—choose hot ones in particular. Fruit juice, warm water, or black currant tea will not only quiet a dry cough but also help loosen any phlegm. Avoid drinks containing caffeine and alcohol, however, as these are diuretics—flushing fluid from the body via the urine—and fluid loss makes mucus harder to cough up. It's also wise to eat a healthy diet (see p. 9) with five servings a day of vegetables and fruits.

From the vegetable bin: Many vegetables form the basis of traditional cough remedies, such as juices, teas, and poultices.

Croup in children

A child with croup has a harsh, barking cough and difficulty breathing as a result of inflammation and congestion of the voice box and windpipe. Croup is often worse at night and is most prevalent in winter. Although distressing, this condition, caused by a viral or bacterial infection, is not usually dangerous. Steam is the best home remedy. Create a steamy atmosphere by keeping a kettle of water safely boiling, running a hot shower or bath, or using an electric vaporizer. The homeopathic remedy Aconite may be effective. Belladonna can also be used for croup.

Seek emergency medical help if treatment is ineffective and the child is struggling to breathe and getting bluish around the lips.

- Make a juice from carrots, which help shift phlegm, or turnips, which boost immunity and have an antiseptic effect on the respiratory system. To draw out the juice from a turnip, slice and cover with sugar for a few hours.
- Squeeze boiled leeks through a clean cloth to extract their juice. Drink the juice sweetened with honey according to taste.
- Slice a raw onion, drizzle honey over it, and leave overnight. The next day, take two teaspoons of the juice from the onion every two hours. Or substitute three or four cloves of finely sliced garlic for the onion, and take a teaspoon every two hours.
- Drink cabbage tea or apply a cabbage-leaf poultice (see p. 116) to the chest.

Valuable vegetables
The juices from carrots, onions, leeks, and garlic may reduce or stop coughing.

Herbal remedies: Certain herbs help soothe inflamed breathing passages, break up mucus, counter infection, or bolster immunity. Remedies containing echinacea can bolster immunity, and those containing elderberry help counter the viral infections that are the underlying causes of many coughs.

➤ *continued, p. 152*

Strengthen your resistance to coughs

Asian exercise therapies can help overcome susceptibility to coughs. Consider learning yoga, tai chi, or chi kung. With practice, all these gentle forms of exercise encourage proper breathing and improve posture. They also relax the muscle tension in the shoulders, chest, and abdomen that in many cases accompanies a cough, and they help you cope with stress. Try the chi kung exercise, known as supporting the sky, described below.

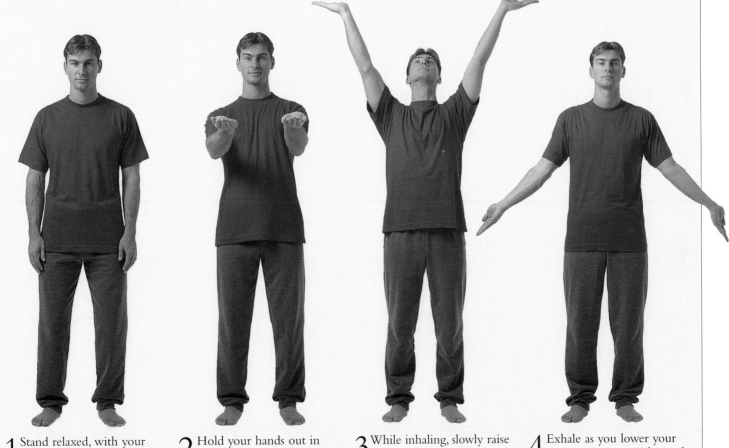

1 Stand relaxed, with your feet shoulder-width apart, knees slightly bent, and your head held lightly and freely.

2 Hold your hands out in front of you, palms upward, as if you were holding a large, light object, such as a ball.

3 While inhaling, slowly raise your arms above your head, palms upward. Stretch your arms and look up.

4 Exhale as you lower your arms out to your sides, and bend your knees slightly. Repeat six times.

151

■ For a cough with phlegm, drink hot teas made from an herb that helps liquefy and bring up the mucus, such as thyme, marshmallow, mullein, or hyssop.

■ For a dry cough, try a tea made from a soothing and antispasmodic herb, such as lungwort.

■ Astragalus and reishi mushrooms, in the form of capsules or tinctures, or as teas or used in cooking, can also provide relief from a variety of types of cough.

Caution: For safety concerns, see pp. 34–37.

Aromatherapy: Essential oils may relieve the persistent cough of such long-term conditions as chronic bronchitis.

■ Try steam inhalations scented with a few drops of eucalyptus oil and/or peppermint oil.

■ Sprinkle a few drops of the above oils on a handkerchief or tissue and inhale the vapor.

■ For a cough caused by a cold or a sore throat, soothe irritation at night by putting two drops of eucalyptus oil on a handkerchief under your pillow. Alternatively, put a few drops of the oil in a vaporizer (see photograph, p. 29).

■ Add oils of cedarwood (three drops), peppermint (two drops), and cajuput (one drop) to two teaspoons of unscented lotion and massage onto your throat and chest. Do not use cedarwood or cajuput oil if you are in the first 20 weeks of pregnancy.

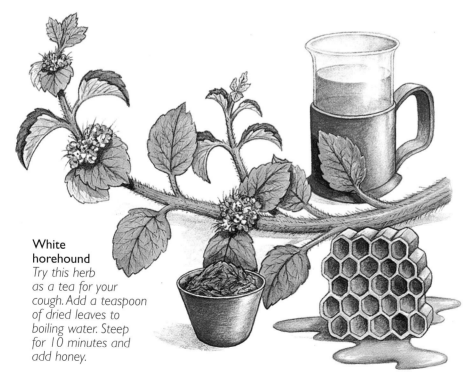

White horehound
Try this herb as a tea for your cough. Add a teaspoon of dried leaves to boiling water. Steep for 10 minutes and add honey.

When to get medical help

● A mild cough is no better after seven days or gets worse after three days.
● A dry cough lasts longer than a month.
● A chronic cough gets worse.
● Any change occurs in a smoker's cough.
● Your cough is painful or produces green or yellow phlegm throughout the day.
● You have a fever.
● The cough develops after taking medication.

Get help right away if:
● You cough up blood.
● You have chest pain.
● You become breathless.
● A baby has a cough.

See also:
ASTHMA, COLDS, SORE THROAT, VOICE LOSS

Cuts and Scrapes

*A*n inevitable part of an active childhood and an occasional occurrence for adults in the kitchen and yard, minor cuts and scrapes can nearly always be dealt with effectively at home by using traditional first-aid remedies. The purpose of treatment is to stop any bleeding, protect the broken skin against infection, and promote healing.

Cleaning a scrape
Wash away any dirt in and around a scrape with a cotton ball dipped in an antiseptic solution.

Cuts to the skin and underlying tissue from a sharp object, such as a knife or piece of glass, will bleed, sometimes profusely, if blood vessels are severed. Scrapes, or abrasions, are superficial wounds that occur when the skin is grazed. They may contain embedded particles of dirt or grit.

TREATMENT

Immediate action: The following steps are designed to remove dirt and stop bleeding:

- Wash hands with soap and warm water and with an antiseptic solution, such as hydrogen peroxide, before touching the wound.
- Gently rinse the wound under tepid running water to remove any dirt.
- Pat dry with a sterile gauze pad or clean cloth, and press the wound gently for a few minutes.
- Hold the edges of a gaping cut together with thin strips of surgical tape.

Cover a small cut or scrape with an adhesive dressing, and a larger one with a sterile gauze dressing, held in place with bandages.

Preventing infection: The following natural remedies reduce the risk of infection.

- Bathe a cut or scrape in a baking-soda solution or cooled cinnamon tea, sage tea, or parsley-leaf tea—all of which are antiseptic. Ordinary black tea, onion juice, and garlic juice are also antiseptic as well as helpful in reducing bleeding. Honey applied to a cut helps prevent infection and promotes healing.
- Apply a solution of distilled witch hazel or hydrogen peroxide on gauze to the wound. This rapidly stops bleeding, helps relieve pain, reduces swelling, and promotes healing.
- Clean a wound with a solution of 10 drops of the homeopathic remedy Hypercal in half a cup of water. If the wound is very painful, apply a temporary dressing soaked in a fresh batch of the same solution.
- Make a mixture of two drops of geranium essential oil, two of lavender oil, and one of peppermint oil, and sprinkle it on the clean dressing before you cover the wound.
- Apply calendula (marigold) ointment to a scrape before putting on the dressing.

Depression

Most people feel "down" once in a while, for short periods of time. A true depressive illness causes persistent sadness, pessimism, and feelings of anxiety and hopelessness. It has both physical and behavioral effects. While severe cases require medical attention, natural therapies may help mild cases and can also support any treatment prescribed by a doctor.

An occasional low mood is a normal part of life. Triggers include stressful events and unresolved problems or disputes. Deeper situational depression may follow a significant loss, such as a marital breakdown, a bereavement, or a business failure. Some people who experience such a loss are unable to recover because they suffer from an imbalance of brain neurotransmitters. An imbalance of neurotransmitters can provoke depression even in the absence of a distressing event. In these cases, professional treatments that deal with both emotional and physical problems usually work best.

More women than men are diagnosed with depression. This is partly because women are more likely to seek professional help for their symptoms and because they may experience hormone-related depression.

CAUSES

Depression can have many causes. These include:

- A genetic and/or biochemical tendency to have fluctuating or depressed moods.
- Depression before a menstrual period—possibly because of changing hormone levels.
- Postnatal depression as a result of hormonal changes and other problems, such as lack of a supportive partner or other close person, isolation, and the loss of work status and income.
- Difficult childhood experiences, such as loss of a parent, leading to depression in later life.
- A food sensitivity. Sufferers may also have other symptoms (see p. 213).
- Sensitivity to lack of bright daylight in the winter, leading to seasonal affective disorder (SAD). Sufferers may crave sugary, starchy foods, gain weight, and feel tired.

Are you seriously depressed?

Listed below are possible symptoms of an illness requiring professional care:

- Inability to work or do everyday tasks
- Little pleasure from activities once enjoyed
- Difficulty in relating to people close to you
- Lack of interest in sex

- Poor sleep and early waking
- Constant fatigue
- Feeling cold
- Anxiety, agitation, or irritability
- Excessive eating or alcohol or drug abuse
- Reduced appetite

- A feeling of worthlessness
- Lack of interest in personal appearance
- Inability to make decisions
- Forgetfulness and poor concentration
- Generalized feelings of guilt

PREVENTION

Since stressful situations make you more vulnerable to depression, reduce their impact by using stress-management strategies. These include:

- Arranging or accepting help and support.
- Eating a healthy, nutrient-rich diet to optimize brain function (see p. 9 and the box below).
- Limiting alcohol to one or two units a day (see "Alcohol Limits," p. 230), and caffeine consumption to the equivalent of one or two cups of coffee a day. A high intake of both of these substances can affect mood adversely over time (see "Treatment").
- Being kind to yourself, allowing yourself to enjoy life's pleasures, and not setting your standards too high.
- Getting enough sleep every night (at least seven hours for most people).
- Practicing yoga, meditation, or another relaxation technique regularly.

TREATMENT

It is not helpful to be told to count your blessings or snap out of it. But there is much you can do to lighten a low mood or to complement professional therapy for a more serious depression.

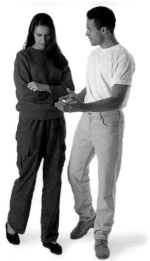

Support from others
Confiding your worries and sad, fearful, or angry thoughts to someone you trust can be comforting.

Nutrients for mind and body

Make sure your diet includes plenty of foods containing these vitamins and minerals, which promote a healthy balance of mood-enhancing chemicals in the brain and ensure that the brain cells are able to operate normally.

Nutrient	Food sources	Benefit for depression
Calcium	Milk products, green leafy vegetables, legumes, nuts, seeds	Activates enzymes needed for normal brain cell activity
Folic acid	Dark green leafy vegetables, such as cabbage	Promotes production of serotonin, a mood-lifting chemical in the brain
Inositol	Brewer's yeast, fruits, vegetables, legumes, meat, milk, whole grains	Helps regulate mood swings
Iron	Meat, fish, egg yolks, beans, dark green leafy vegetables	Boosts the production of a range of chemical transmitters in the brain
Magnesium	Shellfish, beans, whole grains, dark green leafy vegetables, nuts	Promotes normal brain cell activity
Potassium	Whole grains, vegetables, fruits (especially bananas)	Redresses the low levels of this mineral commonly found in depressed people
Zinc	Meat, shellfish, egg yolks, peas, beans, whole grains, root vegetables, nuts	Enhances the release of energy from brain cells, which may help prevent depression
Vitamin B_6	Meat, fish, egg yolks, whole grains, bananas, avocados, nuts, seeds, dark green leafy vegetables	Helps convert tryptophan to mood-lifting serotonin in the brain
Vitamin C	Fresh vegetables and fruits, especially citrus	Enhances iron absorption (see above)

Exercise: Exercise makes you focus on your body, providing relief from difficult feelings and thoughts. If you work your body hard enough, it releases chemicals called endorphins, which may act in the brain to help lift your mood.

If you don't exercise already, you may want to start simply, with a brisk half-hour walk at least three times a week. Once in the habit of exercising, consider something more strenuous, such as aerobic dance. Activities that you share with other people, such as tennis or team games, may be preferable to solitary forms of exercise, such as swimming, which leave your mind free to dwell on negative thoughts. Vary the type of exercise you do, and don't choose something you don't enjoy at all. Be careful not to overdo exercise, or you will feel exhaustion instead of increased energy and improved well-being.

Diet

- You may find it easier to eat several small meals daily than three larger meals.
- Counter a craving for one sort of food—such as sweets or cheese— by eating small, frequent, balanced meals. Cravings may result from a low level of the neurotransmitter serotonin. To increase serotonin levels, eat protein-containing foods that are rich in the amino acid tryptophan.

Boost tryptophan levels
Tryptophan is needed for the production of mood-elevating serotonin. Found in many protein foods, it is best absorbed when eaten with carbohydrates. Good snack choices include milk, turkey or chicken sandwiches, dates, and hazelnuts.

- Occasional treats like chocolate ice cream or French fries and a shake may cheer you up temporarily. Indeed, chocolate contains a compound that is thought to have a positive effect on mood. However, don't eat such sugary or fatty foods too often, and avoid them altogether if you are sensitive to them.
- Don't use alcohol to "drown your sorrows." It may help you relax for a short while, but it also depresses the central nervous system, making depression worse and reducing your ability to deal with problems.
- Limit caffeine consumption. Excessive intake may make depression worse.
- If you suspect that a food allergy is causing your depression, try to identify the food (see p. 214) and then avoid it.

Stress reduction: Practice strategies for minimizing stress. For example:

- Make sure that you and those around you understand that there are limits to what you can do when you don't feel well.
- If possible, delegate tasks that you find too difficult—for example, business trips or organizing the school PTA. People are often willing to assist if you tell them what you need.
- You may find it helps to break down large, daunting tasks into small, manageable steps, listing each one and checking it off when you have completed it.
- Take the time to reflect on your problems and practice activities that will help you cope—for example, yoga, meditation, or prayer.

156

Light therapy

Exposure to bright light may diminish winter depression, or seasonal affective disorder (SAD), by reducing the levels of the sedative brain chemical melatonin and boosting those of serotonin, which is stimulating. You can increase your exposure to light in the following ways:

- Go outside in the middle of the day for a half hour.
- If your doctor approves, try sitting in front of a high-intensity light box for a half hour to two hours every day. Do not use if there is a flickering fluorescent tube in the box, as this could provoke light-sensitive migraine or epilepsy.
- Install a bright, full-spectrum, fluorescent tube in the room where you spend most of your waking hours.
- Make the best use of daylight by adjusting your wake-sleep pattern to dawn and dusk. Alternatively, buy a bedroom lamp specially designed to turn on at dawn and gradually increase in brightness until you rise.

Herbal remedies

- St. John's wort is the best-known herbal remedy for mild to moderate depression. Take it according to the manufacturer's instructions.
- Tea made from a combination of wild oats, vervain, and ginseng may help.

Caution: For safety concerns, see pp. 34–37.

Aromatherapy

- Take a daily warm bath containing a few drops of oils of lavender, chamomile, bergamot, rose, or clary sage oil. Don't use clary sage if you are in the first 20 weeks of pregnancy.
- Ask a friend to give you a massage. Use two drops each of lavender or geranium oil, and one of Roman chamomile oil, in a tablespoon of sweet-almond or grapeseed oil.

Flower essences

- Gorse: for deep pessimism, when you feel that nothing can help you.
- Larch: for feelings of failure and worthlessness.
- Mustard: for depression that comes on for no apparent reason.

Other therapies: A counselor or psychotherapist can work with you to find the causes of your depression and ways of overcoming it. Laughter therapy can also be effective for some people.

When to get medical help

- You feel incapable of trying any of these approaches.
- Your depression lasts longer than two weeks, prevents you from sleeping for more than a few nights, or significantly interferes with your work or relationships.

Get help right away if:
- You have suicidal thoughts.

See also:
ADDICTIONS, ANXIETY, EATING DISORDERS, EMOTIONAL PROBLEMS, FATIGUE, GRIEF, MENOPAUSAL PROBLEMS, PREMENSTRUAL SYNDROME, SEX DRIVE LOSS, SLEEPING DIFFICULTIES, STRESS

Dermatitis

When an allergen or other trigger irritates the skin, the inflammation that results is known as dermatitis. The four main types of dermatitis are eczema, contact dermatitis, photodermatitis, and seborrheic dermatitis. Many cases have no known cause, but you can almost always do something yourself to alleviate the symptoms.

The signs of dermatitis are redness, swelling, heat, and itching, and in severe cases the skin may also blister, crack, and bleed.

- Eczema results from an overactive immune system, but most people never discover the causes of the overreaction. It may develop as an allergic reaction to a substance (allergen) that you have consumed or inhaled. If other members of your family have eczema, asthma, or allergic rhinitis, you may have inherited a tendency to get eczema and to experience other forms of allergic reaction. A few people develop eczema over varicose veins.
- One type of contact dermatitis is an allergic reaction to skin contact with a substance that has no effect on nonallergic individuals—for example, nickel, latex rubber, acrylic polymers, formaldehyde (an ingredient in false fingernails and their glues), and primula plants. Another type of contact dermatitis is a reaction to a skin irritant that is normally damaging only in large concentrations or over long periods of time. Such irritants include detergents, disinfectants, acids, potassium dichromate (used to treat leather), and chemicals in cement. Poison ivy and other plants may also produce an eruption.
- Photodermatitis occurs in those people whose skin is abnormally sensitive to light. When the skin is exposed to sunlight, it erupts into spots or blisters that may itch. Certain prescribed medications, such as tetracycline antibiotics, can trigger this reaction in susceptible people.
- Seborrheic dermatitis (sometimes called seborrheic eczema) most often affects hairy areas, which have a large number of sebaceous (oil-producing) glands. Experts disagree as to whether this type of dermatitis is a response to the over-production of sebum or is a fungal infection. The mild form of the condition may show up as dandruff or, in a baby, cradle cap.

PREVENTION

You can take steps to avoid dermatitis if you know the trigger.

- Some people find that smoking makes eczema worse. Smoking during pregnancy and after the baby is born can make your baby susceptible to such allergic reactions as eczema.
- Stress can aggravate dermatitis, so try to use some effective ways of reducing stress or managing your responses to it, especially if you are going through a difficult time (see p. 347).
- Lack of sleep, infection, digestive problems, temperature extremes, dry air, certain drugs, a diet containing excessive sugar and refined carbohydrates—all these can lower immunity, which increases susceptibility to eczema.
- Many well-known triggers are found in the home, such as dust-mite droppings and dander from cats and other furry pets.

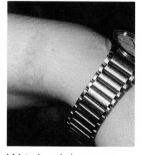

Wristband dermatitis
Contact dermatitis is most likely in areas in which sweaty skin is in contact with metal, such as under a watchband.

■ Allergy to nickel—a metal found in many alloys, including cheap silver and low-carat gold, as well as in stainless steel cutlery, zippers, and keys—is very common. Sweating releases nickel from these alloys, so hot, humid conditions can make this type of eczema worse.

■ Breast-feeding your baby for at least six months will help reduce his or her risk of developing eczema. This is particularly important if either parent has eczema, asthma, allergic rhinitis, or a family history of any of these conditions.

TREATMENT

Aromatherapy: Several essential oils have actions that are useful for treating dermatitis. Roman chamomile has anti-inflammatory properties; geranium and lavender oils encourage new skin cells to grow; lavender and sandalwood oils help soften skin; juniper berry oil has antiseptic properties (but don't use during pregnancy).

■ Make a soothing cold compress using two drops each of Roman chamomile and lavender oils and one of geranium oil (see illustration, above right).

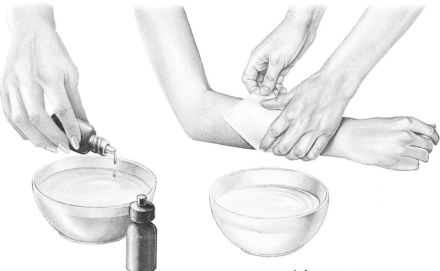

A fragrant compress
Add Roman chamomile, lavender, and geranium oils to cold water. Pick up the surface film of oil with a piece of cloth and apply to inflamed skin.

■ If the skin is oozing and moist, add two drops each of Roman chamomile and lavender oils and one drop of geranium oil to five teaspoons of a simple, unscented lotion. Apply this mixture morning and night to the affected skin.

■ For skin that is inflamed and dry, add one drop of sandalwood oil to four drops each of

Tracking down food triggers for eczema

Eczema resulting from a reaction to a specific food takes up to four days to appear and may last up to three weeks, which makes detective work difficult. You can try a simple elimination (exclusion) diet by avoiding suspect foods one at a time for two weeks each. The most likely eczema-causing foods include wheat, corn, citrus fruits, soy, eggs, and milk. Consumption of coffee, sugar, and alcohol can make eczema worse.

Once you think you have discovered a trigger food, try consuming it again. If the eczema recurs, repeat the test once or twice at weekly intervals for a few weeks to make sure that you are correct. However, unless you are knowledgeable about nutrition, you may want to enlist the help of a physician or dietitian to help you avoid falling short of any essential nutrients. Expert help is vital if a child is involved.

lavender and geranium oils, one drop of juniper berry oil, and five teaspoons of cold-pressed vegetable oil, such as sweet-almond or olive oil. Omit the juniper berry oil if you are or might be pregnant. Apply this mixture each morning and night. If stress aggravates your dermatitis, use the same mixture to massage your shoulders and neck, or ask a friend or partner to do this for you.

- Make a mixture of four drops each of sandalwood, chamomile, and tea tree oils, and six tablespoons of jojoba oil. Add two tablespoons of this scented mixture to the water in your tub.
- To treat cradle cap, add two drops each of cedarwood and sandalwood oils to two teaspoons of olive oil. Gently massage the mixture into the scalp and leave overnight. This helps loosen scales, which can be rinsed or shampooed away or gently rubbed off the following day. You may need to repeat this treatment daily for several days to remove all the scales from your baby's scalp.

Diet: Eat a healthy diet (see p. 9) that supplies all the nutrients needed by your skin and your digestive and immune systems to help them counter allergy or irritation. In addition:

- Try eating watercress regularly to reduce the severity of eczema.
- Drink a glass of one part beet juice, one part carrot juice, and one part water each day.
- Consider taking daily supplements of vitamins A and B complex and zinc. These nutrients may help relieve inflammation. Vitamins C and E and flavonoids can also help counter allergic dermatitis.

Herbal remedies

- Make a compress for inflamed skin by soaking a towel in a bowl of marigold (calendula) or chickweed tea, then squeezing it out. Marigold tea helps reduce inflammation and chickweed tea helps soften dry skin and relieve itching.
- Make a poultice (p. 73) from borage leaves, but use sparingly and only on unbroken skin. Avoid if breast-feeding.
- Bathe oozing dermatitis with tea made from yellow dock, a common weed.
- To possibly ease itching, bathe the affected skin with the water in which carrots have been boiled. Carrots contain vitamin A, which often has a powerful healing effect on the skin.
- Apply the juice squeezed from a length of cucumber to calm inflamed skin.
- For eczema or psoriasis, make a paste of gotu kola powder, available at health-food stores, and spread over the affected area.

Caution: For safety concerns, see pp. 34–37.

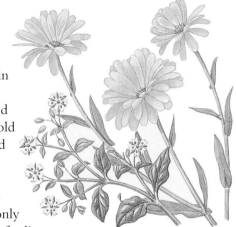

Marigold and chickweed
The anti-inflammatory properties of these plants can soothe irritated skin.

Healing foods
Flavonoids present in red, orange, and dark green vegetables, such as beets, carrots, and watercress, work against the effects of eczema.

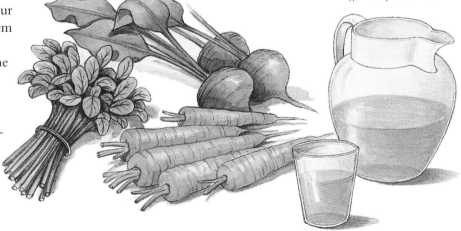

Living with dermatitis

Simple changes in the way you carry out every-day activities can often have a big impact on the severity of dermatitis. Try incorporating the following tips into your daily routine:

- Avoid wool and synthetic fibers, which can irritate inflamed skin. Wear cotton (preferably organic) as often as possible.
- Humidify the air in your home with houseplants and with a humidifier or bowls of water on or near radiators.
- Turn down the heat in your home.

When bathing

- Always rinse and dry your hands thoroughly after washing them.
- Use tepid water when bathing, since hot water can sometimes provoke dermatitis.
- Add some unscent-ed bath oil to the water to help mois-turize your skin.
- Wash yourself with an emulsifying oint-ment from the drugstore or with a soap-free cleanser instead of soap.
- To calm itching, add two cups of powdered oatmeal (sold in drugstores as colloidal oat-meal) or two tablespoons of baking soda to your bathwater.
- After your bath, apply a lanolin-free emollient cream, such as petroleum jelly or even olive oil. This prevents moisture from evaporating,

helps keep inflamed skin from becoming dry and cracked, and replaces some of the skin's natural oils.

- If antiperspirants or deodorants make your skin inflamed, try using baking soda and/or cornstarch, or try a medicated powder.

When doing housework

- When washing clothes or dishes, use only tepid water and wear rubber gloves (or plastic if you are allergic to latex rubber). Rinse clothes thoroughly to remove all traces of detergent and fab-ric softener.

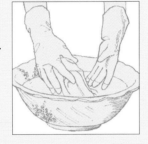

- If you suspect that you are allergic to dust-mite droppings, keep your home as free of dust mites as possible by improv-ing ventilation, damp-dusting, washing bed linens at very high temperatures, and using a vacuum cleaner with an efficient filter.

Sunlight

Some people find that avoiding sunlight on the skin improves their dermatitis, while others say that the sun makes it better. If you suffer from the condition and find that sunlight helps, you can heighten its effect by eating celery, parsnips, or a handful of fresh parsley each day. These foods contain substances called psoralens that can magnify any healing properties of ultraviolet rays. However, be aware that too much exposure to these rays has been shown to cause skin cancer. Always protect your skin from burning and avoid sun exposure at times of day when it is at its strongest.

When to get medical help

- Your dermatitis does not improve with home treatment or gets worse.
- Your skin becomes tender or redder.
- Your skin oozes, has an odor, or is crusted.
- The condition affects a young child.

See also:
DIAPER RASH, DRY SKIN, SKIN PROBLEMS

Diabetes

The hormone insulin enables our cells to use glucose, mainly derived from carbohydrates, as a form of energy. When insufficient insulin is produced or the hormone does not function normally in the body, diabetes mellitus results. Diabetes can usually be controlled by attention to diet, weight control, and physical activity, in addition to any medical treatment prescribed.

There are two types of diabetes mellitus. With insulin-dependent (type I) diabetes, the more severe form, specialized cells within the pancreas cease to produce an adequate amount of insulin. Body cells are therefore unable to utilize sugar in the blood, and the blood-sugar level rises. The onset of this condition usually occurs before the age of 35—most commonly between the ages of 10 and 16. Type I diabetes develops rapidly, and without regular insulin injections, it is fatal. Type I diabetes results from immune cells mistakenly destroying the insulin-producing cells in the pancreas. Susceptibility to the condition may be inherited. Suggested—but unproven—triggers include Coxsackie virus infection and a reaction to cow's-milk protein.

Non-insulin-dependent (type II or adult-onset) diabetes is much more common. It usually develops gradually, and it mainly affects those over 40. Some people with type II diabetes make insufficient insulin, but most suffer from insulin resistance—in which the body's cells don't respond to the insulin produced. People with high blood pressure and "central obesity"—excess weight carried mainly around the waist—are especially susceptible to this type of diabetes.

The glycemic index

Some carbohydrate-containing foods are transformed into sugar by digestion faster than others. These foods are said to have a high glycemic index.

Diabetics should opt mainly for slowly digested foods—those with a relatively low glycemic index. If you do eat a high-glycemic-index food, have some fat or protein as well, to lower the overall glycemic index of the meal. Consult your dietitian or physician before making any major changes to your diet.

Very low	Green vegetables, kidney beans, soybeans, lentils, peanuts, butter, cheese, eggs, fish, seafood, meat, barley, fructose (fruit sugar)
Low	Baked beans, butter beans, black-eyed peas, chickpeas, nuts, yams, sweet potatoes, corn, apples, grapes, oranges, pears, milk, yogurt, pumpernickel, oatmeal, bulgur wheat, pasta
Moderate	Beets, watermelon, raisins, bananas, whole-grain and white bread, rye crackers, rice, muesli, white sugar
High	Potatoes, parsnips, carrots, French bread, rice cakes, cornflakes, puffed rice, honey

SYMPTOMS

Without insulin, the body is unable to store or use glucose, a form of sugar, for energy. This causes fatigue, dizziness, and hunger. It also leads to tissue damage and, with type I diabetes, to weight loss. Sugar accumulates in the blood and is expelled into the urine, drawing water with it and leading to abundant urination and thirst. Untreated type I diabetes rapidly worsens, with the high blood-sugar level causing mental confusion and then a coma. This does not happen with type II, but if untreated, the disorder may lead to such complications as cataracts, neuralgia, leg ulcers, kidney disease, and heart and other arterial disease.

PREVENTION

Breast-fed babies seem to be less likely than bottle-fed babies to develop type I diabetes, according to Australian research. Losing excess weight lowers the risk of developing type II. If a close relative has the condition or if you have high blood pressure or tend to accumulate fat around the abdomen, it's especially important to maintain a normal weight. Regular aerobic exercise also lowers the risk.

Diet: If you think you may have a high risk of developing type II diabetes, change your diet in the following ways:
- Get about 50 percent of your calories from carbohydrates, especially unrefined products, such as whole-grain bread and brown rice. Avoid foods made with white flour and sugar and those with a high glycemic index (see box, facing page). This regimen provides plenty of fiber, which slows the absorption of sugars from the intestine and prevents excessive swings in the blood-sugar level. It also reduces high levels of the blood fats called triglycerides, which are associated with diabetes.
- Limit the proportion of fats in your diet to 30 percent of total calorie intake, and get a maximum of 20 percent of calories from protein. (As a rough guide, one ounce of butter contains approximately the same number of calories as three or four slices of bread or three ounces of grilled lean steak.)

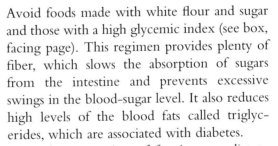

Chromium for blood-sugar control
Eat plenty of foods, such as those pictured above, that are rich in chromium, a mineral needed for insulin to work properly.

➤ continued, p. 164

163

TREATMENT

Diabetes treatment aims to keep the blood-sugar level within the normal range. Type I requires daily injections of insulin. If you have type II, you are unlikely to need insulin injections, but you may need oral medication. Whichever type you have, you can help manage your condition by improving your diet, losing any excess weight, and exercising regularly.

Diet: Space your food intake evenly throughout the day. Four or five small meals enable the body to better regulate blood sugar than three large ones. Follow the dietary guidelines outlined under "Prevention." Carbohydrates should come mainly from legumes, whole grains, fruits, and vegetables. Limit your intake of saturated fats (found mostly in meat and full-fat dairy products), but, if necessary, increase your intake of omega-3 and omega-6 fatty acids (found in oily fish and cold-pressed nut and seed oils respectively) as well as monounsaturated fats (such as olive oil) to help keep your arteries healthy. Eat three servings of oily fish a week, a few nuts and seeds every day, and five daily servings of vegetables and fruits (to supply antioxidants). Special "diabetic foods" are unnecessary. Using your knowledge of the glycemic index of the foods you eat can help stabilize your blood-sugar level. Keep sugary foods to a minimum: they cause fluctuations in blood-sugar level and encourage weight gain.

You may be able to drink some types of alcohol in moderation, but check with your doctor first. If you do drink,

Preventing hypoglycemia
Keep some candy or a sugary drink with you in case you experience a dangerous drop in blood sugar (hypoglycemia), and tell friends how to recognize this and what to do in such a situation.

always eat something at the same time, especially if you are on insulin treatment or take medication to lower blood sugar.

Exercise: Regular exercise helps keep weight down and therefore can work to control type II diabetes. If your diabetes results from insulin resistance, you may find that exercise also increases your sensitivity to insulin and helps improve blood-sugar control. Exercise increases the amount of sugar taken up by the muscles for up to 72 hours. If you are sedentary or have stopped exercising for a while, get advice from your doctor before you start.

If you are on insulin or another drug treatment, guard against a sudden drop in your blood-sugar level by checking it before and after each exercise session and by learning to balance exercise with your food intake. You may need to adjust your dose and/or food intake to allow for the energy expenditure during exercise and to prevent a drop in blood sugar.

Smoking: Since the risk of heart disease and other complications increases with diabetes, and smoking further increases that risk, it is especially important not to smoke.

Herbal remedies: The following therapies are no substitute for orthodox treatment, but they may improve your sense of well-being. Check with your doctor, however, before taking herbs.
- Eat raw garlic, cooked onions, or onion juice daily to enhance circulation and help reduce your blood-sugar level.
- Drink a cup of dandelion-root tea daily.

Dandelion root is believed to stimulate the pancreas and encourage insulin production. Burdock leaves and roots are another traditional remedy for an elevated blood-sugar level, as is bilberry leaf tea.

- Take Siberian ginseng. This is an "adaptogenic" herb, which means that it helps the body regulate aspects of metabolism, perhaps including a fluctuating blood-sugar level.
- Evening primrose oil, rich in gamma linolenic acid, may reduce pain and tingling from nerves damaged by diabetes.

Caution: For safety concerns, see pp. 34–37.

From the drugstore: Certain vitamins and minerals may help your body cope with diabetes. These can usually be obtained from food, but ask your doctor whether you should also take supplements.

- Vitamins A, B, C, and E and flavonoids may help you avoid long-term complications of diabetes.
- Chromium helps boost the action of insulin. As a supplement, chromium picolinate may be beneficial in regulating the blood-sugar level.
- Magnesium may decrease insulin resistance and lead to better blood-sugar control.
- Manganese is often lacking in those with diabetes. This mineral can improve arterial health.
- Those with type II diabetes may need to increase their intake of zinc.

Bilberry benefits
Bilberry works two ways for diabetics: it strengthens the blood vessels, which are often weakened by the disease, and helps prevent related eyesight problems.

Aromatherapy: Eucalyptus and lemon oils are believed to influence the pancreas. Add these to your bathwater, individually or in combination, or add five drops to four teaspoons of grapeseed or sweet almond oil for a massage.

When to get medical help

- You have any of the symptoms described on page 163 or slow-healing wounds, blurred vision, or numbness or tingling in the hands or feet.

Get help right away if:
- You are diabetic and develop persistent light-headedness, repeated vomiting, prolonged fever, severe shortness of breath, or acutely worsening pain or ability to think clearly.
- A person with diabetes loses consciousness.

See also:
ARTERIAL DISEASE, HIGH
BLOOD PRESSURE, OVERWEIGHT,
PREGNANCY PROBLEMS

Diaper Rash

Keeping a baby's skin clean and healthy when it is covered most of the time with a diaper is a real challenge. Most babies—however well cared for—occasionally experience soreness. Diaper rash can mean anything from slight redness to severe inflammation with infected sores, but the condition is usually mild and easily treated at home.

Dry and happy
Expose the diaper area to air as often as you can.

The most common type of diaper rash results from ammonia, a skin irritant formed by the action of intestinal bacteria on the urine. The wet diaper chafes the skin and makes it sore, and the ammonia makes the soreness worse. Some babies develop psoriasis in the diaper area; others have dermatitis, seborrhea (overly oily skin), or an allergy (for example, to the rubber in elastic). Broken skin encourages infection with yeasts (candida), bacteria, or viruses.

PREVENTION

The best way to prevent diaper rash is to keep your baby's skin as dry as possible by changing a diaper as soon as it's wet or dirty. Also:

- When changing a diaper, wash your baby's bottom with water and dry it thoroughly, then smooth on a thick, waterproofing layer of ointment or cream. Use a zinc cream, or stir a few drops of lavender oil into a tablespoon of unscented cream. Don't use talcum powder; fine particles can irritate the lungs and prevent the umbilicus from healing properly. If you want to use a powder, choose a product made from cornstarch.
  - Plastic pants retain moisture and may harbor infection. If you use them, wash frequently.
  - Sterilize, wash, and rinse cloth diapers thoroughly. Use the highest temperature possible and the minimal amount of nonbiological washing powder (available from health-food stores).
- Avoid fabric conditioner.

TREATMENT

- Use the preventive methods above, but instead of your usual cream, apply calendula (marigold) or chamomile cream at each diaper change, or use a soothing oil made from four drops of lavender oil, two drops of Roman chamomile oil, one drop of sandalwood oil, and 10 teaspoons of calendula oil.
- Give your baby a long soak, morning and evening, in a warm bath to which you have added two drops of lavender oil. This is calming and stimulates the growth of new skin cells.
- When washing cloth diapers, add six drops of lavender oil to your washing machine during the rinse cycle.

When to get medical help

- Mild diaper rash persists after trying the above treatments for a few days.
- The skin is very inflamed or broken.

See also:
DERMATITIS, FUNGAL SKIN INFECTIONS

Diarrhea

Attacks of frequent and loose or runny bowel movements affect most people at some time. They occur when food residues travel too rapidly through the digestive tract, most commonly because of an infection in the tract. In healthy adults, bouts of diarrhea generally clear up with rest and fluids. There is usually no serious underlying problem.

Acute attacks of diarrhea, lasting from a few hours to seven days, are most often the result of food poisoning caused by viral or bacterial infections. The microorganisms (or the toxins they produce) cause gastroenteritis, inflammation of the lining of the stomach and intestines. Diarrhea resulting from infection may be accompanied by vomiting, abdominal cramps, bloating, gas, and a slight fever. Sometimes diarrhea is caused by food sensitivity (such as an intolerance to cow's-milk sugar, or lactose) or it may be a side effect of drugs—for example, antibiotics. Poisoning with lead, pesticides, or certain plants can also cause attacks of diarrhea.

Long-term and recurrent diarrhea may indicate a chronic problem, such as irritable bowel syndrome, inflammatory bowel disease, diverticular disease, an overactive thyroid gland, or a stress-related disorder. In rare cases, diarrhea is a symptom of intestinal cancer.

Poisonous plants
Yew, deadly nightshade, and laburnum are among the plants that may cause diarrhea if ingested.

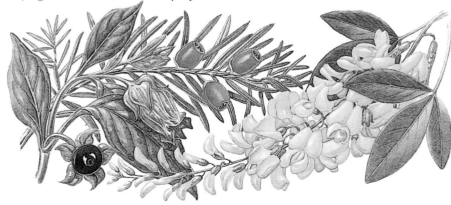

PREVENTION

Personal hygiene: Paying attention to the basic rules of hygiene is the best way to prevent diarrhea caused by infection.

- Always wash your hands thoroughly with soap after using the bathroom and before preparing food or eating.
- In public washrooms, dry your hands with a clean paper towel rather than under a hot-air drier, which may harbor germs.

Kitchen hygiene: Care in choosing, using, and storing food is important for avoiding diarrhea from food poisoning.

- Use only fresh eggs (check the date label) and discard cracked ones. Cook thoroughly.
- During pregnancy, prevent diarrhea from infection with listeria bacteria by avoiding soft and mold-ripened cheeses; unpasteurized milk; cheeses made with unpasteurized milk; soft ice cream; precooked, refrigerated foods, unless thoroughly reheated; precooked poultry; pâtés; deli meats; rare or undercooked meat; and prepackaged salads, unless washed thoroughly.
- Don't buy cans that are swollen or dented at the rim or seam. Don't buy any food that is past its "sell by" date.
- Consume food before any "use by" date.
- Cook raw meats and reheat leftovers thoroughly. Be especially careful with chicken.

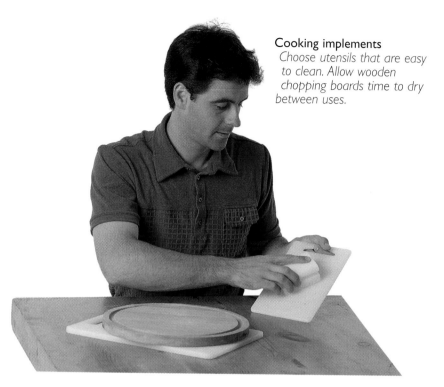

Cooking implements
Choose utensils that are easy to clean. Allow wooden chopping boards time to dry between uses.

- Defrost frozen food completely in the refrigerator, not the kitchen counter, before cooking, unless package instructions advise otherwise. Do not refreeze.
- Store cooked and uncooked meats on separate refrigerator shelves. Make sure that raw meat does not come into contact with other foods.
- Regularly clean your refrigerator, freezer, kitchen surfaces, and utensils.
- Wash dishcloths, sponges, and dishwashing utensils frequently, and disinfect them with a bleach solution (one teaspoon of chlorine bleach in one quart of water).
- Don't handle or prepare food for others if you have gastroenteritis.

Stress: Stress can readily disrupt the digestive system and cause diarrhea. If you feel too pressured, find effective ways of preventing stress or managing your reaction to it (see p. 347).

TREATMENT
Preventing dehydration: One of the dangers of diarrhea is dehydration, especially if you are also vomiting. Particularly at risk are young children and people who are frail, elderly, or have a weakened immune system. Take the following measures to prevent this problem:

- Drink plenty of water or water-based fluids, but avoid alcohol and caffeine. If vomiting is one of your symptoms, take frequent sips to help keep some fluid down.
- Replace the salts and sugars lost through diarrhea, especially if you can't eat or keep much food down. Make a specially balanced drink by squeezing out the juice of two fresh oranges, adding a half-teaspoon of salt and two teaspoons of honey, and then adding water until you have a pint. Drink a glass every half hour until your symptoms improve.

Avoiding traveler's diarrhea

In some foreign countries, you may be vulnerable to local bacteria. When in doubt, take these measures:

- Use only chemically sterilized, boiled, or bottled water for drinking or brushing your teeth.
- In restaurants ask for bottles of water to be opened in front of you (some establishments may refill bottles with tap water).
- Avoid ice.
- Peel all fruit and avoid raw vegetables and salads.
- In restaurants eat only cooked foods served hot. Don't eat food that has been kept warm for a long time.

Acupressure to relieve diarrhea

Use the point (St 37) eight finger-widths below the lower border of the kneecap, one finger-width outward from the crest of the shin-bone. Apply thumb pressure for two minutes on each leg.

- Drink such herbal teas as chamomile, thyme, ginger, peppermint, and fennel. These soothing herbs are mildly antiseptic and help relieve the cramping abdominal pains that often accompany diarrhea caused by infections of the digestive tract.
- Drink unsweetened black currant or elderberry juice to reduce inflammation in the intestines. The vitamin C in these juices also helps fight infection.
- Mix one tablespoon of arrowroot with a little water to make a smooth paste, then add a pint of boiling water and stir as it thickens. Flavor with honey or lemon juice. Drink at regular intervals throughout the day to thicken the bowel contents.

Getting back to normal: Once you start feeling better, you can gradually resume a normal diet if you've been eating little or nothing. Start with rice, which is nonirritating and helps bind the bowel contents. Eating some yogurt with live cultures each day will help restore the balance of microorganisms in your intestines, and a daily vitamin and mineral supplement will help restore your body's nutrient balance.

Homeopathy: If you still have diarrhea after 24 hours, try a homeopathic remedy.
- Arsenicum: for food poisoning involving vomiting and nausea.
- Colocynthis: for diarrhea accompanied by severe abdominal cramps.

Aromatherapy: Astringent (drying) oils, such as ginger and geranium, can be helpful for the relief of diarrhea, as can oils, such as peppermint and Roman chamomile, that calm muscular contractions in the intestines. Tea tree oil is also good, because it is an antiseptic.
- Sprinkle three drops each of geranium and ginger oils and two of peppermint oil into your bathwater. Relax in the tub for 15 to 20 minutes. Be sure to keep the water warm.
- Make a massage oil with three drops of tea tree oil, two drops each of peppermint, geranium, and sandalwood oils, and five teaspoons of sweet almond oil, olive oil, or another cold-pressed vegetable oil. Warm the oil (see illustration, right) and use it to massage

Warm massage oil
Heat your aromatherapy massage oil by immersing the container in hot water for a few seconds. This helps release the healing vapors and makes the oil feel pleasant on the skin.

169

your abdomen, as described on page 70. Repeat the massage every few hours.

Yoga: Deep relaxation while lying on the floor (see p. 69) can reduce the mental and physical tension that can sometimes provoke attacks of stress-related diarrhea.

Special advice concerning young children: Infants and toddlers are at an increased risk of dehydration from fluid loss. If your baby or young child has diarrhea:

■ Check whether the child could have eaten anything poisonous. Call a poison control center or hospital if this is a possibility.

■ Check the child's diet for irritating foods. Hot spices, peppers, onions, tomatoes, rhubarb, and too much fruit may provoke diarrhea. Reduce your own intake of these foods if you are breast-feeding.

■ Give your breast-fed baby as much time at the breast as desired, and offer more feedings than usual both day and night. Your milk supply will increase naturally; drinks of cooled boiled water are needed only rarely. Give your bottle-fed baby extra diluted formula or cooled boiled water.

■ Give a weaned child extra drinks, including pasteurized apple juice or well-diluted orange juice that you've squeezed yourself. The water in which rice has been boiled is also suitable.

■ Wash your hands thoroughly after touching your child and before eating, serving, or preparing food.

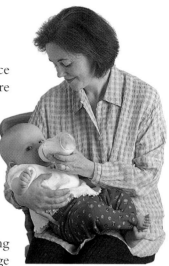

Extra fluids
Bottle-fed babies who are suffering from diarrhea may need additional drinks of cooled boiled water.

When to get medical help

Babies and young children
● Mild diarrhea has lasted longer than 24 hours or severe diarrhea longer than 12 hours.

Get help right away if:
● The child is vomiting and can't keep fluids down or won't nurse or eat.
● The child seems dehydrated, with a dry mouth, sunken eyes, loose skin, and fewer wet diapers than you usually expect. Dehydration may also cause the soft spot (fontanelle) on top of a baby's head to become depressed.
● The child won't stop crying or is unusually sleepy or listless.
● There is fecal blood, or the child has a fever or other symptoms.
● You think your child may have eaten or drunk something poisonous.

Older children and adults
● You are normally fit and healthy and have mild diarrhea for more than three days or severe diarrhea for more than two days.
● You are elderly or frail.
● You suffer from frequent infections or are taking steroids, antibiotics, or any other medicine that may be a possible cause.
● Others who share your home are affected by similar symptoms.
● You have severe diarrhea and are taking oral contraceptives.
● There is red or black fecal blood.

Get help right away if:
● You have signs of dehydration—including drowsiness, glazed eyes, loose skin, and very small amounts of dark urine or no urine at all.

See also:
ABDOMINAL PAIN,
DIVERTICULAR
DISEASE, FOOD
SENSITIVITY,
IRRITABLE
BOWEL
SYNDROME,
NAUSEA AND
VOMITING

Diverticular Disease

Commonly occurring in people over 50, diverticulosis is a disorder in which many small pockets (diverticula) form in the wall of the large intestine. When the lining of one or more of these pockets becomes inflamed, the condition is called diverticulitis. Both forms of the condition are less likely to develop if you eat plenty of fiber.

Most cases of diverticular disease probably stem from a diet low in fiber and high in refined carbohydrates. The condition is rare before the age of 20, but in the United States nearly one-third of 50- to 60-year-olds is affected, and possibly as many as 60 percent of those over 70. Many people with diverticular disease also have symptoms of irritable bowel syndrome.

When you eat a refined diet, the muscles of your colon have to work harder than normal to push along sticky, dry food residues, and they may temporarily go into spasm. Pressure builds up, causing the colon to dilate and forcing pockets of its lining (known as diverticula) out from the stretched wall. These distended segments usually cause little trouble, but they can lead to constipation or diarrhea, together with a nagging ache—usually on the left side and sometimes relieved by passing gas. Possible complications include diverticulitis (when a pocket becomes inflamed or infected), bleeding from a burst pocket, and an obstructed intestine.

PREVENTION

Diverticular disease is rare in countries in which the normal diet is high in fiber. You are unlikely to develop the condition if you adopt similar eating habits. This means eating five servings of vegetables (including peas and beans) and fruits daily, as well as some nuts and seeds (chewed

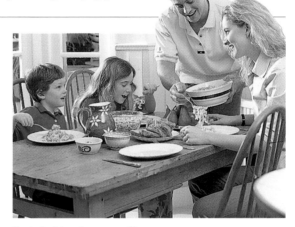

Early habits that pay off
A high-fiber diet starting in childhood can reduce susceptibility to diverticular disease in later life.

well). You should also choose foods made with whole grains rather than white rice or flour. However, do not add wheat bran or other insoluble fiber to your diet, as it can be irritating to the intestines. A high-fiber diet requires plenty of fluids—at least eight glasses a day.

Another important way of preventing the disease is to exercise every day. This massages the intestines and helps prevent constipation (a major risk factor for diverticulitis). Taking fresh garlic (preferably raw) or garlic tablets three times daily counters abnormal bacterial activity and may help prevent diverticulitis.

➤ continued, p. 172

TREATMENT

Diet: During a bout of pain, help your colon relax and recover by avoiding dairy products (except yogurt) and foods made with wheat and other cereal grains. You may, however, be comfortable with oatmeal made with oats soaked overnight and cooked with soy milk. Eat vegetables, soups, applesauce, fruits, and yogurt for two days, then add fish, brown rice, and legumes. Return to a normal diet when your symptoms have subsided. For the long-term health of the intestines, have one tablespoon of walnut, flaxseed, or olive oil daily, which provides essential fatty acids that help reduce inflammation.

Acupressure: For persistent pain, apply firm pressure with your fingertips for up to five minutes on the following points: the inside of the calf four finger-widths above the ankle bone (Sp 6, see p. 276), the pair of points two thumb-widths from either side of the navel (St 25), and the point four thumb-widths below the navel (CV 4, see p. 276). Do not use Sp 6 during pregnancy.

From the drugstore
- Take a multiple vitamin and mineral supplement daily to counter inflammation.
- Take acidophilus as a supplement or in yogurt with live cultures to add to the beneficial bacteria in the intestines.

Homeopathy: For abdominal pain from diverticular disease, take one of the following remedies every half hour for up to five hours:
- Belladonna: for a sharp, throbbing vicelike pain; a red, hot face; and a tender abdomen.
- Bryonia: for a pain in your left side that is so severe that it keeps you from moving or talking.
- Colocynthis: for a cutting pain that makes you double up or cry out, and for gas. This especially suits someone prone to bouts of anger.
- Magnesia phosphorica: for severe, sudden pain that makes you cry out but is eased by warmth and by rubbing your abdomen.

Herbal remedies
- To reduce muscle spasms and promote healing of inflamed intestines, drink peppermint or chamomile tea after meals, but no more than three or four cups daily.
- To protect inflamed intestines, have a slippery elm drink (see illustration) or, if you dislike the taste, take the herb in tablet form.
- To soothe the intestines, drink a daily half-cup of aloe vera juice.

Caution: For safety concerns, see pp. 34–37.

A protective coating
Slippery elm helps constipation and soothes the intestinal lining. Mix one teaspoon of pure slippery elm bark with a little cold water to make a paste; then add boiling water and honey (to taste). Drink before each meal.

When to get medical help

- Your symptoms are new, requiring diagnosis.
- Natural therapies fail to improve your symptoms.

Get help right away if:
- You have severe abdominal pain, especially if accompanied by fever or vomiting.
- You notice fecal blood.

See also:
BLOATING, CONSTIPATION, DIARRHEA, IRRITABLE BOWEL SYNDROME

Dizziness

The feeling of lightheadedness and unsteadiness—dizziness—is usually a mild sensation that passes quickly. Sometimes this symptom is more prolonged and serious, requiring investigation, but natural home remedies and lifestyle changes can often complement medical treatment or, in milder cases, make it superfluous.

Most attacks of dizziness are caused by a momentary drop in pressure in the arteries that transport blood to the brain. This reduces the brain's blood supply, leaving it low in oxygen. Dizziness often happens after rising from a lying or sitting position (postural hypotension); it usually lasts only a few seconds. It can also occur if the blood-sugar level drops too low as a result of not eating or of poor control of diabetes. Dehydration resulting from low fluid intake or fluid loss, as from diarrhea, is also a possible cause. Vertigo (see box, p. 174) may ensue from a condition affecting the inner ear.

PREVENTION
■ Avoid postural hypotension by taking a few deep breaths before getting up from a sitting or lying position. Then move slowly, rising in stages rather than in one rapid movement.

Yoga for the circulation
Regular yoga practice can help prevent low blood pressure, which can cause dizziness, because of its toning effect on the blood vessels. Avoid any postures that worsen your symptoms.

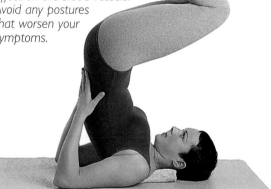

■ Maintain a stable blood-sugar level by eating regular meals that include high-fiber foods. Limit your intake of foods containing white flour and added sugar.
■ Improve the efficiency of your heart and lungs and help maintain a good oxygen supply to your brain by getting at least 30 minutes of aerobic exercise daily. Appropriate exercise includes walking and swimming.
■ Tone your blood vessels and boost your circulation by taking alternate hot and cold showers or sitz baths (see p. 49), repeating several times. This stimulates blood flow and prevents attacks

Other causes of dizziness

Below are some of the reasons dizziness may occur. Be aware that it can be a symptom of a serious underlying problem.

- Arterial disease
- Abnormal heart rhythms
- Stroke
- Osteoarthritis in the neck joints
- Sudden emotional stress
- Epilepsy
- Intoxication with alcohol or other recreational drugs
- Eye strain
- Food allergies
- Hormonal changes
- Brain infection

Put your feet up
Whenever you start to feel dizzy, take deep breaths and sit down. Relax with your feet propped up, which helps restore normal blood flow to the brain.

Acupressure

- To boost circulation, apply firm pressure in a circling movement with your thumb on the point (CV 6) two finger-widths below your navel.

- To counter vertigo, apply thumb pressure with a press-and-release action in the hollow between the jaw and the skull (TH 17), just behind the earlobe.

of dizziness. Be careful not to make the bath-water too hot, since this might dilate the veins in your legs and lower your blood pressure, making you feel dizzy when you get out.

TREATMENT

Your priority if you feel dizzy is to put your feet up (see above). Eat something nutritious, such as a sandwich made with whole-grain bread, if it has been more than two hours since you last ate.

Exercises: Certain head and body exercises can be successful for vertigo (see box, below left). An ear specialist can arrange for you to learn these "vestibular rehabilitation exercises."

When to get medical help

- Dizziness recurs.
- You also have a painful or stiff neck, fever, an earache, or a headache.
- You are taking prescribed medication.

Get help right away if:
- You also experience a change in vision, numbness in the face or limbs, palpitations, chest pain, breathlessness, or confusion.
- Dizziness persists despite self-care.

The vortex of vertigo

With the severe attack of dizziness called vertigo, you feel as though your surroundings are spinning around you. Closing your eyes to shut out the sensation may not be enough to stop the feeling that you or your environment is unstable. If the spinning sensation continues for more than a minute or so, you may feel nauseated or even vomit. You may also be unable to stand up, or you may faint. This symptom is usually caused by a disorder affecting the organs of balance in the inner ear, such as viral labyrinthitis or Ménière's disease.

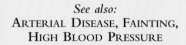
See also:
ARTERIAL DISEASE, FAINTING,
HIGH BLOOD PRESSURE

Dry Skin

When the sebaceous—oil-secreting—glands in the skin fail to produce enough oil, called sebum, to protect the skin from atmospheric conditions, the skin becomes dry, flaky, and sometimes sore. Following simple rules for skin care and choosing from a range of natural formulas and other treatments generally alleviate the problem.

You may have dry skin because your sebaceous glands are relatively inactive. This could be an inherited tendency, the result of a temporary hormonal imbalance (as during pregnancy), or a nutritional deficiency. The skin also tends to become drier with increasing age.

Extremes of temperature and strong winds deplete moisture from the skin. The hands, feet, and elbows are particularly vulnerable, since they have relatively few sebaceous glands, and the face and neck are also readily affected because they are usually exposed to the environment. Dry skin may also result from such conditions as eczema, psoriasis, and diaper rash, as well as from dehydration caused by low fluid intake.

A beneficial garden weed
Tea made from chickweed can soothe and soften dry skin.

PREVENTION

Use a high-factor sunscreen outdoors, wear warm socks and gloves in cold weather, and apply lip salve and moisturizer regularly. Indoors, keep the temperature comfortably cool. Turn down the heat by day; wear extra clothing instead.

Air conditioning, heating, and electrical appliances, including TVs and computers, increase the air's concentration of positive ions, which have a drying effect on the skin and remove moisture from the air. Reduce the positive ion count by keeping a window open,

Protecting dry skin
- Use cleansing lotion or cream, not soap.
- Avoid alcohol-based astringents or toners, since these remove skin oil.
- Use light moisturizer in the morning and a richer one at night.
- Lubricate the skin around the eyes—which contains few sebaceous glands—with eye cream, lotion, or gel.
- Apply ointment or cream to your hands before doing housework or manual work.
- Wear rubber gloves when using detergents or other cleaning products.

humidifying the air (by using a humidifer or placing bowls of water on or near radiators), and introducing houseplants.

Avoid sleeping under an electric blanket. Exercise regularly to improve your circulation and ensure that your skin is supplied with plenty of nutrients and oxygen.

TREATMENT
Diet: A healthy diet that includes raw fruits and vegetables helps keep the skin moist and supple. Prevent dehydration by drinking at least six glasses of noncaffeinated beverages daily.
- Eat foods rich in essential fatty acids (see p. 12).
- Increase your intake of foods containing vitamins A and D (see p. 12). (Be aware, however,

175

that most vitamin D comes from the action of sunlight on the skin.)

- Eat foods rich in vitamin E and zinc (see p. 12).
- Take supplements of fish oil.

Kitchen cabinet remedies

- There's no need for expensive skin creams. Many dermatologists consider solid vegetable shortening to be the best moisturizer. An ordinary cold cream from the drugstore is also often very helpful.
- Oatmeal has healing and soothing properties. To soften skin, put a muslin bag containing two cups of coarse oatmeal in a lukewarm bath, and soak for no more than 15 minutes. Pat yourself dry and apply moisturizer immediately to seal in moisture.
- Honey, which draws moisture from the air, makes an effective, if sticky, mask for dry skin.

Herbal remedies

- Aloe vera gel is emollient, improving the condition of rough facial skin.
- Chickweed has soothing properties. Make a compress (see p. 37) with cooled

Feeding your skin
Nourish your skin from within by eating foods rich in essential fatty acids and vitamins A, D, and E.

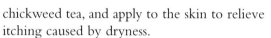

Hydrotherapy for blood flow

Stimulate the flow of nutrients to the skin of your hands and feet by bathing them in hot and then cold water for one minute each. Also apply alternate hot and cold compresses between your shoulder blades and the base of your neck to treat dry hands. Apply compresses to your lower back for dry feet.

chickweed tea, and apply to the skin to relieve itching caused by dryness.
- Take evening primrose oil, which contains essential fatty acids.

Caution: For safety concerns, see pp. 34–37.

Aromatherapy

- Geranium oil: add a few drops to a warm bath.
- Sandalwood and rose otto oils: mix two drops of each with one tablespoon of wheat germ oil and the contents of a capsule of evening primrose oil. Apply to dry skin at night.

When to get medical help

- The dryness gets worse.
- You have soreness or inflammation.

See also:
CHAPPED LIPS, DERMATITIS, DIAPER RASH, ITCHING, SKIN PROBLEMS

Earache

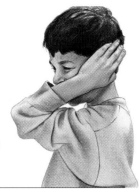

*M*ost of us can remember having earaches as a child, but the symptom occurs in adults, too, often in conjunction with a viral infection of the nose and throat. In some cases, simple home remedies may not only help ease the pain and promote healing but also make earaches less likely.

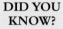

DID YOU KNOW?

Earache is often worse at night. The middle ear does not drain as well when you lie down, especially if you lie on the side of the affected ear, and swallowing, which encourages the eustachian tube to open, occurs less often during sleep.

Earache frequently results from conditions that affect the outer or middle ear (see illustration, p. 238). Among the causes of pain in the outer ear are infection or inflammation, either localized in the form of a boil or as a generalized area of redness and swelling. The latter may result from irritation resulting from an allergic reaction or from frequent immersion in water (a condition known as swimmer's ear). Pain may also be caused by a foreign body lodged in the outer ear canal. This is especially likely in young children, who sometimes insert small objects, such as beads, into their ears. If an object gets stuck, it can cause soreness and inflammation. If an infection then develops from bacteria or fungi, there may be a discharge. Wax blockage may be painful if it puts pressure on the eardrum.

The most common painful condition affecting the middle ear is infection (otitis media), a possible complication of colds and other nose and throat infections, especially in children. This occurs when inflammation in the nasal passages blocks the eustachian tube, allowing fluid to accumulate. Viruses and bacteria may then multiply in the fluid, causing increased pressure on the eardrum. Discomfort, along with hearing loss, may also result from allergic rhinitis. Other causes of earache include referred pain from a dental problem, and air pressure changes when diving or flying (see box).

PREVENTION

Help protect your baby from future earache by breast-feeding, preferably for at least one year. The antibodies and other substances in breast milk that boost immunity and counter infection play an important role in preventing ear trouble. Both children and adults should avoid smoke-filled air, which encourages congestion of the lining of the eustachian tube and middle ear.

If you are prone to swimmer's ear, insert lamb's wool covered in petroleum jelly into your ears before you swim. Avoid public pools and polluted lakes and rivers.

Diet: Boosting immunity with a healthy diet helps prevent earache from infection or allergy.

When you fly

To help prevent earaches caused by pressure changes in a plane, take the following measures during take-off and landing:

- Yawn frequently.
- Swallow repeatedly, chew gum, or sip water.
- Unless you have an infection, hold your nose, close your mouth, and try to blow out through the back of your nose and throat (see photograph).

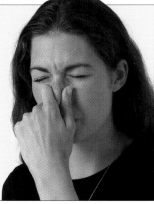

Eat some raw garlic each day, and consider taking a supplement of beta-carotene, vitamins C and E, and flavonoids. If you think your (or your child's) earaches may result from a food sensitivity, try to identify the culprit food (see p. 214).

TREATMENT

A foreign body in the outer ear should be removed only by a doctor. For advice on removing earwax, see page 239. An earache from an inflamed or infected ear can sometimes be relieved by the following simple remedies:

■ Sleep with an extra pillow to encourage your eustachian tube to drain.
■ Apply some heat. Either hold a covered hot-water bottle to the painful ear, or use a hot salt bag (see illustration, right).

Aromatherapy: Essential oils inhaled in steam (see p. 141) or diluted in oil and applied to the skin can help relieve pain in the ear. Avoid cajuput oil in the first 20 weeks of pregnancy.

■ Add five drops of lavender, cajuput, or chamomile oil to a pint of steaming hot water. Inhale the steam for 10 minutes.
■ Add three drops of cajuput or lavender oil to two teaspoons of warmed olive oil, or use mullein or St. John's wort oil undiluted. Lean your head to one side with the affected ear uppermost. Put a few drops of the oil into your ear, then gently plug your ear with

Soothing warmth
Fill a cotton bag with three or four tablespoons of sea salt. Heat it in the oven or microwave until it's hot but still comfortable to the touch. Hold it against your ear until it cools.

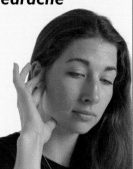

Acupressure for earache

Open your mouth and locate the point (SI 19) between the jaw joint and the middle of the front of your ear. Press gently and steadily with your fingertip for a few seconds. Release and repeat several times.

cotton. Never put oil in your ear if there's a discharge, whether clear fluid, pus, or blood, as this may indicate that the eardrum has perforated; oil might then enter the middle ear, causing further irritation.

■ Add three drops of any of the previously mentioned oils to two teaspoons of sweet almond oil, and use a few drops of this to smooth gently into the skin of your ear and throat.

When to get medical help

● The earache is severe or continues for more than a few days.
● There is a foreign body or pus in the ear.
● You have a high fever.

Get help right away if:
● The ear discharges blood or clear fluid.

See also:
ALLERGIC RHINITIS, COLDS,
HEARING LOSS, TOOTHACHE

Eating Disorders

Anorexia nervosa, bulimia, and compulsive eating are most common in female adolescents and young adults with emotional problems. Professional help may be essential, but developing insight into eating disorders and using practical tips may prevent a minor problem from getting worse as well as complementing any expert help.

There are a number of different types of eating disorders, but all are characterized by an abnormal relationship with food. Anorexia nervosa, in which a person—usually a female—rejects food, often because she falsely believes herself to be overweight, usually begins in the early teenage years. Bulimia, in which the sufferer sometimes binges and induces vomiting after eating, is most common between the ages of 15 and 30. Compulsive eating may happen at any age.

An eating disorder usually causes great distress to the person concerned and to family members. Since food satisfies unconscious emotional needs and desires as well as hunger, an eating disorder represents an attempt to deal with unmet needs that are causing stress, anxiety, or depression. Those who suffer from eating disorders are often tense, have low self-esteem, and tend to interact poorly with the outside world.

Anorexia and bulimia sometimes reflect an intense fear of putting on weight, often triggered by emotional problems. A person with an eating disorder may eat too little, induce vomiting, or overeat to blot out painful feelings or to feel more in control of what seems like a frightening, chaotic, or dangerous life, or, perhaps, to punish herself for angry or negative thoughts. Some people with anorexia develop nutritional deficiencies, which reduce their appetite further.

SYMPTOMS

Anorexia nervosa: This disorder is characterized by a refusal to eat adequately, including, at times, restricting the range of foods; severe, possibly life-threatening, weight loss; restlessness; fatigue; weakness; and thinning hair. Some anorexics increase weight loss by exercising excessively and obsessively.

Bulimia: The key symptoms of bulimia are bouts of excessive eating followed by self-induced vomiting, or the use of laxatives to prevent food from being digested and absorbed. Body weight may be normal. Repeated episodes of vomiting may cause fatigue, dental decay,

Recognizing the signs

A person who has an eating disorder is likely to have several of the following symptoms or behavior traits:

- Excessive concern about weight
- Strict dietary restraint
- Viewing foods as good or bad
- Eating only a few types of food
- Regularly skipping meals
- Intense fear of gaining weight or being fat
- Distorted perception of body weight, body fat, size, and shape
- Continuous weight loss
- Dramatic weight fluctuations
- Guilt or shame about eating
- Secret binges
- Self-induced vomiting
- Inappropriate use of laxatives
- Excessive exercising
- Irregular menstrual cycles or missed periods
- Withdrawal from friends and family
- Irritability, depression, or anxiety
- Tiredness, fainting, or dizzy spells

persistently sore throat, abdominal pain, bloating, digestive disturbances, and various metabolic disorders. Excessive use of laxatives can disturb the muscle action of the intestines, leading to chronic constipation. It may also cause fluid, electrolyte, and nutritional deficiencies.

Compulsive eating: People with this disorder, who are likely to be overweight, have the urge to eat even when they are not hungry. Binge eating is a type of compulsive disorder that involves eating an enormous amount of food at one sitting, often in a very short time. The sufferer feels completely out of control while eating and eats rapidly—but fails to feel full. Some binge eaters spend a great deal of time planning meals and buying food. However, they feel embarrassed and guilty about their bingeing, and they usually eat secretly.

Helpful diversions
To overcome a compulsive eating disorder, look for new, pleasurable ways of relieving stress. Listening to music, for example, can provide a valuable alternative to using food as a source of comfort.

TREATMENT

Stress management: Since stress and anxiety play a large part in many eating disorders, finding ways to deal with these problems can be very helpful. You need emotional support from someone with whom you can talk openly about your condition. Some people find that creative activities, such as keeping a journal, painting, and sculpting, help them express feelings they can't verbalize. If you are eating too much, make a list of interesting and enjoyable things to do instead, whenever you crave food. For example, have a relaxing, fragrant bath, go for a walk, or phone a friend to arrange a visit.

Flower essences: To help counter negative feelings about yourself and your body, choose one or more essences that most closely match your emotions. Take four drops in a little spring water, four times a day on an empty stomach. The following essences may be especially appropriate:

- Crab Apple: if you dislike your appearance.
- Rock Water: if you are very hard on yourself—for example, by denying yourself food.

Crab Apple
This flower essence may help those who are overly concerned with cleanliness and hate the way they look.

Diet: Compulsive eaters often eat high-sugar, starchy foods, which make their blood-sugar level rise quickly. The pancreas responds by

producing excess insulin, which can make the blood-sugar level drop too low. This can trigger a craving for yet more sugar or refined carbohydrates. Try to reduce your intake of these types of foods, and also do the following:

■ Increase the fiber in your diet.

■ Keep blood sugar stable by eating small amounts several times during the day, rather than two or three big meals.

■ Eat more chromium-rich foods (see p. 12). Chromium helps regulate blood-sugar levels.

■ Reduce your intake of alcohol and caffeinated beverages, since these can produce energy dips that encourage food cravings.

■ Identify any food sensitivity that may be to blame for food cravings and weight fluctuation. Try an elimination diet to identify the foods that may be responsible (see p. 214), but consider professional help in doing this, especially if your weight is low.

Vitamins and minerals: Appetite is controlled by neurotransmitters in the hypothalamus. The efficiency of these chemicals is influenced by the blood levels of sugar, fatty acids, and hormones, which, in turn, are affected by anxiety, depression, and deficiencies of vitamin B or zinc. To help keep your neurotransmitters in balance, eat foods rich in the following nutrients (or take them in the form of a multiple vitamin and mineral supplement):

■ Calcium (milk, cheese, nuts, seeds, green leafy vegetables, legumes)

■ Magnesium (shellfish, nuts, whole grains, legumes, green leafy vegetables)

■ Manganese (tea, nuts, seeds, whole grains, organic green leafy vegetables, pineapple, raisins, blueberries)

■ Potassium (fruits, vegetables)

■ Selenium (fish, whole grains, organic fruits and vegetables)

■ Vitamin B complex (lean cuts of meat, milk, whole grains, fresh vegetables)

■ Zinc (lean cuts of meat, poultry, shellfish, egg yolks, nuts, seeds, whole grains, hard cheeses, root vegetables)

Yoga: Regular yoga practice can relieve tension and depression, helping you meet emotional needs in other ways besides eating. It works by:

■ Giving you more self-control, which will allow you to master the urge to gratify your desires instantly or in an unhealthy fashion.

➤ continued, p. 182

Fresh and nutritious
Foods carefully selected for freshness and variety are likely to provide the balance of nutrients you need to regulate appetite and control blood sugar.

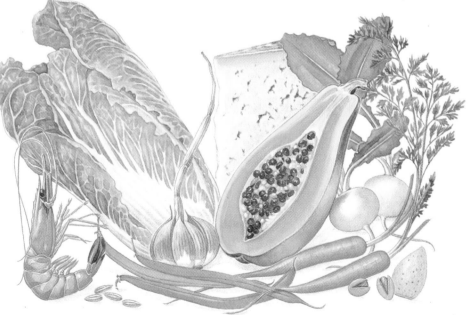

Color breathing for inner harmony

This technique helps you relax, clear your mind of negative thoughts, and feel at peace with the world around you. As you breathe, you focus on each of the body's so-called energy centers (known as chakras in Ayurvedic medicine), the colors they are associated with, and the emotions and qualities they are said to govern.

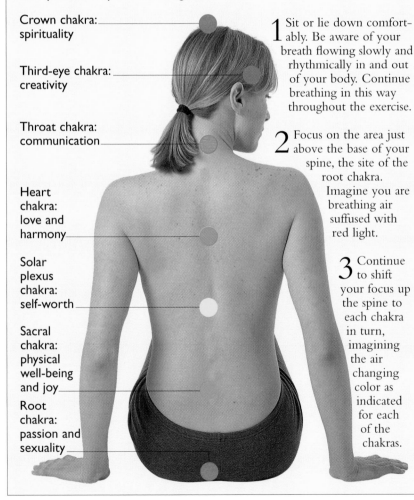

Crown chakra:
spirituality

Third-eye chakra:
creativity

Throat chakra:
communication

Heart
chakra:
love and
harmony

Solar
plexus
chakra:
self-worth

Sacral
chakra:
physical
well-being
and joy

Root
chakra:
passion and
sexuality

1 Sit or lie down comfortably. Be aware of your breath flowing slowly and rhythmically in and out of your body. Continue breathing in this way throughout the exercise.

2 Focus on the area just above the base of your spine, the site of the root chakra. Imagine you are breathing air suffused with red light.

3 Continue to shift your focus up the spine to each chakra in turn, imagining the air changing color as indicated for each of the chakras.

■ Helping you feel relaxed.
■ Providing an alternative to abnormal eating as a way of feeling in control of your life.

Emotion culturing: This technique aims to cultivate a positive state of mind and to control the urge to binge without inducing a sense of guilt when around food. When you feel a craving for food, say to yourself, "I am going to eat, but why hurry? Be slow, be easy—let me enjoy this food." Then take five deep breaths and start to eat slowly, savoring the flavors in each morsel.

Other therapies: Ask your physician to refer you to a psychiatrist or psychotherapist who specializes in eating disorders. A nutritionist will be able to provide advice on eating behaviors and on choosing a good balance of foods to help combat your eating problem.

When to get medical help

● Your eating pattern has been abnormal for longer than four weeks.
● You are continuing to lose or gain a significant amount of weight.
● You are abusing laxatives, diuretics, or emetics.

Get help right away if:
● You develop bulimia or stop eating completely.

See also:
ANXIETY, APPETITE LOSS,
DEPRESSION, EMOTIONAL
PROBLEMS, FOOD SENSITIVITY,
OVERWEIGHT, STRESS

Emotional Problems

Psychological distress, whether arising from personality traits, biochemical imbalances, or difficult or uncomfortable circumstances or events, can have a profound effect on your physical well-being and quality of life. Sympathy and support from a trusted person, together with home remedies and lifestyle changes, can often ease difficulties.

The constant stress of living with unresolved emotions—such as sadness, anger, fear, and anxiety—can affect you physically, because it changes levels of hormones and neurotransmitters (chemicals that convey messages between nerves). These changes can make you sluggish and tired and may depress your immune system, increasing your susceptibility to infection and illnesses, such as rheumatoid arthritis, that are triggered by attack from your own immune cells.

The way you respond emotionally to problems in life is shaped by your personality, experience, and circumstances. You may become ill as a result of a problem that someone else copes with relatively easily. However, you can learn how to better manage emotional problems.

PREVENTION

Your customary responses to difficult situations are not unchangeable. You may have emotions that are uncomfortably close to the surface, last too long, and disrupt your well-being and relationships; however, you can learn to deal with situations in a different way. Or if you are emotionally restrained, bottling up your feelings, you can learn to become more open.

- Aim to develop self-knowledge, accept your strengths and weaknesses, and recognize and commit yourself to your primary goals in life.
- If decision-making upsets you, practice clarifying your options and objectives. Don't be afraid to recognize your sense of loss or other feelings about the possible life choices you have rejected.
- Remember that total control of all

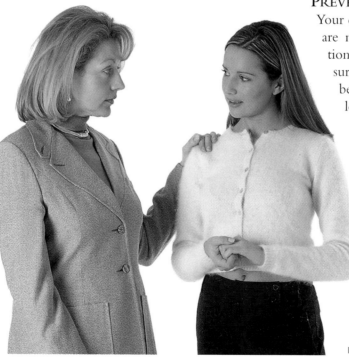

Sharing your feelings
Let others around you help you through difficult times. You may benefit from practical help they can offer, but it is equally important to have someone tell you they understand how you're feeling.

183

aspects of your life is neither possible nor desirable, and adjust your expectations accordingly.

TREATMENT

Mind games: A growing body of evidence suggests that optimism gives some protection against mental and physical ailments. If you tend to see only the worst aspects of situations, make an effort to take a more balanced view. For example, if a relationship breaks down, the disadvantages may be all too clear, but there are potential benefits, too: you might have the opportunity to move to a different area or follow interests that your partner didn't share.

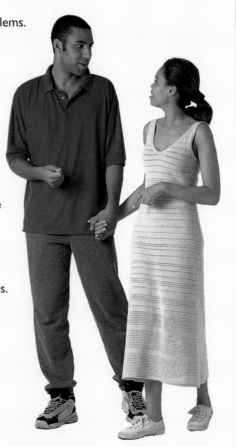

Express yourself

Emotional distress sometimes results from relationship problems. Try the techniques described below to improve your communication skills.

Problem-solving

If a misunderstanding with another person is causing you anxiety or distress, try the following:
- Arrange a meeting at which both people take uninterrupted turns to say how they feel.
- State your case in the first person. For example, "I feel hurt when you do that," rather than "You make me feel hurt when you do that." By doing this, you take responsibility for your response to the other person's actions. You also comment on the behavior, but not on the person. The person can then—if able or willing—take responsibility for the behavior and modify it in the future.
- Next, listen to the other person's response (see below).

Empathic listening

This type of listening focuses on the other person's emotions. It helps to be aware of your own feelings, so you should get into the habit of listening carefully to yourself. Empathic listening has three stages:
- Put your own feelings to one side for a while.
- Try to identify the other person's emotions by using your ears, eyes, and intuition.
- Tell the person what you think those emotions are. This generally has the powerful effect of imparting a feeling of understanding. At the least, the person will know you're trying to see things from his or her point of view.

Even if you are unable to see things in a positive way, you may find a situation more bearable if you try to move on, accepting that nothing stays the same in life, rather than dwelling on your emotional pain. Losing your job may feel like a disaster, but if you acknowledge your feelings of anger and bitterness without letting them overwhelm you, it may then be possible to consider future plans more constructively.

Communication: One of the main reasons we have emotional problems is that we sometimes find it difficult, if not impossible, to express our feelings clearly, especially during stressful times. Instead of explaining what we are feeling and why—as well as listening to the other person— we may shout, argue, accuse, or stop talking completely. Try to communicate your emotional responses clearly. The more uncomfortable or embarrassing this is, the more important is good communication. It is often better to deal with upset feelings sooner rather than later. (See also the box on the facing page.)

- Don't wait until anger or resentment has built up and both parties have become entrenched in their positions.
- Before discussing a problem, make a list of the points you want to raise, so you don't lose track of them.
- Tell the other person clearly and in a non-confrontational way what you want, and listen when it's his or her turn to do the same.
- Be careful to avoid falling into the trap of inappropriate sharing of emotions. Choose your confidant and the time and place for such confidences with care.

Improving self-understanding: Gaining a good understanding of your emotional responses and behaviors is a key to overcoming emotional difficulties. Some people find it useful to keep a diary to record their feelings. Try noting each day how you have felt, the events or circumstances that you think contributed to your feelings, and how you coped with any challenging emotions. Gradually you may begin to see patterns of feelings and behavior and may then be able consciously to alter any habitual negative responses. For example, if you always respond to insults or criticism by becoming upset and blaming yourself, it may be helpful to try focusing instead on other possible explanations for the person's behavior. You thereby avoid taking responsibility for the behavior of others (see also "Affirmation," p. 88).

Aromatherapy
- Put a few drops each of clary sage and juniper berry oils in a warm bath, to clear thoughts and promote a good night's sleep. (Do not use these oils if you are or might be pregnant.)
- When you feel unhappy, scent your room by using six

Time of serenity
Try meditation to achieve a clearer, calmer view of yourself and any distress you're feeling.

drops of clary sage (omit if you're pregnant), three of rose otto, and one of sandalwood oil in a vaporizer (see p. 29).

Flower essences: These are used to treat mental and emotional problems, and each flower essence is said to help alleviate a particular negative emotional state. Choose one or more remedies based on your personality or the way you normally respond to difficulties. Useful remedies include the following:

■ Cherry Plum: if you find it difficult to control your temper.
■ Holly: if you feel jealous or full of hate.
■ Larch: if you lack belief in your own abilities.
■ Mimulus: if you are shy or anxious.
■ Pine: if you have a tendency to blame yourself for past actions.
■ Scleranthus: if you are not able to make decisions easily.
■ Star of Bethlehem: if you are mourning the loss of a loved one.

Flower power
Flower essences are extracted from many common plants, including (left to right): willow, star of Bethlehem, holly, pine, and scleranthus.

■ Willow: if you are feeling sorry for yourself or are bitter and resentful.

Homeopathy: You should ideally take into account your personality type, as well as your symptoms, when choosing the most appropriate remedies. The aim of treatment is not to suppress your emotions, but to help you achieve a state of emotional balance so that you can express your feelings without being overwhelmed by them.

■ Arsenicum: for extreme anxiety, exhaustion, and restlessness.
■ Ignatia: for emotional upsets, sadness and grief, hysteria, mood swings, excessive weeping, or inability to cry.
■ Nux vomica: for irritability and explosive anger when you cannot take any more stress.

Other therapies: A trained counselor or psychotherapist can help. Many other therapies can be of benefit, including biofeedback, cranial osteopathy, and creative therapies.

When to get medical help

● Your emotional problems are affecting your relationships or otherwise disrupting your usual lifestyle.

Get help right away if:
● You have suicidal thoughts.

See also:
ADDICTIONS, ANXIETY,
DEPRESSION, EATING DISORDERS,
GRIEF, SEX DRIVE LOSS, STRESS

Eye Irritation and Discharge

Conjunctivitis, or pink eye, is the most common form of eye irritation, causing soreness, redness, or discharge. Blepharitis produces similar symptoms, and both conditions may be a result of injury, infection, a foreign body in the eye, allergy, or exposure to irritating chemicals, such as those in cigarette smoke and vehicle exhaust fumes.

Conjunctivitis involves inflammation of the conjunctiva, the transparent membrane covering the whites of the eyes and lining the lids. The eyes look red, feel gritty and itchy, and produce a discharge that in infective conjunctivitis may cause the eyelids to stick together during sleep. In allergic conjunctivitis—often associated with allergic rhinitis—the discharge is clear, and the eyelids are often swollen. There may be abnormal sensitivity to light.

Blepharitis, an inflammation of the eyelids, causes redness, irritation, and scaly skin at the lid margins. There may be crusty beads of dried discharge on the lids and lashes. The condition, which is sometimes associated with dandruff or eczema, tends to recur.

PREVENTION

Reduce your chances of catching eye infections by never sharing towels or washcloths and by encouraging any household member who is affected to seek treatment. Protect your eyes with goggles when performing tasks that generate dust or smoke and when swimming in pools if you are sensitive to chlorine.

If you are susceptible to eye infections, build up your resistance by eating five servings of fruits and vegetables daily, including berries and yellow and orange produce. Avoid foods made with white flour and sugar.

Foreign body in the eye

Dust particles are usually easily removed by blinking. Larger objects can sometimes be removed using the methods below. Seek medical help if a foreign body is on the pupil, embedded in the eye, or if first aid fails.

1 **Lower lid:** Try flushing out the object with water or lifting it out by touching only the white part of the eye with the dampened corner of a clean cloth or tissue.

2 **Upper lid:** Holding the lashes, gently pull the lid outward and downward over the lower lid, or try flushing the object out by blinking underwater.

TREATMENT

If you have an eye infection, avoid touching your eyes, and wash your hands often. Also, wash towels, washcloths, and bedsheets frequently. If you have blepharitis and dandruff, treat the dandruff at the same time.

➤ continued, p. 188

Diet: Persistent eye irritation that may result from an allergy may improve if you exclude dairy products, tea, and coffee from your diet.

From the drugstore: To help fight infection and soothe irritation, take supplements of evening primrose oil, vitamins A, B, and E, and flavonoids, as directed on the bottle. For infectious conjunctivitis, try a boric-acid eyewash.

Homeopathy

- Aconite: if eyes feel hot, dry, and gritty and look red and inflamed, with swollen lids. The symptoms may have been caused by cold wind.
- Apis: if eyelids are red and puffy.
- Belladonna: if eyes are dry, bloodshot, and sensitive to light, and symptoms develop quickly.
- Euphrasia: if eyes water and burn. Bathe the eyes with a few drops of the tincture in an eye bath of sterilized water. Use fresh solution for each eye.
- Pulsatilla: if you have a yellowish discharge that does not burn or irritate, but the eyelids are sore and, perhaps, sticky.

Herbal remedies: Bathing the eyes in eyebright tea soothes many symptoms. Simmer the tea for 10 minutes to sterilize the liquid, then cool and strain (through a sterile gauze pad or cheesecloth) into a sterile eyecup. Use fresh tea for each eye and do not store any leftover tea.

To boost your immune system, drink tea made from a combination of eyebright, echinacea, cleavers, burdock, and licorice. Drink a cup once or twice daily for two weeks.

Caution: For safety concerns, see pp. 34–37.

Acupressure for eyes

Soothe irritated eyes by pressing one or more of the points described below steadily for about two minutes. Release and repeat every few breaths.

- The point (*tai yang*) one thumb-width away from the outer bony margin of the eye, level with the top of the ear.

- The point (B 1) immediately above the inner corner of the eye, at the inner end of the eyebrow.

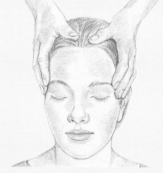

- The point (Liv 3) on the top of the foot between the first and second toes, along with the point (GB 37) on the shin five thumb-widths directly above the outer ankle tip, in front of the bony ridge on the outside of the leg.

When to get medical help

- Your eye problem is causing pain.
- There is a profuse, colored discharge.
- Your vision is gradually affected.
- Your symptoms fail to improve within two days.

Get help right away if:
- Your eye has been injured.
- Your vision is acutely affected.

See also:
ALLERGIC RHINITIS, EYESIGHT PROBLEMS, HAIR AND SCALP PROBLEMS

Eyesight Problems

*W*hen your eyes are unable to focus images accurately, the result is blurred vision. Glasses or contact lenses are the conventional way of correcting the problem, but simple home remedies, dietary measures, and exercises may be able to arrest the rate of deterioration and in some cases even improve your existing eyesight.

The causes of blurred vision include too long or too short an eyeball (nearsightedness and far-sightedness) and discrepancies in the curvature of the surface of the eye (astigmatism). In middle age the lenses start to harden (presbyopia), so that it becomes more and more difficult to bring close objects into focus. Other conditions that cause increased blurring of vision include a clouded lens (cataract), excess fluid in the eyes (glaucoma), and changes in the retina resulting from aging (macular degeneration).

PREVENTION

Some eyesight problems are inherited, so prevention is impossible, but for others you can safeguard the health of your eyes.

- Wear sunglasses in strong light to reduce the risk of cataracts from cumulative ultraviolet damage. Protect your eyes with goggles when doing haz- ardous jobs.
- Nourish your eyes and the blood vessels and nerves that supply

them by eating a diet containing plenty of veg- etables and fruits. Those shown below (see illustration) and dark green leafy vegetables are especially beneficial.

- Limit consumption of saturated fats and stay away from cigarette smoke to help keep free radicals from forming in the retina and causing macular degeneration.

➤ continued, p. 191

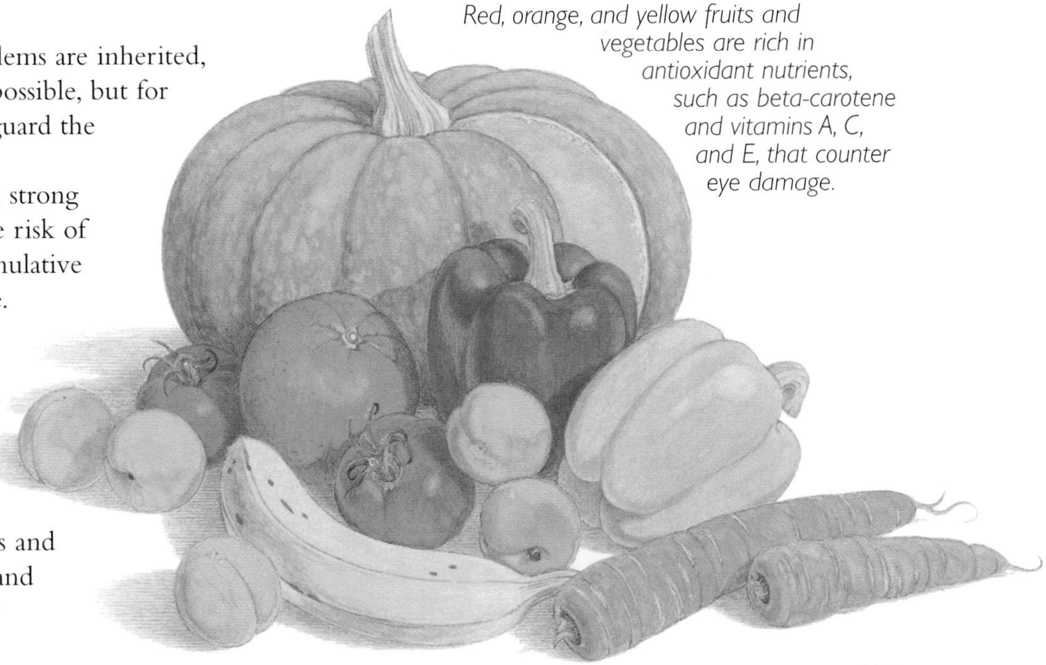

Vision vitamins
Red, orange, and yellow fruits and vegetables are rich in antioxidant nutrients, such as beta-carotene and vitamins A, C, and E, that counter eye damage.

Yoga-based eye exercises

Practiced daily, the exercises below help relax and strengthen the eye muscles. The first sequence, known as candle *gazing, is also good for steadying the mind. The second sequence helps train the eyes to make the adjustments* *needed during everyday activities, such as reading, driving, and working at a computer screen.*

1 Position a candle three feet away from your eyes at eye level.

2 Gaze at the flame for 10 seconds, then palm your eyes for 30 seconds (see "The Bates Method" on the facing page), while observing the after-image of the flame.

3 Next, gaze at it with one eye at a time, then with both eyes while turning your head from side to side. Palm between each stage to avoid eye strain.

4 Repeat, gazing first for 10, then 20, then 30 seconds. Increase the times by 10 seconds each week, until you are gazing for one, two, and three minutes.

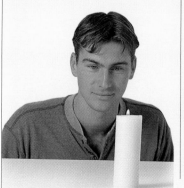

1 With your forefinger, touch the spot between your eyebrows. Gradually move your finger away, focusing on it as it moves and continuing until your arm is fully extended. Hold the position for a few seconds, then bring the finger back between your eyebrows. Cover your eyes with your palms, then repeat the whole sequence.

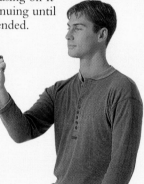

2 Extend your right arm in front of you, with the thumb pointing upward. Focusing on the middle of your thumb, move your arm gradually to the right, following the thumb with your eyes without moving your head. When you have followed it as far as you can, hold the position for 15 to 30 seconds. Move your arm slowly to the front again, following your thumb with your eyes. Cover your eyes with your palms. Repeat with the left arm, and palm once more.

3 Hold both arms out in front of you, with the thumbs pointing up. Gaze at both thumbs and gradually move your arms apart. Continue until you are about to lose sight of the thumbs. Hold the position for one minute, then bring your arms slowly back to the starting position. Cover your eyes with your palms.

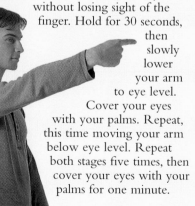

4 Hold out your right arm, pointing with your forefinger to the left. Without moving your head, slowly raise your arm while focusing on the finger. Move your arm as far as you can without losing sight of the finger. Hold for 30 seconds, then slowly lower your arm to eye level. Cover your eyes with your palms. Repeat, this time moving your arm below eye level. Repeat both stages five times, then cover your eyes with your palms for one minute.

TREATMENT

Although natural therapies may not cure problems with vision, there is much you can do to slow deterioration of eyesight.

- Do close work, such as reading, in good light. Position yourself so that the light comes over your left shoulder if you are right-handed and over your right shoulder if you are left-handed.
- When reading a newspaper, start with the largest type, such as headlines, before reading the small print.
- If you have a cataract, take bilberry extract. Research has shown that this herbal remedy, which contains antioxidant pigments called proanthocyanidins, can help slow the development of cataracts.

Homeopathy: Use Ruta for tired eyes when it's hard to focus—for example, after spending too much time in front of a computer screen.

The Bates method: This technique aims to "re-educate" the eye muscles and improve the eyesight. Bates teachers use such exercises as the following (do not wear glasses or contact lenses while you are doing these exercises):

- Every morning, close your eyes and splash them 20 times with warm water, then 20 times with cold. At bedtime, repeat the exercise, starting with cold water.
- Throughout the day, blink frequently— about 15 times per minute.
- Cover your eyes with your palms to rest them completely three or four times a day. Sit with your elbows resting on a table and place the palms of your hands over your eyes, with the base of your little fingers on the bridge of your nose. Do this for several minutes. Listening to music will help you relax.
- Hold your forefinger 6 to 10 inches from your eyes. Move it from your left shoulder to the right, and follow it with your eyes, keeping your neck relaxed and allowing your head to move with your finger. Focus on the finger, but be aware of the moving background too. Do this at least once a day.
- Do the same exercise, but focus on the moving background instead.

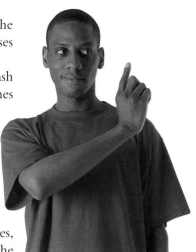

Focusing
Exercises in which you follow your finger with your eyes are a key element of the Bates method.

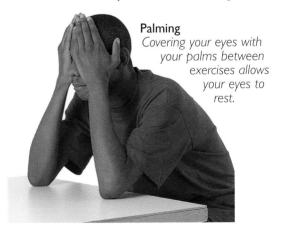

Palming
Covering your eyes with your palms between exercises allows your eyes to rest.

When to get medical help

- Your eyesight deteriorates.
- You experience eye pain.
- You have a vision change in one eye only.

Get help right away if:
- You lose vision suddenly.
- You have headaches along with loss of vision.

See also:
EYE IRRITATION
AND DISCHARGE

Facial Pain

Many people experience aching or other pain in the face at some time. Facial pain can range from a continuous dull ache to a sharp, intense spasm, depending on the cause. Simple home remedies often make all the difference, but some causes of facial pain, such as an inflamed temporal artery, are potentially serious and require medical attention.

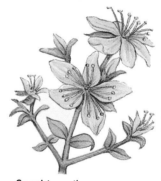

Soothing oil
For nerve pain, add three drops of St. John's wort oil to two teaspoons of olive or sweet almond oil. Smooth onto the painful area every three hours.

Understanding why your face hurts can help you plan what to do. Possible reasons include dental problems, migraine, sinusitis, upper respiratory infections, and mumps. Another cause is a dysfunctional jaw joint (temporomandibular joint syndrome, or TMJ), which may be triggered by dental problems, stress, poor posture, or injury.

An inflamed temporal artery (temporal arteritis) creates persistent pain in one or both temples. This serious condition, affecting mainly people over 50, requires prompt medical treatment. A damaged trigeminal nerve (trigeminal neuralgia), also more common in older people, brings about attacks of brief but severe pain in the face.

Shingles, an infection of the facial nerves caused by the varicella zoster virus, produces discomfort and sensitivity in the affected side of the face. Several days later, a blistery rash occurs. Pain may persist after the rash has disappeared.

Prevent facial pain by practicing good dental hygiene, reducing stress, and treating any infections promptly.

TREATMENT

Home treatments can help relieve pain, boost immunity, and manage the stress that may underlie the condition or result from long-term pain.

Heat or cold: Place a hot-water bottle wrapped in a towel or other cover over the painful area,

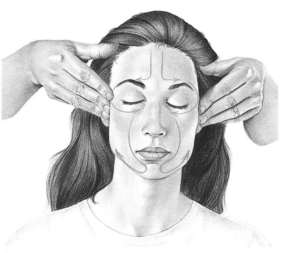

Gentle massage
Stroke both sides of the person's face with the fingers. Use only light pressure, following the direction of the arrows shown above. Start at the center of the forehead and finish with sweeping movements along the jawline and up toward the ears.

or apply a hot, damp washcloth repeatedly. If you find the application of cold more soothing, use a washcloth wrung out in cold water instead.

Massage: Massage encourages the release of natural painkillers called endorphins, and a gentle facial massage also releases tension in the muscles. You can either give yourself one or ask a friend to do it (see illustration, above). Use five drops of lavender or peppermint oil in two tablespoons of

192

sweet almond oil or another cold-pressed vegetable oil. If the pain is so severe that you cannot bear for your face to be touched, massage the tops of both big toes instead. Reflexologists call this the pituitary reflex; the pituitary gland affects many parts of the body.

Acupressure: The point (LI 4) between the base of your forefinger and thumb, used for treating colds (see p. 140), can also be helpful for relieving facial pain. Press this point several times on each hand. Do not use this point if you are pregnant. Alternatively, press with both thumbs along the base of your skull. Use small circular movements and work from the center outward.

Immune-boosting remedies: Increasing immunity may help relieve sinusitis and shingles. Eat a healthy diet, with five daily servings of vegetables and fruits. Include some fresh garlic, or take garlic capsules. Consider supplements of vitamins B and C and flavonoids. Make an herbal tea of echinacea, goldenseal, and licorice; drink a cup three times a day. Or take echinacea and astragalus as capsules or tincture.
Caution: For safety concerns about herbal remedies, see pp. 34–37.

Stress management: Continual stress makes pain worse and depresses immunity. Use stress-management strategies (see p. 347).

For TMJ: Eating soft foods puts less stress on your jaw. Keep your jaw muscles relaxed. If you work at a desk, check your posture, and don't lean forward. Avoid propping up your chin with your hands or cradling a telephone between your shoulder and chin. Do not carry heavy shoulder bags; instead use a backpack.

Finding the cause of your facial pain

Symptoms	Possible cause
Pain in forehead, nose, ears, cheekbones, or behind eyes	Sinusitis
Aching cheeks	Stress-induced tension
Pain and a rash on the upper half of one side of face	Shingles
Pain in jaw and mouth	Dental problems
Sensitivity on one side of face and, possibly, in one eye, followed by severe pain	Migraine
Intense shooting pain on one side, often provoked by even a light touch	Trigeminal neuralgia
Swelling and tenderness in temple, possibly with headache and, at worst, vision problems	Temporal arteritis
A stiff, clicking jaw joint and dull ache or pain in the jaw muscles	TMJ

When to get medical help
- You also have an earache, eye pain, headache, toothache, or a facial rash.
- The pain is severe.
- The pain has lasted longer than a week or is worsening after one or two days.

Get help right away if:
- You have had a head injury,
- You have a throbbing ache in your temple, vision problems, or a rash near your eye.

See also:
COLDS, HEADACHE, MIGRAINE, TOOTHACHE

193

Fainting

When insufficient oxygen reaches the brain, a brief loss of consciousness, known as fainting, can result. Recovery is usually quick, because falling to the ground places the head at the same level as the heart, thus restoring blood flow and oxygen to the brain. Prolonged loss of consciousness—for more than a minute—requires emergency treatment.

Fainting is caused by a sudden reduction in the blood supply to the brain, which leaves it short of sugar and other nutrients, as well as oxygen. Simply being in a hot, stuffy room is enough to make some people pass out, but fainting can also indicate a serious medical condition. Other causes include the following:

- Standing still for a long period, which makes the leg veins dilate and fill with blood, leaving less circulating blood available for the brain.
- Hunger, which leads to low levels of sugar in the bloodstream.

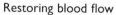
Restoring blood flow
If you feel you are about to faint, place your head below the level of your heart as quickly as possible. If it is difficult to lie down, sit with your head between your knees.

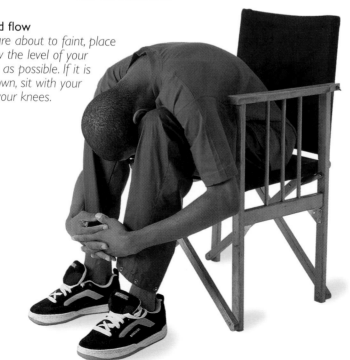

- Breathing too fast, or hyperventilating, because of anxiety. This reduces the blood's carbon-dioxide level and the amount of oxygen available to the brain cells.
- A shock—for example, from witnessing an accident or hearing bad news—which affects the nerve that controls blood pressure.
- Severe anemia, fever, uncontrolled diabetes, heart and circulatory disease, and certain other medical disorders.
- New medication.

Fainting is often preceded by such unpleasant sensations as dizziness, sweating, clamminess, and nausea. Other warning signs or symptoms include repeated yawning, feeling hot, shaking, pallor, and breathlessness. You may feel that you are suffocating and need fresh air, and some people experience an overwhelming sense of impending disaster.

Most people feel well again quickly after fainting, unless they are injured from falling against a hard object. If you have hit your head hard enough to cause a cut or a large bump, have the injury examined by a doctor; you may have a concussion or a fracture.

PREVENTION

- Eat regularly. If you miss a meal, at least have a nutritious, high-fiber snack, such as a whole-grain sandwich, a cereal bar, an apple, a banana,

or some nuts to prevent low blood sugar. Most important, don't skip breakfast.

- Eat a well-balanced diet, with plenty of fiber-rich foods and limited amounts of refined carbohydrates, such as white flour and sugar. Over the years this protects your pancreas—the gland that produces insulin, the blood-sugar regulating hormone—from becoming overstimulated by excess sugar. An overstimulated pancreas can react to the intake of refined carbohydrates by producing too much insulin. This leads to a sudden dip in the blood-sugar level, which makes fainting more likely.
- Open a window or turn up the air conditioning if a room is hot or stuffy.
- Check your breathing. Hyperventilation is a common response to stress. Practice slow, deep breathing every day (see p. 87).
- When standing still for a long time, stimulate your circulation by rocking back and forth on your heels and the balls of your feet, or by alternately tightening and relaxing your calf muscles—just as sentries do on guard duty.
- To avoid feeling faint after rising from a lying-down position, sit upright for a few moments, then get up slowly.
- If your blood pressure is low, drink a daily cup of hawthorn tea to help normalize it, but first see pp. 34–37 for safety concerns.

TREATMENT

Posture: Occasionally, fainting results from a sudden compression of the blood vessels in the neck—for example, from a sudden or violent sideways or backward jerk of your head. If you think this compression may have happened,

When someone has fainted

If the person is breathing normally and no serious injury has occurred, raise the legs above head level for a few moments, and loosen any tight clothing. This allows more blood to get to the brain. Discourage people from crowding around. When the person regains consciousness, encourage him or her to sit or lie quietly until fully recovered.

For prolonged unconsciousness

If the person does not revive after a minute, summon medical help, and follow the steps below.

1 Make sure that the unconscious person is breathing easily, and tilt the head back slightly to keep the airway open.

2 If you saw the person faint and know that there is no neck or spinal injury, place the victim in the recovery position: While kneeling down beside the person, bend the leg that's close to you and fold the arm on the same side across the body. Raise the other arm above the head.

3 Gently roll the person over so that his or her cheek is resting on the hand of the bent arm and the upper leg stabilizes the body. Lift the chin to improve the airway.

stand up straight and imagine that the top of the back of your head is attached by a taut string to the ceiling. Allow your head to rise up out of your neck, and keep your shoulders relaxed.

Breathing: If you are hyperventilating (breathing too rapidly), try to take slow, deep breaths into your abdomen, or cup your hands over your mouth and nose as you breathe; this raises your carbon-dioxide level and helps restore alertness. Or breathe in and out of a paper bag (see photograph).

Diet: Don't accept any medicinal alcohol, which could make you choke or vomit—and inhale the vomit because of a reduced level of consciousness. Once the faintness passes, sip some cold water. Upon regaining full consciousness, have something sweet—candy, a cookie, a teaspoon of honey, fruit juice, or sweetened tea or coffee. As soon as possible, eat something more nutritious and fiber-rich, or you may start to feel faint again when the raised blood-sugar level induced by the sugary snack passes its peak.

Homeopathy: Take your chosen remedy every 10 minutes while feeling faint or after reviving, then use as necessary. Helpful remedies include:
- Arnica: for an emotional shock.
- Aconite: for fright that remains after a shock.
- Gelsemium: if you feel weak and shaky after an emotional shock.

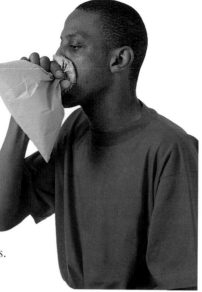

Regulating breathing
Breathe steadily through your mouth into a paper bag (never use plastic) so that it deflates and inflates as you breathe in and out.

An instant lift
The application of lavender oil to the temples can provide rapid relief from faintness. You can also add a few drops of this oil to sweet-almond or wheat-germ oil for a reviving massage after an episode of faintness.

- Ignatia: if you have had bad news or another shock and you feel you are losing control.
- Pulsatilla: after an emotional shock, when you are tearful and feel better from being comforted or getting fresh air.

Aromatherapy: Smelling salts (ammonium carbonate crystals) are a traditional remedy. You can achieve a similar result by inhaling the aroma from certain essential oils if you are feeling faint.
- To revive yourself and clear your head, rub a few drops of undiluted lavender oil into your temples and over the backs of your hands.
- To calm yourself and restore vitality, pour a few drops of lavender oil onto a tissue, and inhale the vapor for several minutes.

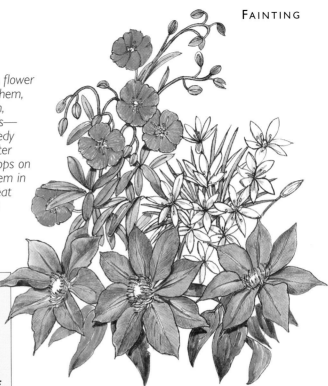

Herbal remedies: The following teas help speed recovery after fainting. Do not drink anything if you feel you are about to faint, because this could make you choke.

- After regaining consciousness, sip tea made from ginger, rosemary, or elderflowers.
- If fainting resulted from emotional shock and you continue to feel tense or stressed, have up to four cups daily of tea made from lemon balm and chamomile.

Caution: For safety concerns, see pp. 34–37.

Flower first aid
The combination of the flower essences Star of Bethlehem, Rock Rose, Cherry Plum, Impatiens, and Clematis—known as Rescue Remedy—helps you recover after fainting. Place a few drops on your tongue, or take them in a little cold water. Repeat every few minutes until you feel better.

Acupressure for a fainting victim

Use these points to help revive a person who has fainted, but not if there is a head, neck, or spinal injury.

- Press firmly with your thumbnail on the point (GV 26) in the furrow between the nose and upper lip. Continue until the person revives, keeping your other hand on the forehead just above the hairline.

- As the person is reviving, apply firm pressure to the point (Sp 6) four finger-widths above the tip of the ankle bone on the inside of the calf, just behind the shinbone. (Do not use this point on a pregnant woman.)

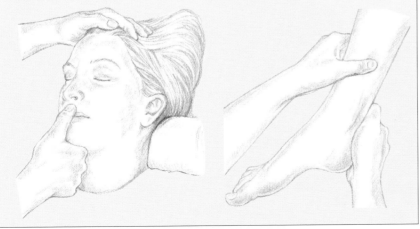

When to get medical help

- You faint frequently from a known cause.

Get help right away if:
- You experience first-time or unaccustomed fainting.
- Fainting results in a head injury or another possibly serious injury.
- The victim remains unconscious for longer than one minute.
- You have confusion, numbness, or loss of vision or movement upon recovery.

See also:
ANEMIA, ARTERIAL DISEASE, DIABETES, DIZZINESS, SHOCK, STRESS

Fatigue

It is normal to feel tired at the end of the day or after strenuous mental or physical exertion. Rest, relaxation, and a good night's sleep are usually all that are needed to restore energy levels. However, persistent fatigue or fatigue that seems out of proportion to the energy you have expended may indicate the presence of an underlying illness or the need for lifestyle changes.

So many people feel constantly fatigued that the complaint "tired all the time" (TATT) has now entered the medical vocabulary—albeit as a description rather than a diagnosis. Fatigue resulting from insomnia, or that is unrelieved by rest and sleep, has many possible causes. Overwork and anxiety are the most common. Other physical and/or emotional causes of persistent fatigue include anemia, chronic fatigue syndrome, stress, depression, an eating disorder, an infection, low blood pressure, obesity, malnourishment, an underactive thyroid gland, and certain medications. Frequently, more than one factor is involved.

A healthy balance
Maximize your energy level by complementing strenuous physical activity with adequate rest and sleep.

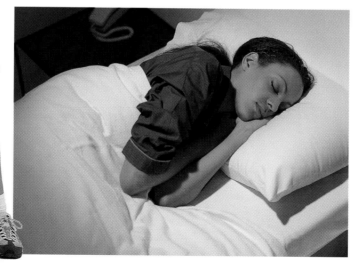

PREVENTION

Eat a nutritious, mainly fresh-food diet and get enough sleep (most people need at least seven hours a night). Get regular exercise and develop sound stress-management strategies (see p. 347).

Diet: To obtain the nutrients needed for physical and mental energy, eat foods rich in vitamins B (meat, fish, milk, whole grains), C (fresh vegetables and fruits), and E (oily fish, nuts, seeds, vegetable oils), iron (meat, fish, egg yolks, green leafy vegetables), magnesium (nuts, whole grains, legumes, green leafy vegetables), and potassium (vegetables and fruits).

If you often eat junk food, your pancreas may eventually overreact to the resulting surge in blood sugar by producing too much insulin. After you eat refined carbohydrates, your blood-sugar level will first rise steeply, then dip to an abnormally low level (see graph, facing page). This is likely to make you feel faint, irritable, headachy, and tired. Low blood sugar can raise the risk of developing a food sensitivity. To avoid unnecessary drops in your blood-sugar level:

■ Include high-fiber foods in your regular diet. You digest and absorb these more slowly than foods that

contain refined carbohydrates, and this helps keep your blood-sugar level within the optimum range.

- Opt especially for foods that are rich in soluble fiber, such as apples, oats, and legumes.
- Limit foods made with refined carbohydrates —those containing white flour or added sugar, for example.
- Limit your caffeine intake. Although caffeine can provide a temporary energy boost, it is generally followed by increased fatigue as a result of a drop in blood sugar.
- Limit your alcohol intake. Alcohol is a central nervous system depressant and also reduces the blood-sugar level.
- Check that you are eating enough chromium-rich foods. This mineral is necessary for good blood-sugar control. Such foods include liver, cheese, and whole grains.

Exercise: Physical activity is usually energizing because it dissipates the unhealthy bodily changes brought on by inactivity or by physical or mental stress. Over time, regular exercise speeds up body processes, increasing your energy level. Inactivity makes you more likely to gain weight, and carrying extra pounds is tiring. However, you should exercise only within the limits of your ability (see p. 13).

Stress management: Try to do the following every day:

- Find time to relax. Your body and brain can cope with only so much before demanding a rest. If you are constantly on the go, trying to fit as much as possible into your schedule, then

Managing low blood pressure

Low blood pressure may cause fatigue. If you have this disorder:

- Eat a healthy diet (see p. 9).
- Use more salt in your diet.
- Tone up your circulation with a daily cup of herbal tea or a dose of herbal tincture, made from a combination of ginger, angelica, hawthorn, and nettles.
- Add a few drops of ginger, marjoram, rosemary, or cinnamon oil to a bathtub of warm water.

overdoing it just a little more than usual may suddenly and unexpectedly lead to exhaustion.

- Vary your activities. Working long hours at a desk or on a production-line can deplete both physical and mental energy. If this is your problem, try to get a change of scene during the day, such as an occasional walk outside.

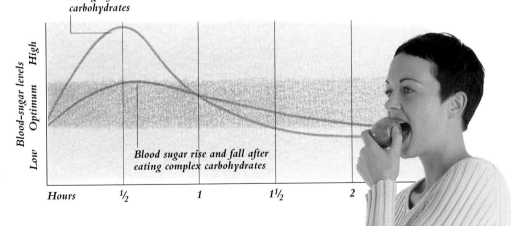

Blood sugar rise and fall after eating refined carbohydrates

Blood sugar rise and fall after eating complex carbohydrates

Blood-sugar levels — High / Optimum / Low

Hours — ½ 1 1½ 2

Blood-sugar levels after eating
The chart above compares the dramatic rise and fall in blood-sugar levels after eating refined carbohydrates with the gradual changes that occur after consuming complex carbohydrates, such as whole grains and most fruits and vegetables.

TREATMENT

Diet: When energy flags, eat a nutritious meal or a restorative snack to keep you going until your next good meal. Choose protein foods or complex carbohydrates (such as whole-grain crackers or an apple) rather than foods containing sugar and white flour, such as cookies or cake—which may give you a quick energy boost but will soon leave you feeling tired again. Cut out alcohol and caffeine completely.

Stress management: If you are weary because you are doing too much at work, at home, or in the community, decide whether the pressure comes from other people or from yourself. Then think of practical ways to reduce the load that is sapping your vitality.

Have a change of scenery, or do something interesting or recreational to counteract the fatigue that accompanies boredom or the "cabin fever" that often arises after being cooped up in the same place for too long.

Exercise: When your energy is low after a day in which you have had little physical activity, take a brisk walk, go for a swim, or try a workout at the gym.

Yoga and tai chi: These specialized forms of exercise are helpful in increasing energy, through deep breathing, stretching, and gentle, conscious movements. Yoga-based techniques for deep relaxation (see p. 69) can be especially reviving if practiced at the times when you feel most tired, such as when you get home from work in the evening.

Aromatherapy

■ Have a friend give you a massage with essential oils. Take a tablespoon of sweet-almond or grapeseed oil, and add four drops of lavender oil to relax you or four drops of lemon oil to invigorate you, according to your need.

■ Massage your face, feet, legs, abdomen, hands, or arms yourself, using three drops each of lavender and ylang ylang oils, plus two drops of Roman chamomile oil, in a tablespoon of grapeseed or sweet almond oil.

■ Add a few drops of rosemary oil—or a combination of clary sage, juniper berry, and lemongrass oils—to a vaporizer. The effect is calming, and thus may reduce the fatigue resulting from mental stress. Avoid these oils during pregnancy.

Herbal remedies

■ Ginseng is thought to be one of nature's greatest cures for people who are feeling run-down. Its adaptogenic properties mean that it can either stimulate or relax the central nervous system, depending on your needs. It also increases resistance to stress and acts as a general pick-me-up. Ginseng is available from health-food stores as tablets, a tincture, and in herbal tea mixtures.

■ When you feel exhausted and tense, a cup of herbal tea makes a soothing nightcap. Try catnip, chamomile, hops, lemon balm, and lime tree flower, all of which have sedative and relaxant properties that enable you to rest better and wake up invigorated. Experiment to find which herbs suit you best.

Energy-boosting vapors
Sprinkle a few drops of rosemary oil onto a tissue, and tuck it inside your clothing. The aroma released by your body heat will stimulate both body and mind.

■ Gotu kola, an herb with stimulant properties, can help relieve fatigue.
Caution: For safety concerns, see pp. 34–37.

Hydrotherapy
A warm bath can help with tiredness brought on by stress. A cold shower or swim can revitalize you if your sense of fatigue results from boredom or inactivity. Alternate hot and cold showers, or a sauna followed by a cold shower or dip, are especially invigorating.

Homeopathy: Tailor your choice of remedy to your specific symptoms and to the suspected cause of your fatigue.

■ Arnica: if your tiredness results from excessive physical exertion.
■ Arsenicum: if you are suffering from extreme anxiety and restlessness.
■ Kali phosphoricum: if you are suffering from mental strain.
■ Valerian: if you can't sleep because you can't stop thinking.

Flower essences: Use these remedies when emotional difficulties make life stressful and

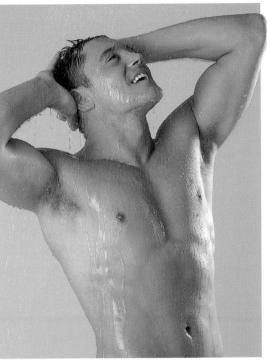

Reviving water
A cool shower may help release the physical and mental tension at the end of the day.

tiring. Choose from one or more of the following essences according to your need:

■ Olive: when you feel fatigued or tired.
■ Centaury: when you feel under pressure to do more than you can cope with.
■ Oak: when you keep going even though you feel you've reached the end of your strength.
■ Hornbeam: when you feel tired at the thought of the day ahead.

Counseling: Emotional problems—such as grief, suppressed anger, and frustration—can take the form of constant tiredness. You may be unable to deal with this kind of difficulty by yourself, because it is often hard to analyze a situation to which you have become accustomed and to work out strategies for improving it. Discuss your problem with a good friend, or seek professional counseling.

Other therapies: Acupuncture, reflexology, yoga, and craniosacral osteopathy are among the types of treatment that may help cases of persistent fatigue. You may also want to consult a practitioner of Chinese or Ayurvedic medicine.

When to get medical help

● Fatigue worsens, or it persists in spite of home treatment.
● You experience breathlessness, chest pain, severe headache, dizziness, visual changes, or abdominal pain.

See also:
ANEMIA, CHRONIC FATIGUE
SYNDROME, DEPRESSION,
JET LAG AND IN-FLIGHT HEALTH,
SLEEPING DIFFICULTIES, STRESS

Fertility Problems

Infertility affects millions of people and has many possible causes. One couple in five takes more than a year to conceive a child, and one in ten couples takes more than two years. One in six couples seeks medical help for infertility, but some of these might conceive without medical aid if they followed simple lifestyle changes and used natural treatments at home.

The three most common fertility problems are:
- Reduced sperm count, or sperm of abnormal structure or motility.
- Ovulation problems, which often result from polycystic ovary syndrome, a hormonal imbalance associated with cysts in the ovaries.
- Blocked fallopian tubes, sometimes resulting from pelvic inflammatory disease.

Other causes include uterine disorders, endometriosis, and cervical mucus that tends to block the entry of sperm. Smoking, drinking alcohol, and being exposed to pesticides or other poisons can also affect fertility, as can taking certain medications. For females, fertility declines with age; the older a woman is when trying to conceive, the more difficult success is likely to be.

PREVENTION

Some fertility problems can be prevented with self-help measures. Improving your general health boosts your chances of producing healthy eggs and sperm and conceiving when you want. It also gives your newly conceived baby the best prospect of developing normally.

Many apparently infertile couples actually conceive numerous times, but each time the fertilized egg or the embryo dies. This problem is often due to an actual miscarriage or the fact that the fertilized egg hasn't been successfully implanted in the uterus, not infertility.

PROMOTING CONCEPTION

Starting at least six months before you wish to conceive, take the following simple steps in order to give sperm, eggs, and unborn baby the best possible start. The advice below applies whether or not you and your partner have been experiencing difficulty with conception.

Diet: Some dietary deficiencies are associated with fertility problems, particularly a lack of folic acid, selenium, zinc, essential fatty acids, and vitamins C, E, and the B complex family. Eat a diet rich in these substances (see p. 12). Wash, scrub, or peel vegetables and fruits to remove traces of pesticides, or buy organic produce, if available.

Too much caffeine may reduce both male and female fertility. Limit your intake to a maximum of 300 milligrams a day—and be aware that some doctors recommend only 100 milligrams. One average cup of ordinary-strength brewed coffee contains about 100 milligrams of caffeine, a cup of instant coffee 60 milligrams, and a cup of tea or can of cola 40 milligrams. However, a recent study, though not conclusive, suggests that women who drink more than a half cup of black or green tea a day greatly increase their chances of becoming pregnant.

Nutritional supplements: Because it may be hard to obtain the amounts of nutrients you need

from food sources, supplements are often advised. Ask your doctor about those described below.

- Women should generally take extra folic acid (400 micrograms daily) from the time they start trying to conceive until the end of the 12th week of pregnancy, or, as some experts suggest, throughout pregnancy. If you have ever had (or miscarried) a baby with spina bifida or another neural tube defect, the dose should be increased to 4 milligrams daily.
- Iron may also be needed and is present in prenatal vitamin supplements.
- If you are a woman who eats poorly, is underweight, smokes, drinks alcohol, or has ever miscarried, take a multiple vitamin and mineral supplement formulated for women trying to conceive. Also check with your doctor to see if you need additional nutrients. Any multipurpose supplement is suitable for a man.
- For men, L-carnitine, an amino-acid-like chemical related to the B vitamins, can raise sperm count and improve sperm motility.
- The herbs ginseng and Siberian ginseng can be rotated every three months to aid sperm formation and sperm count; take 100–250 milligrams of ginseng or 100–300 milligrams of Siberian ginseng twice a day.

Body weight: Both men and women should ideally attain or maintain a healthy weight for their build and height (see p. 302). An overweight woman is less fertile, partly because of a higher risk of polycystic ovary syndrome, and also is at higher risk of miscarriage if overweight leads to diabetes. A seriously underweight woman is more likely to ovulate infrequently or to fail to ovulate at all. An overweight man is less likely to be fertile, since excess fat can interfere with sperm production.

Alcohol: Too much alcohol reduces fertility by damaging sperm and eggs. It also makes miscarriage more likely. Some experts recommend giving up alcohol completely. Others suggest having at most five units of alcohol a week (for example, five small glasses of wine), and to abstain the remaining two days. To avoid the risk of fetal alcohol syndrome, women trying to conceive should not drink at any time during their cycle when they might be pregnant.

Exercise: Both men and women should get a half hour of moderately strenuous exercise at least five days a week. Besides being generally beneficial, this boosts circulation to the reproductive organs. For women it is especially

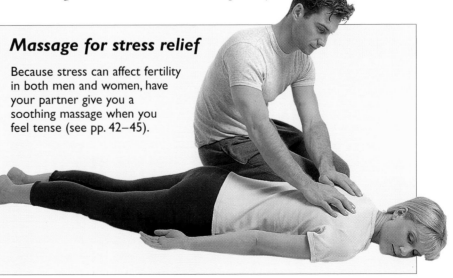

Massage for stress relief

Because stress can affect fertility in both men and women, have your partner give you a soothing massage when you feel tense (see pp. 42–45).

important to maintain a good blood supply to the ovaries: poor circulation can in some cases lead to reduced fertility. However, be aware that excessive exercise can reduce a woman's fertility.

Contraception: At least three months before you plan to conceive, stop taking oral contraceptive pills, or have your intrauterine device or hormone implants removed. Use a barrier method of contraception, such as a diaphragm, until you wish to conceive.

Ovulation and sex: Find out the time in the month when you normally ovulate by using an ovulation prediction kit or by taking your temperature each morning and noting the slight rise that accompanies ovulation. Then each month, during the week before you expect ovulation and for a day or two after your temperature rises, have sexual intercourse once a day, ideally just after waking in the morning. At other times, have sex whenever you wish.

Smoking: Smoking reduces fertility and increases the risk of miscarriage. Smoking during pregnancy can also affect the health of your baby. If you can't stop immediately, try cutting down, and seek help in quitting.

Stress management: Feeling stressed can suppress ovulation and reduce sperm count. Practice stress-management strategies and relaxation techniques (see p. 347). You may also want to try yoga or meditation.

Concerns at work: The workplace can be hazardous if you are hoping to conceive.
■ Check that your employer enforces any necessary safety precautions, for example, having to do with exposure to chemicals or radiation.
■ Sitting for very long periods (especially with your legs crossed) or being exposed to direct heat may overheat the testes, depressing sperm production. If low sperm production is a problem, consider whether your occupation—for

Advice for men

Men with fertility problems should:
● Avoid beer, since its natural estrogen content may lower sperm count.
● Reduce consumption of meat, dairy products, beans, and peas, which may also contain estrogens.
● Avoid hot tubs. Sperm production is more efficient when the testes remain cool.

Precautions for women

Tell your physician or pharmacist that you are trying to conceive before accepting any medications; some can damage a newly conceived baby. Before agreeing to an X ray, inform your physician, dentist, and X-ray technician that you are trying to become pregnant so that appropriate precautions can be taken, or so that the X ray can be rescheduled.

Drugs
Avoid all unnecessary drugs, including non-prescription medicines (except on medical advice) and so-called "recreational" drugs, such as marijuana.

Immunization
If possible, women should avoid immunization with live vaccines, such as those for measles, mumps, rubella, polio, and yellow

fever, during pregnancy and in the six months before conceiving. Tell your doctor if you become pregnant soon after such an immunization.

Herbal remedies, essential oils, and supplements
Always seek the advice of a qualified practitioner before using these remedies while trying to conceive or when pregnant.

example, bus driver or welder—may be the cause. If so, it may be worthwhile to change to another type of work, if possible, until your partner conceives.

- Some occupations are statistically linked to lowered female fertility. Examples include being a dental assistant, and jobs involving exposure to textile dust.

- Some office buildings have poor supplies of fresh air; elevated levels of extra-low-frequency electromagnetic radiation (from computers and other electrical equipment); and heightened concentrations of chemicals in the air, such as formaldehyde, which vaporize ("outgas") from synthetic wall and floor coverings. Such an environment could theoretically affect fertility. The same may also apply to some homes. If you live or work in such conditions, spend as much time outdoors as possible.

House and garden: Many household products contain chemicals that can inhibit fertility.

- Don't breathe organochlorine pesticide vapor —for example, from pet flea sprays—or touch any pesticide-containing product.

- Don't inhale smoke from burning plastic that contains polyvinyl chloride (PVC).

- Don't strip old paint that may contain lead.

- Don't inhale the vapor from solvents, glues, felt-tip markers, and paints.

Avoiding infection: Because the mother's state of health can affect a developing baby, it is important to try to avoid contracting infections of all kinds when trying to conceive and throughout pregnancy.

- Both partners should stay away from people who have colds, coughs, the flu, childhood infections, or other viral illnesses.

- At least six months before attempting to conceive, a woman should check her immunity to rubella and be immunized, if necessary.

- Consult your physician about precautions against toxoplasmosis, a protozoal infection that can damage a developing baby. If you own a cat, ask someone else to clean the litter box. If you must do it yourself, wear a mask and rubber gloves or look for a kitty-litter processing box. Wash your hands after handling raw meat and eat only well-done meat.

- Take measures to avoid infection with listeria, an organism that can harm a fetus and may cause miscarriage. Don't eat pâté; soft, mold-ripened cheeses, blue-veined cheese, and feta cheese; soft ice cream; unpasteurized milk; precooked poultry; prepackaged salads (unless washed again); and—unless thoroughly reheated—precooked, refrigerated foods.

When to get medical help

- You are a woman who has been trying unsuccessfully to conceive, using the above guidelines, for one year if under 35, or six months if over 35.

See also:
FIBROIDS, FOOD SENSITIVITY, OVERWEIGHT, PELVIC INFLAMMATORY DISEASE, STRESS

Fever

Having a fever—usually defined as a temperature of 99°F or above—is generally a sign that your body's immune system is doing its best to combat an infection. But if your temperature is so high that it makes you uncomfortable, you'll benefit from using some simple home remedies. You will also need to find out what is causing the rise in temperature.

Normal body temperature varies from person to person, ranging from 96.5°F to 99.5°F. Body temperature is affected by food, drink, exercise, sleep, time of day, and the menstrual cycle. A fever is an abnormally raised body temperature. It can be a sign of any of several common ailments, including influenza, tonsillitis, and the childhood infectious illnesses, such as chicken pox, as well as rarer infections, such as malaria and typhoid fever. Heatstroke caused by prolonged exposure to heat is another possible cause.

A rise in temperature may be heralded by bouts of shivering and by feeling alternately sweaty and chilled. Once a fever begins, it may also be accompanied by a headache and rapid breathing. In certain illnesses, such as malaria, the episodes of shivering are so severe that they are described as rigors. The feverish stage of an infection usually lasts no more than three days.

TREATMENT

If you feel unexpectedly cold and shivery, it is likely that you are developing a feverish illness. It is best to rest, but it is not necessary to go to bed unless you want to. A lukewarm bath may also make you feel better, but take care not to become chilled.

Reducing a fever: There is no need to take special action to bring down your temperature unless it is above 100°F or is hard to tolerate. However, if you do want to do this, turn room heat down or off, open windows and doors, if necessary, and turn on an electric fan or air conditioning (on low). Dress in light clothes, and if you feel too hot in bed, remove blankets or replace a duvet with a single blanket or sheet. Most people are more comfortable when lightly covered than with no bed covers at all. Clothes and bed covers made of natural fabrics allow sweat to evaporate more easily and aid cooling.

Compresses: You can use cold, wet compresses on your forehead, back of the neck, wrists, and calves. Keep the rest of your body covered.

Cooling by sponging
An adult with a high fever may benefit from sponging. Use lukewarm water to which you have added a few drops of lavender, Roman chamomile, or eucalyptus oil. Treat the skin a little at a time. If necessary, cover the parts of the body that aren't being sponged to avoid becoming too cold.

206

Change the compresses as they become warm. Continue until your temperature falls and you feel better.

Body wrap: A body wrap (see p. 50) is an effective means of bringing down a high temperature, but take care not to reduce the temperature too much. Wrap the feverish person firmly in a cold, wet sheet or several cold, wet towels, and then with a dry woollen blanket. Change this wrap every 15 to 20 minutes, until the person feels comfortably cool.

Replacing fluid: Consume enough liquids to enable you to pass plenty of pale urine. Choose water and drinks with a high vitamin C content, such as black currant, orange, or lemon juice.

Herbal remedies: Drink teas made from white willow bark, lime tree flower, lemon balm, elderflower, echinacea, ginger, or peppermint. Echinacea tincture may also be helpful.
Caution: For safety concerns, see pp. 34–37.

Homeopathy
For a high fever
- Aconite: if thirst and sweating are pronounced, perhaps due to a sudden chill.
- Belladonna: if you feel a dry, burning heat and you have a red face.

For a slowly developing low fever
- Bryonia: if you are noticeably irritable and experience intense thirst.
- Gelsemium: if fever is accompanied by marked shivering and shaking.
- Pulsatilla: if a child is clingy as well as feverish.

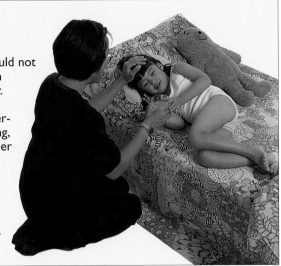

Fever reduction in children
A child with a fever should not be sponged or bathed in cool or lukewarm water. This may result in an excessive drop in temperature, leading to shivering, which may cause a further rise in temperature. If your child has a fever, remove all but a light layer of clothing and make sure the room is cool and well-ventilated. Offer plenty of fluids.

When to get medical help
- You have vomited, coughed up phlegm or blood, or passed blood during bowel movements.
- You have a condition, such as heart disease or diabetes, that requires medical monitoring.
- You have a temperature of 101°F or 102°F that has lasted more than 72 hours.

Get help right away if:
- You have a fever of 103°F or more.
- You also have a severe headache, a stiff neck, a rash, or a sensitivity to bright light.
- You also have severe abdominal pain or urinary problems.
- You experience confusion, unusual drowsiness, irritability, and/or labored breathing.
- A baby under three months has a temperature of 100°F or more.
- A baby three to six months has a fever of 101°F or more.
- A child older than six months has a fever of 103°F or more.

See also:
CHILDHOOD VIRAL INFECTIONS, COLDS, CONVULSIONS, COUGHS, INFLUENZA

Fibroids

A benign tumor of the uterus, a fibroid consists of muscle and fibrous tissue that grows slowly in the uterine wall. Fibroids may be as small as a pea or as big as a grapefruit. They may occur singly, or several may develop within the uterus. Fibroids pose few serious risks to health and usually produce no symptoms unless they are quite large.

One in four Western women has fibroids. They are most common in childless women over the age of 35 and before menopause. The specific cause of fibroids is unknown, but it is thought to be related to an abnormal response to the hormone estrogen. Estrogen stimulates fibroids to grow larger, so they may become more troublesome during pregnancy, when estrogen levels are higher than normal. Fat cells produce estrogen, which may account for fibroids being more likely in obese women. The association with estrogen also explains why fibroids shrink and disappear after menopause, when estrogen production falls, unless estrogen (hormone) replacement therapy is undergone. Surgery to remove fibroids is necessary only if the growths cause severe symptoms and other treatments fail.

PREVENTION

Keep your weight within recommended limits (see p. 302). Eat relatively little saturated fat and animal protein. Instead, emphasize vegetable protein and fiber. Such a diet may discourage fibroids by lowering your estrogen level.

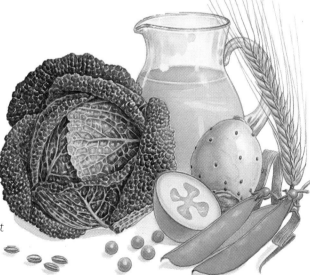

Anti-fibroid foods?
Some researchers believe that plant hormones help counteract the high estrogen level that encourages fibroids. They are present in beans, peas, seeds, whole grains, and most fruits and vegetables.

Do you have fibroids?

Fibroids may be discovered only when you have a physical examination, and if they produce no symptoms, they need no treatment.

If a fibroid grows, it may erode the uterine lining and cause prolonged or heavy menstrual periods or bleeding between periods. If you lose a lot of blood month after month, you may eventually become anemic and experience symptoms of that disorder, such as fatigue and shortness of breath.

Other possible symptoms include:
- Severe cramps and a dull ache or feeling of uncomfortable pressure in the lower back and thighs during menstruation.
- Constipation or a need to urinate more often than usual (a fibroid may be pressing on the intestines or bladder).
- Very light menstrual flow (a large fibroid near the cervix may be partially blocking it).
- Pain during sexual intercourse.

TREATMENT

Aromatherapy

- A gentle abdominal massage may soothe painful symptoms and reduce tension. Make a massage oil with four drops each of clary sage and lavender oils, and two of true melissa or rose otto oil, to one tablespoon of sweet almond or a cold-pressed vegetable oil.
- To ease abdominal pain or backache, add four drops each of clary sage and sweet marjoram oils and three of Roman chamomile oil to a bowl of hot water. Use this to make a warm compress (see p. 295) to hold against the painful area. Do not use clary sage oil in the first 20 weeks of pregnancy.

Exercise: If fibroids cause cramps or heavy bleeding during menstruation, you may not feel like being active. However, exercise at other times of the month stimulates uterine circulation and may therefore make pain from fibroids less likely.

Herbal remedies

- For fibroids with heavy periods, drink a cup of tea twice daily—or 15 drops of

Herbs for severe symptoms
When fibroids cause painful periods, a tea made of blue cohosh, black currant leaves, cramp bark, raspberry leaves, and wild yam may help.

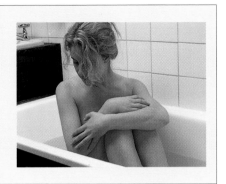

Improving circulation with hydrotherapy

Blood flow in the wall of the uterus may be sluggish if you have fibroids. Increase uterine circulation by sitting in cool water up to your hips for two or three minutes every morning. This may reduce the severity of your symptoms.

tincture in a little water—made from agrimony, beth root, chasteberry, and raspberry leaves. You can also add nettles, which are rich in vitamin C and iron, to soups, stews, and salads, and drink a cup of nettle tea twice daily.

- For fibroids with painful, heavy periods accompanied by blood clots, drink a cup of tea twice daily—or 15 drops of tincture in a little water—made from the herbs shown at left.

Caution: For safety concerns, see pp. 34–37.

When to get medical help

- You feel excessively tired or weak.
- You have irregular or problematic periods.
- You're due for your gynecological checkup—to ensure that any growth is not cancerous.

Get help right away if:
- You have any unaccustomed severe pain.

See also:
ABDOMINAL PAIN, ANEMIA, MENSTRUAL PROBLEMS

209

Flatulence

*H*aving excessive gas in the digestive tract can be annoying as well as embarrassing. Many people are able to overcome or at least reduce the problem by avoiding gas-producing foods and improving their eating habits. Flatulence may be accompanied by indigestion or constipation. It can be a sign of underlying disease, but this is rare.

Flatulence is often accompanied by a bloated sensation. This discomfort is generally relieved when the gas is expelled, either via the mouth—belching—or the anus. Belching is more likely when you're standing or sitting, and expelling gas from the anus is more likely when you're lying down. Excessive gas production may lead to obvious distension of the abdomen.

Flatulence occasionally results from gastritis (an inflamed stomach lining), irritable bowel syndrome, gallbladder disease, or a peptic ulcer. It can also occur as a result of long-term stress.

PREVENTION

Adjusting your diet usually eases the problem. Flatulence results from the action of bacteria or fungi in your intestines causing certain digested foods to ferment and produce gas. Common culprits include cabbage, onions, peas, and beans. You may find that fatty foods, carbonated drinks, sugar, drinks containing caffeine, or uncooked vegetables and fruits make the problem worse. Flatulence can also result from sensitivity to a particular food or foods, or from combinations of certain foods, notably starch with protein or fruit. Examples are dough with fruit (as in apple pie), and bread with meat (as in a ham sandwich).

Eating habits: It isn't just *what* we eat but *how* we eat that can cause flatulence. Some of us, without realizing it, swallow air along with our food, especially when we are nervous or under stress. This causes gas to accumulate in the stomach and intestines. The same thing can happen if you overeat, eat too fast, don't chew well, or talk

Massage with essential oils

Give yourself a light abdominal massage with a mixture of four drops of peppermint oil and two drops each of juniper berry and caraway oils (omit these oils if you are pregnant) in two and a half teaspoons of sweet almond oil. Massage with sweeping clockwise movements.

The effect of antibiotics

You may develop flatulence as a result of taking antibiotics, which temporarily alter or destroy the normal balance of microorganisms in the intestines. This population of microorganisms, known as the intestinal flora, is essential for healthy digestion. To help restore a healthy balance of intestinal flora, take a supplement of *Lactobacillus acidophilus* or eat yogurt that contains live acidophilus cultures at least once a day.

or drink while eating. The best way to avoid these hazards is to eat slowly and to chew food thoroughly. Try not to leave too much time between meals. Do not eat on the run or at erratic hours, and avoid having a late evening meal.

TREATMENT

Herbal remedies: Chamomile, fennel, lemon balm, wild yam, ginger, or angelica root can ease flatulence. Take the herb in a tea or diluted tincture after meals. For angelica root tea, pour one pint of boiling water over one ounce of chopped root, steep for 10 minutes, and take two teaspoons three times a day before meals.
Caution: For safety concerns, see pp. 34–37.

From the drugstore or health-food store

■ Take charcoal tablets according to the instructions on the label.
■ Take an acidophilus supplement each day for

two to four weeks. Choose a dairy-free product that contains more than one billion organisms in each dose.

Gas-reducing juices: Pineapple juice contains the enzyme bromelain, and papaya juice contains the enzyme papain. Both aid digestion. Juice half a papaya or a third of a pineapple and add an equal amount of uncarbonated water. Drink three times a day for up to three days. Some people find that sauerkraut juice also helps.

Hot and cold compresses: Direct heat sometimes soothes a gassy stomach and relieves distension. Place a covered hot-water bottle on your abdomen and leave for as long as it feels comfortable or until it starts to cool. Or try hot and cold compresses one after the other: put a hot towel (dipped in hot water and wrung out) over your abdomen for three minutes, then a cold towel (dipped in cold water and wrung out) for one minute, and repeat several times.

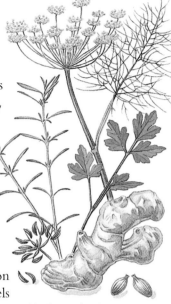

Herbs and spices
Adding herbs and spices to your food can help reduce flatulence by inhibiting the growth of gas-forming bacteria. Try some of the following: parsley, dill, fennel, cayenne, ginger, and cardamom and caraway seeds. Add winter or summer savory when you cook beans to reduce their gas-forming effect.

Acupressure for flatulence

Thumb pressure on the point (St 4) on the inside arch of the foot just behind the ball of the foot can regulate digestion. Sitting comfortably, press this point for 5 to 10 seconds once or twice a day.

When to get medical help

● Flatulence does not respond to natural remedies within seven days, or sooner if it is accompanied by abdominal pain, fever, vomiting, or severe nausea or diarrhea.

See also:
ABDOMINAL PAIN, BLOATING,
CONSTIPATION, INDIGESTION,
IRRITABLE BOWEL SYNDROME

211

Food Sensitivity

An allergic response or an intolerance to a food or food ingredient comes under the general category of food sensitivity. Such reactions cause a variety of unpleasant symptoms, including digestive upsets, headaches, and bloating. In most cases recognizing and avoiding—or at least cutting down on—the offending food is the only effective treatment.

The two basic types of food sensitivity are allergies, which result from immune-system activation, and intolerances. If you have an allergic reaction, your immune system responds to certain foods (allergens, or "culprit" foods) just as to any other invader (see box below). As many as 6 percent of American infants have a food allergy, but only 1.5 percent of adults are affected.

A food sensitivity that does not consist of an immune-system response is termed a food intolerance. It may result from being unable to digest certain foods properly because a necessary enzyme is lacking. Examples include celiac disease, which involves gluten intolerance, and lactose intolerance (inability to digest sugars in cow's milk). Some people react to monosodium glutamate, or MSG, with faintness, flushing, headache, and abdominal pain (known as Chinese restaurant syndrome). Certain artificial food colorings (especially the orange and yellow food colorings) can trigger eczema or asthma, and caffeine can lead to insomnia and shaking. Some individuals develop abdominal pain after eating fruits and other carbohydrates. The stomach is slow in emptying such foods, and they then produce gas from bacterial fermentation, which distends the stomach and intestines.

It is thought that damage to the intestinal lining—for example, by irritation from certain foods, infection, or antibiotics—can cause a "leaky gut" and allow traces of undigested foods to enter the blood, triggering a food allergy in susceptible people.

Symptoms

Immediate-onset allergy: In this form of allergic response, symptoms appear within one to two hours of eating even a small amount of the culprit food. The immune system produces inflammatory substances and a type of antibody known as IgE. Blood tests and skin tests for IgE are most likely to identify immediate-onset allergy. Symptoms may include:

- Hives
- Allergic rhinitis (hay fever)
- Asthma
- Swelling of the lips, mouth, and the lining of the respiratory tract

The allergic response

When you have a food allergy, the immune system reacts by releasing antibodies, which attack the culprit food, from white cells. Their attack releases other substances from white cells, such as histamine and leukotrienes, that cause inflammation. This inflammation results in the production of reactive oxygen particles (free radicals), which can damage the body.

The immune system may also manufacture antibodies. These "mop up" the food in the intestines, blood, or elsewhere in the body, creating tiny particles called immune complexes. These can also lead to harmful physical effects.

Delayed-onset allergy: Symptoms appear up to 72 hours after eating the culprit food. They're usually provoked by eating a large amount of it or having it frequently. The immune system produces IgG (and, perhaps, IgE) antibodies and in some cases inflammatory substances as well. Identifying the culprit can be difficult because symptoms tend to be vague, take time to appear, and often result from foods that are common in the diet (see "Common Culprits," p. 214). You may be more susceptible to this form of reaction

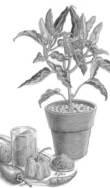

Hot tip
If you have allergy symptoms, experiment by avoiding paprika, cayenne pepper, and chili pepper. Evidence suggests that these spices irritate the intestines, encouraging food sensitivity.

A healthy start
Reduce your baby's risk of developing food sensitivities later in life by selecting first foods with care. Fruit and vegetable purées are the best starter foods.

Anaphylactic shock
This is a potentially fatal allergic reaction that includes breathing difficulty, a rapid fall in blood pressure, and, in some cases, loss of consciousness. If you experience shortness of breath or feelings of faintness after eating a suspected food allergen, seek urgent treatment. An epinephrine injection could save your life.

when physically or mentally stressed, and you may crave the very food that makes you ill. In addition to the symptoms listed for immediate-onset allergy, possible symptoms include:

- Flushing
- Fatigue
- Muscle weakness, aching, and stiffness
- Eczema
- Nausea and vomiting
- Diarrhea
- Abdominal pain
- Joint pain
- Palpitations
- Bloating
- Weight fluctuation

PREVENTION
- Help prevent damage from allergic reactions by eating a healthy diet that includes foods containing flavonoids, copper, iron, magnesium, selenium, zinc, essential fatty acids, and vitamins A, B (especially B_6), C, and E (see p. 12).
- If you are sensitive to wheat, don't use cookies and cakes as "comfort foods" unless you know that they are wheat-free.
- If you have an attack of gastroenteritis, you may

suffer from temporary food intolerance to gluten or sugar, so take care as you recover to reintroduce only gradually foods containing wheat, barley, oats, rye, or added sugar into your diet.

■ To reduce your baby's risk of an allergy or other food sensitivity developing in later life, breast-feed for at least a year, and wait until the infant is four to six months old before introducing any other foods.

■ Withhold those foods most frequently implicated in allergies (see illustration below) until a baby is at least six months old—longer if there is eczema or asthma in the family.

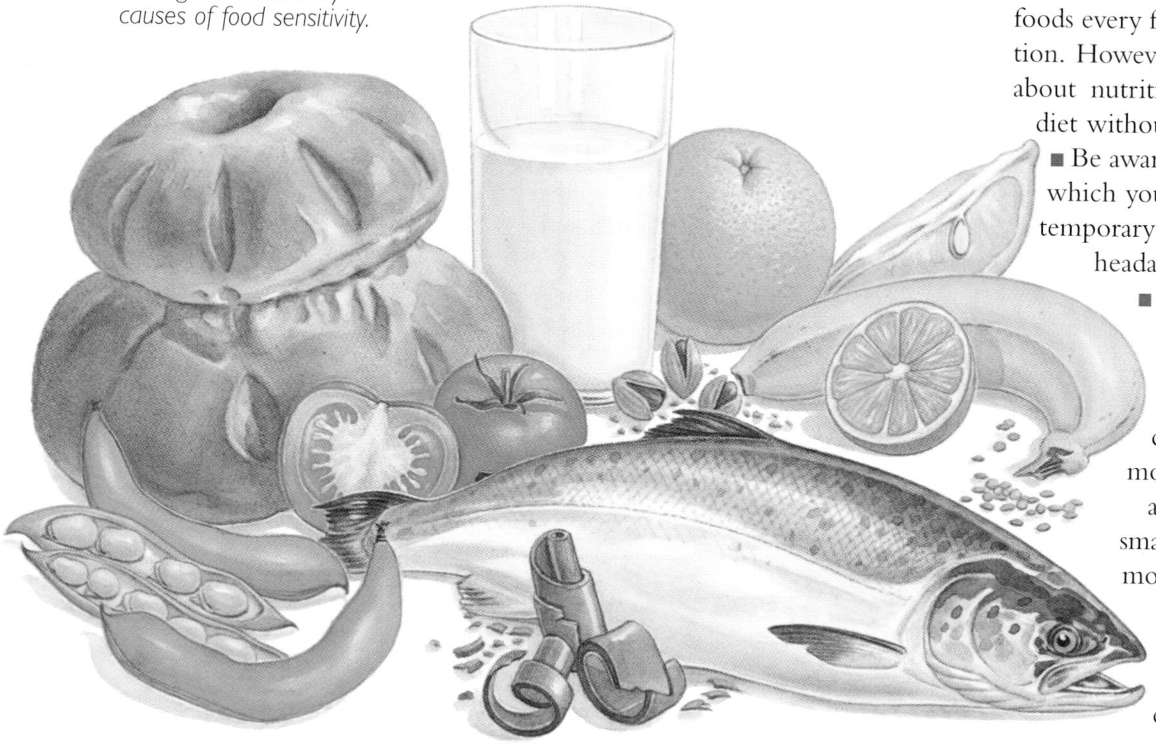

Common culprits
Wheat, milk, soy, bananas, eggs, fish, shellfish, nuts, seeds, beans, peas, lentils, tomatoes, citrus fruit, yeast, chocolate, and food additives are among the most likely causes of food sensitivity.

TREATMENT

Diet: Try to identify your culprit foods. People with an immediate-onset allergy generally react to one or two foods, while those with a delayed-onset sensitivity may react to up to 15.

■ Keep a food diary for three months, recording everything you eat and any symptoms. This may allow you to identify an obvious relationship between a food and an adverse reaction.

■ If you suspect a certain food, don't eat it for three weeks, then reintroduce it to see if it causes problems.

■ If this single-food elimination doesn't work, exclude all the most likely culprits for three weeks. Then try a small amount of one of these foods every four days to see if it triggers a reaction. However, if you are not knowledgeable about nutrition, don't attempt this exclusion diet without medical supervision.

■ Be aware that when you give up a food to which you are allergic, you may experience temporary withdrawal symptoms, such as headaches, fatigue, and irritability.

■ Once you identify your culprit foods, you can omit them from your diet altogether, in which case all your symptoms should disappear within three to six months. Or, if you are not severely allergic, see whether you can eat a small amount once every four days or more without trouble. You may need to exclude the culprit foods completely for six months before you gradually reintroduce them in this way.

214

Supplements

■ If you have digestive problems, take *Lactobacillus acidophilus* tablets (as directed on the package), along with vitamins A, C, and E, as well as flavonoids and zinc, to help heal the lining of the intestines.

■ If your food sensitivity results from a lack of a specific digestive enzyme, try taking a supplement of that enzyme.

Herbal remedies: Herbs cannot cure an allergy, but some may help soothe symptoms while you are searching for culprit foods. They may also aid in healing after withdrawing the problem food from your diet.

■ Drink a cup of an herbal tea or a few drops of a tincture made from echinacea, licorice, and red clover three times daily.

■ Drink a cup of yarrow or chamomile tea every four hours—or combine both herbs in a tea. Yarrow and chamomile contain substances that act as natural antihistamines and therefore counter food allergies.

Caution: For safety concerns, see pp. 34–37.

Anti-allergy salad

Nettles are especially rich in vitamins A and C and iron and other minerals, and their astringent properties can reduce the inflammation associated with allergy. Add nettle leaves to salads, stews, and soups. Or drink a cup of nettle tea twice a day or half a teaspoon of tincture daily.

When to get medical help

● You are uncertain about the cause of your symptoms.
● You suspect lactose intolerance or celiac disease.
● Symptoms from a suspected food allergy do not improve after self-help measures.

Get help right away if:
● You suffer a severe allergic reaction, such as a rash, shortness of breath, fainting, or swelling of the mouth, tongue, or throat.

See also:
ABDOMINAL PAIN, ALLERGIC RHINITIS, ARTHRITIS, ASTHMA, BLOATING, CONVULSIONS, DEPRESSION, DERMATITIS, DIABETES, DIARRHEA, FATIGUE, HEADACHE, HIGH BLOOD PRESSURE, INDIGESTION, IRRITABLE BOWEL SYNDROME, ITCHING, MIGRAINE, NAUSEA AND VOMITING, OVERWEIGHT, STRESS

Foot Problems

*C*orns, calluses, bunions, and ingrown toenails are not only unsightly and uncomfortable, but they also make it difficult to buy shoes that fit. These problems are preventable, and many natural home remedies can ease them. By caring for your hard-working feet, you make sure that walking and other forms of exercise remain pain-free and pleasurable.

Prolonged friction or pressure from ill-fitting shoes is the main cause of most foot problems. The following descriptions are of the most common foot conditions:

- Corns are raised areas of thickened skin, usually on the toes. Each corn has a hard center formed from a cone of tightly packed dead skin that points downward into the underlying tissue. If you press a corn, this hard point puts pressure on the nerve endings beneath the skin, causing pain. Corns between the toes are usually softened by sweat, and corns on the soles are generally very small—the size of a grain of rice. People with high arches are most likely to be affected, because when they walk, they put greater pressure on the toes, increasing the risk of rubbing against the shoes.

- Calluses are raised patches of thickened skin on the sole. Unlike a corn, a callus is insensitive. Calluses may be caused by any disorder of the foot or leg that prevents the sole from accepting the body's weight evenly. (Calluses can also occur on the hands, as a result of excessive pressure or friction.)

- A bunion is a fluid-filled pad (bursa) on the side of the big toe, overlying the joint between the toe and the foot. It may become red and tender. The natural shape of the big toe joint in some people makes it more likely to be damaged by shoes that compress the toes or don't match the shape of the feet.

- An ingrown toenail develops if pressure on the nail—usually that of the big toe—forces its growing edges into the adjacent skin, leading to pain, inflammation, and sometimes infection. The condition is most likely to occur if the nails are cut incorrectly or if the skin is continually damp from sweating—for example, because of shoes or socks made from synthetic materials that do not allow moisture to escape or that are too tight.

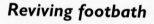

Reviving footbath

A regular herbal footbath not only helps keep your feet clean and fresh, but also improves circulation. Add a tablespoon of dried rosemary leaves (for their antiseptic and stimulating properties) to some hot water in a large basin—big enough to allow you to immerse your feet—and let stand for five minutes. Fill another basin with cold water, and place both basins on the floor by a chair. Sit with your feet in the hot, herb-scented water for one minute, then put them into the cold water for about 20 seconds. Repeat several times, ending with a brief plunge of the feet into the cold water. Pat your feet dry.

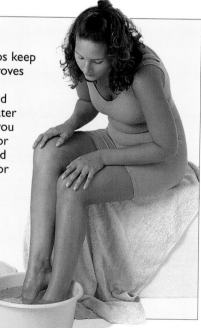

PREVENTION

Go barefoot as often as you can. In cultures in which this is the custom, there are few deformed feet and no corns or bunions. Wear shoes made from materials that allow the feet to "breathe," such as leather, canvas, or certain synthetic products. Make sure the shoes fit well, with space for the toes to move but without so much room that the feet slip. The heel should be well supported. Socks should not be too tight.

Wearing properly fitting shoes is crucial during infancy and childhood, when growing feet are so flexible that they feel no pain if shoes don't fit correctly. The wrong shoes can, over the years, lead to foot problems and even deformity. Babies don't need anything on their feet until they begin to walk outdoors. Children's feet should be measured for length and width by a trained fitter. They should be remeasured and shoes replaced (if necessary) every three months in the first seven or eight years, then less often as foot growth slows.

Make certain that you cut your toenails correctly (see illustration, left). Before cutting, let your nails grow long enough to allow their edges to clear the skin. Avoid digging into the sides of the nail to clear away dead skin and other debris.

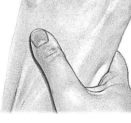

Pedicure pointers
Prevent ingrown toenails by cutting the nails straight across. Do not cut into the corners, but be sure to remove any protruding spikes at the nail edges.

TREATMENT
General measures

■ Remove any source of pressure or friction on your feet and toes by buying better-fitting footwear. Avoid high-heeled shoes. If necessary, stretch tighter-fitting leather shoes. Ask your shoe-repair store to do this, or buy shoe-stretching liquid or an expandable wooden shoe-stretcher from a shoe-repair store. Consider wearing shoes that are designed for walking or running; these tend to give more support.

■ Prevent fungal infection by keeping your feet clean and dry.

■ For an ingrown toenail, make a small, V-shaped cut in the center of the nail to ease the pressure at the sides.

➢ continued, p. 219

Aromatherapy foot massage

Self-massage with aromatherapy oil is relaxing, reduces a tendency toward excessive sweating, and suppresses the bacteria that act on sweat and cause foot odor. Add three drops of lemon, tea tree, peppermint, or rosemary oil to two teaspoons of soya or sweet almond oil, and rub the mixture into your feet. (Avoid rosemary oil during the first 20 weeks of pregnancy.) Use slow, smoothing strokes and/or firm kneading, depending on what feels most comfortable to you.

Foot massage

A massage brings relief for tired and aching feet. You can massage your feet yourself (see p. 217), or have a friend or partner do it for you while you lie on your stomach, with one lower leg lifted from the knee. Do not massage the foot if the joints are swollen or inflamed, and stop any massage that causes pain or discomfort.

1 Holding the toes and ankle, slowly rotate the whole foot first one way, then the other.

2 Press down on the heel with one hand, and with the other push the front of the foot back for about 15 seconds.

3 Hold either side of the Achilles tendon (just above the heel), then with the other hand press downward on the ball of the foot, while pushing the heel upward.

4 Holding each side, push the foot toward one side, then the other, several times.

5 Roll the ball of the foot firmly between the heels of your hands, working across the foot, below the toes.

6 Stretch each toe in turn by grasping the two adjacent toes and pulling them slowly apart, stretching the skin between them.

7 Rotate and pull each toe by holding the foot in one hand, grasping each toe in turn between your thumb and forefinger, and gently rotating it several times, then pulling it gently for a few seconds.

8 Stretch all the toes at once by grasping the four small toes with one hand and holding the big toe in the other, then lifting the leg up and shaking it slightly. Perform this sequence on both feet.

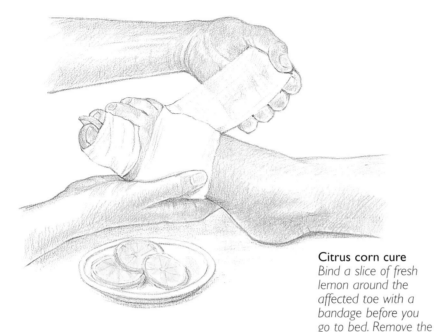

Citrus corn cure
Bind a slice of fresh lemon around the affected toe with a bandage before you go to bed. Remove the next morning, and repeat each night for a week or two.

From the drugstore

- For corns or bunions, apply felt or sponge corn pads or rings to ease pressure and pain.
- For a callus, soften by soaking in water or with a product containing salicylic acid. Then use a pumice stone or callus file to remove the thickened skin. Repeat once or twice a week.
- Castor oil also softens corns and calluses, as does pure lanolin (do not use if you're allergic to wool).
- For smelly feet, try bathing them daily in a solution of Kosher salt and water.

Kitchen cabinet remedy: For an ingrown toenail, soak your foot in a basin of warm water to which you have added about three tablespoons of salt. Do this for five minutes twice a day. Cut the nail only when inflammation has subsided.

Aromatherapy

- Rub a corn with a few drops of lemon oil, then cover in plastic wrap for 20 minutes. Repeat this procedure daily for a week or two.
- For an ingrown toenail, soak the affected foot for five minutes twice a day in a basin of warm water to which you have added six drops of tea tree oil. This will help prevent infection.

Herbal remedies

- For an ingrown toenail, soak your foot in two pints of warm water containing two teaspoons of marigold (calendula) tincture. Because marigold has antiseptic properties, this solution will also help cleanse and soften the nail. Or, instead of marigold, add a tablespoon of witch hazel extract to the water.
- Thuja may help clear corns or verrucas. Apply thuja ointment to the sore area, and cover with an adhesive bandage overnight.

When to get medical help

- You have pain, a sore, or swelling that persists longer than seven days.
- You have a fluid- or pus-filled swelling.
- No shoes are comfortable.
- Calluses remain painful.
- You experience numbness or tingling.
- An ingrown nail remains embedded.

See also:
COLD HANDS AND FEET,
FUNGAL SKIN INFECTIONS,
STRAINS AND SPRAINS,
WARTS

Fungal Skin Infections

*A*thlete's foot (Tinea pedis) *and ringworm of the body* (Tinea corporis) *are examples of skin conditions caused by a group of funguslike organisms. Tinea infections are highly contagious and can be acquired from people, animals, soil, wet places (such as showers and swimming pools), and household objects. They don't usually clear up without treatment.*

Clean and dry
Wash your feet regularly, and be sure to dry especially carefully between your toes.

Certain types of tinea, the fungus responsible for athlete's foot and ringworm of the body or scalp, thrive in warm, moist areas, such as the skin between the toes, beneath the breasts, and in the groin area (*Tinea cruris* or "jock itch"). Symptoms include a red, itchy rash. The affected skin then peels and may become very sore. The fungal spores are spread through contact with infected animals and humans.

Ringworm is associated with circular patches of white, itchy skin with a well-defined red margin—hence its name. (Contrary to popular belief, it is not caused by worms.) It most often affects the trunk and scalp. Ringworm of the scalp (*Tinea capitis*) occurs mainly in children and causes round, itchy, bald patches. *Candida albicans*, a yeastlike fungus, can also affect the skin and is associated with the flaking of the scalp known as dandruff.

PREVENTION

Fungal infections thrive in warm, moist conditions, so dry your skin properly after washing, especially in hot weather. To prevent athlete's foot or ringworm from spreading, have family members use individual, frequently laundered towels and washcloths, and make sure that those with an infection wash their hands after touching affected areas.

For athlete's foot

- Change your shoes and socks daily. Give your footwear time to air out thoroughly between each wearing.
- Use foot powder to help keep sweaty feet dry.
- Wear socks made of natural fibers that absorb moisture or those designed to draw moisture away from the foot. Allow your feet to "breathe" by choosing shoes made of leather or another natural material, or with ventilation holes if the materials are synthetic.
- Always wear footwear around swimming pools, in public changing rooms, or in any other place where people who might have athlete's foot walk barefoot.

For ringworm: Vacuum carpets and upholstery frequently if you have pets to minimize the risk of catching an infection from infected animals.

TREATMENT
Aromatherapy

- For athlete's foot: In the evening, before you go to bed, soak your feet for 10 minutes in a bowl of warm water containing two drops each of marigold (calendula), lavender, and tea tree

oils. Alternatively, apply a warm compress soaked in this mixture to each foot. Cover with plastic wrap and wear socks to keep the compresses in place overnight. In the morning, mix the same oils with half a teaspoon of marigold oil and apply between your toes.

■ For athlete's foot or ringworm: Dilute three drops of eucalyptus oil in two teaspoons of jojoba oil and apply to the affected skin.

Herbal remedies

■ Apply burdock tea or diluted marigold (calendula) or chamomile tincture to the affected areas twice a day.

■ Apply diluted tincture of myrrh (avoid if you are pregnant), oregano, or echinacea three times a day.

■ Drink a cup of tea made with a mixture of echinacea, nettles, dandelion root, burdock, and peppermint once or twice a day. This boosts immunity and helps counter infection.

Kitchen cabinet remedies

■ Soak a piece of cotton in honey and secure with a bandage to the sore area. Leave on overnight. This soothes the skin and speeds the healing process.

■ Use apple-cider vinegar in the same way. (It stings when first applied.)

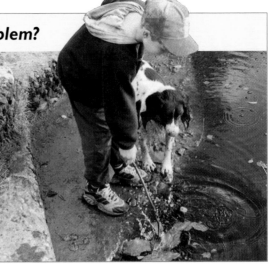

Is your pet a problem?

Take a pet that is scratching a lot to the veterinarian to determine whether it has developed a fungal infection. Also have any animals examined if a family member develops ringworm. A pet may have passed along the condition and may itself need to be treated.

Healing herbs
Marigold and chamomile tinctures and creams can help eliminate ringworm and athlete's foot.

■ Rub crushed garlic over the sore area each day to help combat the infection.

Homeopathy

■ Sulfur: for an infected scalp, every four hours for up to 10 doses, followed by Sepia if there is no improvement.

■ Tellurium: for ringworm on the torso, every four hours for up to 10 doses.

When to get medical help

● You have extreme redness, swelling, or pain.
● The condition persists despite treatment.

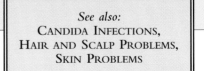

See also:
CANDIDA INFECTIONS,
HAIR AND SCALP PROBLEMS,
SKIN PROBLEMS

Gallbladder Problems

The principal disorder of the gallbladder is gallstones. In many cases, these solid lumps of matter are so small that they can pass out of the body unnoticed, but in others, they measure up to an inch in diameter. Some 10 percent of the U.S. population (at least two-thirds of them female) has gallstones, but only one sufferer in five experiences symptoms.

Bile, a digestive juice produced by the liver, is concentrated and stored in the gallbladder. Consuming fats stimulates the gallbladder to squirt bile into the duodenum, part of the small intestine, where the bile helps break down fats so that they can be digested. Eating extremely bland or infrequent meals provides little stimulation, and stagnant bile may then encourage the formation of stones. However, too much fat in the diet may also be a cause of gallstones. Most stones contain cholesterol, as well as bile pigments, bile salts, and minerals, such as calcium.

Digestive helpers
Bitter foods—such as watercress, chicory, endive, and artichokes—and bitter herbs and spices, such as rosemary and turmeric, may contribute to healthy gallbladder activity.

Contraceptive pills and hormone replacement therapy increase the risk of stones, as do certain cholesterol-lowering drugs. People who are overweight or suffer from constipation or food sensitivity (to eggs, pork, onions, chicken, milk, or coffee) are more likely to get gallstones. The problem may also be associated with a tendency to other digestive problems: One in two people with gallstones makes too little stomach acid, which can cause indigestion. Flatulence may accompany gallstones as well.

Occasionally, the gallbladder squirts out a stone along with some bile, and a big or rough one may become lodged in the bile duct—causing biliary colic (pain in the abdomen or back), nausea, vomiting, and fever. This requires prompt medical treatment. The lining of the gallbladder may become inflamed because of a stone or an infection. This condition, called cholecystitis, usually requires antibiotics.

PREVENTION

- Limit your intake of foods containing animal fats (whole milk, cheese, egg yolks, butter, fatty red meat, cookies, cakes).
- Cut down on animal protein and added sugar.
- Eat plenty of vegetables, fruits (including grapefruit, grapes, and pears), and other foods rich in vitamins C and E, and foods, such as nuts, containing essential fatty acids.

- Choose brown rice and whole-grain cereals.
- Eat regular meals, especially breakfast.
- Have bitter drinks, such as tonic water, to promote sound digestive action.
- Every day, drink the juice of half a lemon in a glass of hot water approximately an hour before you eat breakfast.
- Don't drink coffee.

TREATMENT
Kitchen cabinet remedies
- To lessen the risk of over-concentrated bile, drink at least six glasses of water a day.
- To stimulate bile flow, which may help flush out small gallstones, take one tablespoon of cold-pressed olive oil and one of lemon juice daily.

Herbal remedies: Dandelion and other bitter herbs may aid bile flow.
- Make tea from dandelion root, wild yam, fumitory, lemon balm, and licorice. Drink a cup every hour until the pain eases.
- As an alternative, drink chamomile or peppermint tea.
- If fatty meals cause pain, make tea from dandelion root, agrimony, yarrow, fumitory, peppermint, and wild yam, and drink a cup three times daily.

Caution: For safety concerns, see pp. 34–37.

Supplements
- If you have indigestion and medical tests reveal a stomach acid deficiency, take a

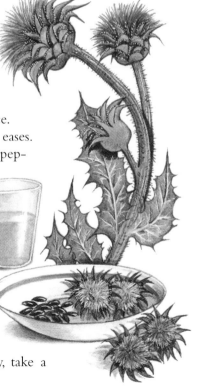

A bile stimulant
Have tea made from the seeds of milk thistle three times a day. This encourages the flow of bile and also helps protect the liver from damaging substances.

Soothing warmth
Ease the discomfort of biliary colic by holding a covered hot-water bottle over the area.

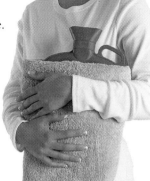

daily supplement of betaine hydrochloride.
- To help emulsify fats, sprinkle a tablespoon of lecithin granules on your food daily.
- Take a supplement of vitamin C (1,000–2,000 milligrams) daily.

Homeopathy
- Chelidonium: take daily as a general support remedy for gallbladder problems.
- Colocynthis: to help with the pain of biliary colic that is better from doubling up.

When to get medical help
- Your skin or eyes turn yellow.

Get help right away if:
- You experience severe pain, especially in the right upper part of the abdomen, or pain accompanied by nausea, vomiting, or fever.

See also:
ABDOMINAL PAIN, FOOD
SENSITIVITY, INDIGESTION,
OVERWEIGHT

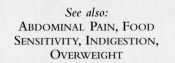

Grief

The painful emotional response to the death of a loved one, grief is an unavoidable part of life. A similar sense of loss may follow other traumatic life events, such as divorce, miscarriage, or loss of a job or home. People express grief in different ways, but recognizable stages of bereavement are common to all. Gentle natural therapies can provide support and comfort at such times.

Feelings of grief vary in intensity according to the depth of the loss and the pre-existing state of mind of the bereaved. It's difficult to know what to say to a grieving person, but most bereaved people find support in the mere presence and listening ear of a friend or relative.

PREVENTION

There is no way of preventing grief, but it is possible to lessen its more distressing effects. For example, we can all try to improve poor relationships with family members and friends while they are still alive. This can prevent the bitter and protracted pain stemming from sorrow, anger, or frustration over "unfinished business."

TREATMENT

Take care of yourself during this emotionally fragile and challenging time. Although the future may seem bleak, hold on to the hope that things will one day get better.

Diet and supplements: If you find eating difficult, arrange for company during at least one meal every day, and take a multiple vitamin and mineral supplement.

Herbal remedies: A daily dose of St. John's wort can relieve depression. For anxiety, try kava, valerian, passionflower, or chamomile.
Caution: For safety concerns, see pp. 34–37.

Stages of mourning

Many people experience four distinct stages of grief, which may occur one after the other or may overlap.

1 Feelings of numbness usually characterize the first stage of grieving, when the death or loss seems unreal. There may also be an unconscious denial of the event. This stage may last a few days or a few months.

2 Once the numbness wears off, you may experience an overwhelming maelstrom of emotions, as you confront the reality of the loss.

3 These turbulent feelings may eventually give way to prolonged depression, perhaps with physical symptoms, such as sleeping difficulties, headaches, and disturbed appetite.

4 Slowly and unpredictably, occasional and then more frequent glimpses of your old self will return, as you come to terms with your loss and begin to think positively about the future. Even years later, however, you may feel distress when, for example, the anniversary of the death triggers memories that make it seem as though the loss were a recent event.

Left column (partially cut off)

Tips

- Choc
  Cons
  and p
  perm
- Avoic
  curlir
  air to
  hair (
  use t
  prod
- Bleac
  hair a
  instru
  profe
  condi
  to co
  henna
  stren

essentia
or swee
- Dry, fla
  three o
  with fi
  oil, or a
- Oily, s
  cedarwe
  you're
  five tea

Massage
sage relie
improves
the scalp
the hair a

---

ble
hyc
wit
wit

He
her
the:
- M
  b
  fc
- C
Cau

Arc
gen

Homeopathy

- Aconite: for severe shock after a sudden death.
- Ignatia: for prolonged mourning, when there are excessive tears or hysteria, or when you can't cry at all.

Exercise: Exercise raises the levels of natural "feel-good" chemicals called endorphins. Walking, perhaps in the company of a sympathetic friend, is a good way of keeping active and getting some exposure to sunlight, which has a beneficial effect on mood.

Flower essences

- Honeysuckle: when you continually dwell on the past.
- Star of Bethlehem: for the sense of loss and for shock.
- Sweet Chestnut: for anguish and despair.
- Walnut: to help you adjust.
- Willow: for bitterness and self-pity.

Massage and aromatherapy: The close contact of massage is comforting and encourages suppressed feelings to surface. Use fragrant oils to add to the effect: mix six to eight drops of essential oil with one tablespoon of sweet almond oil; or put the same amount of essential oil into your bathwater and have a long soak.

- For grief with restlessness, use lavender, ylang ylang, vetiver, or clary sage oil. Avoid clary sage in the first 20 weeks of pregnancy.
- If grief is making you tired and lethargic, try geranium, neroli, jasmine, rose, or bergamot oil.

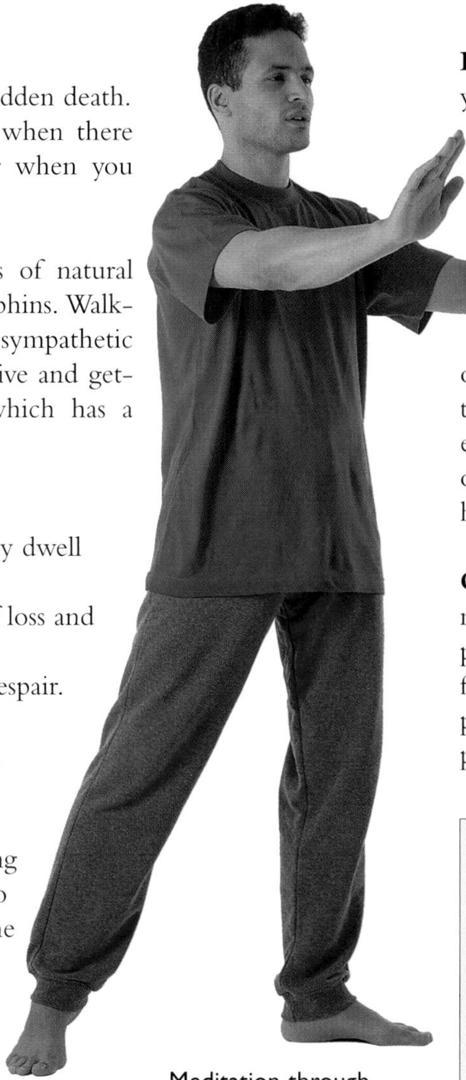

Meditation through movement
The traditional Asian therapy tai chi can promote a sense of emotional perspective, and thus help you cope with your changing life.

Relaxation: You may feel very sad whenever you let your mind go. But it's good to let your feelings surface, especially if you usually hold them back. Set aside time to be alone and quiet. You may find it soothing to practice visualization (see p. 47).

Yoga and meditation: Regular practice of yoga postures, breathing exercises, and meditation can help you rediscover and maintain your emotional equilibrium. Yoga encourages you to open yourself to your painful feelings, which can help you come to terms with your loss.

Other therapies: A psychotherapist, bereavement counselor, or member of the clergy can provide support and help you talk about your feelings, especially if you have no other trusted person to confide in. Creative therapies can also provide an outlet for emotions.

When to get medical help

- Protracted grief negatively affects your work or relationships.
- You experience severe depression.

Get help right away if:
- You have suicidal feelings.

See also:
ANXIETY, DEPRESSION, EATING DISORDERS, EMOTIONAL PROBLEMS, STRESS

Hangover

You may have, at some point in your life, woken up with the throbbing headache that usually signals a hangover. This is not a serious condition in itself, and it generally disappears within a few hours. However, a hangover is a sign that you have been drinking too much and without due care. A range of natural remedies can help your symptoms.

Hangovers vary in severity, depending on the quantity and type of alcohol consumed. Symptoms include headache, nausea, and dizziness. Alcohol dilates the blood vessels, and too much dilatation can cause a headache. It also has a dehydrating effect because it encourages the kidneys to remove more water than usual from the body.

Several factors influence the speed at which alcohol is absorbed from the digestive system into the bloodstream. Food in the stomach can slow absorption. Research also suggests that the more you weigh, the more time it takes for you to absorb alcohol. A woman tends to have a higher level of alcohol in the blood than a man of the same weight who has drunk the same amount. This may be because women produce less of an enzyme that breaks down alcohol.

Frequent or persistent hangovers indicate that you should reduce the amount of alcohol you drink. Regularly drinking large amounts of alcohol is likely to permanently harm your health—for example, by damaging your liver or raising your risk of developing certain cancers.

PREVENTION

Besides simply not drinking too much, there are several strategies to prevent a hangover:

- Always eat something before you drink and/or while you drink to slow alcohol absorption.

Alcohol limits

Drink no more than the officially recommended alcohol limits for men and for women. Consider also your size, weight, health, and metabolism. Your ideal limit may be less than the standard guidelines.

A unit of alcohol is a 12-ounce bottle of average strength beer, a 1.5-ounce shot of hard liquor, or a 4- to 5-ounce glass of wine. For a man, health problems are more likely if you drink more than 14 units of alcohol a week. The limit for a woman is 7 units a week.

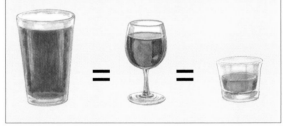

- Reduce your alcohol intake by sipping drinks slowly so they last longer and by alternating nonalcoholic drinks with alcoholic ones.
- Don't mix drinks, and avoid those to which you react badly. Some people find that a hangover is more likely after drinking inexpensive red wine (because of the high additive content) or a fortified wine, such as sherry (because of the high content of natural flavorings and colorings called congeners).

Cleansing cabbage

Raw cabbage, a traditional remedy for hangovers, has been used for centuries because it is believed to detoxify the liver. Its protective effect on the lining of the digestive tract may also counter the adverse effects of alcohol on the stomach and intestines.

- Avoid dehydration by drinking plenty of water before and after drinking alcohol.

TREATMENT

- First drink a large glass of water for immediate replacement of lost fluids.
- Replace lost nutrients, such as magnesium and potassium, with a banana milkshake (see illustration, far right).
- Don't have another drink (the "hair of the dog"). It will worsen or prolong symptoms.
- Don't drink coffee. It won't do any good and may make you jittery. It's also dehydrating.

Herbal remedies: Drink a cup of one of the following teas every hour until you feel better.

- Rosemary tea relieves headaches and is said to help the liver detoxify alcohol.
- Milk thistle or dandelion tea may also aid detoxification of the liver and blood.

- Willow bark tea—made by simmering the bark in a covered pan for 10 minutes—contains natural aspirin-like substances that can soothe a hangover headache.
- Chamomile tea soothes irritation of the stomach and intestines.

Caution: For safety concerns, see pp. 34–37.

Homeopathy: Take the following remedy every 30 minutes for up to six doses.

- Nux vomica: if you feel nauseated but are unable to vomit.

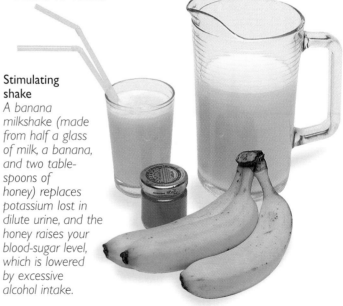

Stimulating shake

A banana milkshake (made from half a glass of milk, a banana, and two tablespoons of honey) replaces potassium lost in dilute urine, and the honey raises your blood-sugar level, which is lowered by excessive alcohol intake.

When to get medical help

- You cannot remember what happened during a drinking session.
- You have regular hangovers.

See also:
ADDICTIONS, HEADACHE

Head Lice

*T*he head louse is a brownish-gray, wingless insect that lives in human hair. Smaller than a match head, the head louse lays its eggs (called nits) along the base of the hair shaft, close to the scalp. Because of concern about the safety of some insecticides, natural methods of eradicating the problem are becoming increasingly popular.

Head lice feed by sucking blood from the scalp. Their bites may itch severely and sometimes become infected. Their brownish eggs hatch within eight days of being laid. The pearly-white, empty egg cases, which look somewhat like dandruff, are carried along the hairs as they grow, so that the egg cases are often found further from the scalp than the lice themselves.

Head lice are easily transmitted by head-to-head contact or by sharing combs, brushes, hats, or towels. Infestations are common in schoolchildren and those who work with children.

PREVENTION

Inspect your child's hair and scalp regularly for lice and nits, paying particular attention to the hairline under bangs, the nape of the neck, and the area above the ears. If there is an outbreak of head lice at your child's school, check even more thoroughly every few days. The best way to do this is to comb your child's hair using the wet comb method (see "Treatment") and see if any lice fall out.

To repel lice, comb the hair twice a week with a comb dipped in a mug of warm water containing 10 drops of tea tree oil.

TREATMENT

If your child gets head lice, he or she should use separate towels and washcloths, and should keep them away from those belonging to the rest of the family. After treating the head lice, wash your child's clothing, sheets, and pillowcases in hot water, and rinse brushes and combs thoroughly. Check all other family members, and treat them in the same way, if necessary.

The "wet comb" method: This is one of the best ways to get rid of head lice without using chemical insecticides. Wash the hair, then apply a lot of silicone-based conditioner evenly through it. Comb the hair first with a wide-toothed comb to remove any tangles. Then, working systematically, use a very fine-toothed comb (one made for the purpose) to remove the lice from one section of the hair at a time. Inspect the comb for lice after each stroke, and rinse them away. Rinse out the conditioner, and comb through again. You won't be able to dislodge the unhatched eggs with the comb because they stick firmly to the hair, but by repeating this treatment every other day for two weeks, you will gradually catch all the lice that hatch from the most recently laid eggs before they reproduce.

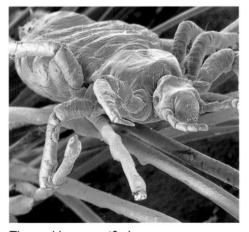

The problem magnified
The head louse, seen here enlarged about 75 times, has three pairs of legs that enable it to cling firmly to the hair shafts.

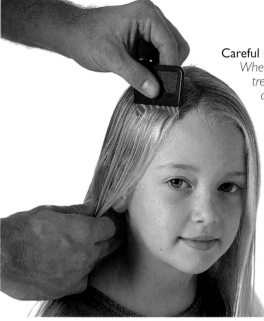

Careful combing
Whether you use herbal treatments, essential oils, or conditioner alone, thorough combing with a specially designed "nit comb" is the key to successful natural treatment of head lice.

Aromatherapy: To kill lice and soothe itching, add two drops of eucalyptus and one drop each of lavender and geranium oils to one teaspoon of unscented body lotion. Massage into the scalp and leave for half an hour. Run a fine-toothed comb through the hair before shampooing out the lotion, then rinse well. Next, apply an antiseptic rinse made by stirring two drops each of eucalyptus, lavender, rosemary (omit if you're pregnant), and geranium oils as well as two and a half teaspoons of vinegar into one cup of water. Rinse the entire head, and let the hair air-dry. Repeat daily. To prevent further infestation, use either

Gentle insecticides
Rosemary, geranium, lavender, eucalyptus, and lemon oils are excellent lice deterrents. During an outbreak, add two drops of eucalyptus and one drop each of lavender and geranium oils to shampoo. After shampooing, add two drops of any of these oils to conditioner or warm water and use as a final rinse.

the same mixture as a final rinse when washing hair, or a blend of six drops each of sweet thyme and rosemary oils with one pint of warm water.

Herbal remedies: Quassia bark and tansy are reputed to have insecticidal properties. Make a double-strength tea from either quassia bark chips (boil the chips in the water for 20 minutes) or tansy. Mix a cup with your usual amount of conditioner, and use as a rinse after shampooing.
Caution: For safety concerns, see pp. 34–37.

An all-round anti-infestation treatment
As well as repelling head lice, tansy is said to combat scabies and intestinal worms. However, it should be taken internally only on the advice of a qualified medical specialist.

When to get medical help
- Treatment is ineffective.
- The scalp becomes inflamed or infected.

See also:
HAIR AND SCALP PROBLEMS

Headache

A headache is not an illness, but a symptom. Rarely a sign of serious disease, headaches are most often caused by muscle tension resulting from a state of mental stress, when hard strands of contracted muscle fibers lead to pain by pressing on nerves or by obstructing the flow of blood, lymph, tissue fluid, or—according to Asian medicine—energy.

Headaches range in severity from mild, short-lived discomfort to a raging pain that makes activity impossible. The site of the pain varies from behind the eyes to the temples, forehead, back of the head, or even the whole head. You may be able to feel the hard, taut muscle fibers responsible for a tension headache under the skin. Migraine is a recurrent severe headache that may be accompanied by additional symptoms. Almost everyone has occasional headaches, but you are likely to have fewer as you get older.

CAUSES

There are many causes of headaches, including:
- Stress
- Dehydration
- A lack of nutrients to the muscles, blood vessels, and nerves
- Flu or other viral infection
- Sinus infection
- Excessive alcohol intake
- Environmental factors, such as a smoky atmosphere or poor lighting
- Prescription and over-the-counter medications
- Hormonal changes, as with premenstrual syndrome (PMS)
- Dental abnormalities
- Temporomandibular joint (TMJ) syndrome
- Eyestrain
- A food sensitivity or allergy
- Blood vessel contraction or dilation (vascular headaches), which can lead to migraine
- Osteoarthritis or a misalignment in the bones of the neck
- In rare cases, brain tumor, meningitis, high blood pressure, or a stroke

PREVENTION

A healthy diet reduces susceptibility to headaches by increasing resistance to infection, improving the condition of the muscles, nerves, and blood vessels, and helping prevent food sensitivity. Drink at least six glasses of water daily to prevent dehydration. Try to respond to stress in as positive a way as possible (see p. 347). Make any necessary changes to your environment, such as avoiding cigarette smoke, moistening dry air with houseplants or a humidifier (be sure to clean thoroughly and regularly), and adjusting the levels and angles of ambient lighting. Some people find an ionizer—a device that removes positively charged ions from the air—helpful.

TREATMENT

Herbal remedies: Take the following herbs as a tea (up to three cups daily) or a tincture (five drops diluted in a little water) drunk during or after eating—every two hours, if necessary, but no more than three times a day.
- Take feverfew tincture for a maximum of two

weeks at a time. Or you can eat feverfew leaves, putting them in a sandwich to disguise their bitterness. Be aware that feverfew leaves cause mouth ulcers or a sore tongue in some people.

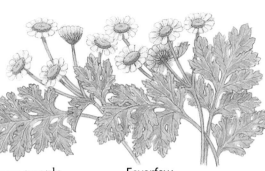

Feverfew
This staple of the herbal medicine cabinet has a marked effect on headaches caused by dilation or contraction of the blood vessels.

- To prevent a headache from worsening, drink a cup of tea or take some tincture made from passionflower, rosemary, or wood betony—or a combination of one or more of these herbs—together with meadowsweet.
- To relax tight muscles, drink a cup of tea or take a tincture made from valerian or cramp bark, with meadowsweet and rosemary. If you feel stressed, include chamomile, vervain, wild oats, or dried pasqueflower.
Caution: For safety concerns, see pp. 34–37.

Aromatherapy: Fragrant essential oils can relieve pain, ease tension, and clear congestion. Put them in your bathtub, in hot water for an inhalation, or in oil for a massage.

- For a tension headache, try lavender, sweet marjoram, and chamomile oils, all of which have relaxing properties.
- If your headache is caused by nasal or sinus congestion, perhaps from a cold or allergic rhinitis, use eucalyptus or peppermint oil.

➤ continued, p. 237

Massage away tension

Smoothing, kneading, or pressing taut muscles in the shoulders, neck, face, and scalp is one of the most effective ways of dealing with a tension headache. Ask a friend to try the following massages, while you are lying down.

Forehead massage

1 Kneel at the person's head and place your thumbs at the center of his or her forehead, just above the eyebrows, with your fingers at each side of the head.

2 Draw your thumbs out toward the temples, then lift them off when you reach the hairline. Repeat the movement, starting a fraction higher each time, until you have massaged the whole forehead.

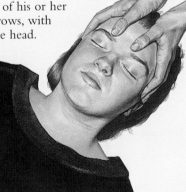

Massaging the temples

1 Place your fingertips on the temples, and press firmly for 10 seconds with the flat ends of your fingers.

2 Release the pressure gradually, and make slow, circling movements with your fingers over the temples.

Yoga for tension

Simple exercises based on yoga techniques may relax tense muscles and thus relieve headaches.

Five-minute relaxation technique

1 Lie on your back on a firm surface, with a cushion under your neck, if necessary, for comfort. To minimize the space between your lower spine and the ground, lift your knees to your chest, then slowly lower them by sliding your feet along the floor. Place your feet 8 to 12 inches apart, and your hands about 18 inches from your sides, with palms upward. Close your eyes.

2 Focus your attention on your body and your breathing. As you breathe, be aware of the movement of your abdomen as it rises and falls. Continue slowly breathing in and out, concentrating on how it feels as the air fills your lungs, and on how your abdomen expands with each inhalation. Notice your abdomen relaxing and sinking toward the floor as you exhale, and feel your whole body sinking into the ground. As you continue this deep breathing, notice the feeling of increasing relaxation as you exhale and of lightness and energy as you inhale.

Neck rolling

This exercise is not suitable if you have neck pain or other neck problems.

1 Get on your hands and knees, and place your hands flat on the floor under your shoulders.

2 Bend your arms until the top of your head touches the floor, then as you exhale, roll your head gently forward. Stop when you feel a gentle stretch down the back of your neck, and hold the position for a few seconds.

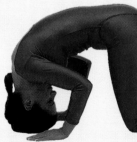

3 As you inhale, slowly roll your head in the other direction until your forehead touches the floor. Repeat this sequence slowly 20 times.

236

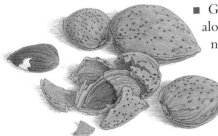

Aid in a nutshell
Eating almonds may help your headache. These tasty nuts contain pain-relieving chemicals.

■ Gently massage two drops of lavender oil along the base of your skull at the back of your neck, on your temples, and behind your ears. Keep the oil well away from your eyes.

■ Sprinkle two drops each of sweet marjoram, lavender, and peppermint oils on a tissue. Inhale deeply three times.

Diet: Reduce your caffeine intake. If you are a heavy consumer, do this gradually—for example, by combining decaffeinated and caffeinated coffee. Be prepared for a withdrawal headache that may last a few days. Eat foods rich in calcium, magnesium, and essential fatty acids (see p. 12). Avoid foods to which you might be sensitive. Some people get headaches from nitrites and nitrates (in cured meats), monosodium glutamate (MSG), tyramines (in fermented foods, certain red wines, processed meats, aged cheeses, beer), sulfites (in dried fruits and relishes), or salicylates (in tea, vinegar, and many fruits).

Hydrotherapy: Apply alternating hot and cold compresses to the nape of the neck. Fold a small towel two or three times, wring it out in hot water, and leave it in place for two minutes; then replace it for one minute with a towel wrung out in cold water. Repeat for 15 to 20 minutes.

Homeopathy: For isolated headaches, try one of the following:
■ Belladonna: for throbbing, hammering headaches that are worse for light and noise.
■ Bryonia: for bursting headaches that are worse for the slightest movement.
■ Ignatia: for headaches arising from acute emotional distress.

Other therapies: Cranial osteopathy, biofeedback, self-hypnosis, meditation, reflexology, and acupuncture may also be helpful.

Acupressure for headache relief

1 Place one hand across the front of your partner's head, while using your other thumb to press the point (GB 12) just behind the bony prominence at the hairline at the back of the ear (see illustration). Direct gently pulsing thumb pressure toward the eye for about two minutes.

2 Put your thumb on the point (GB 20) between the muscles of the side and back of the neck, just under the ridge of the skull. As in the previous step, direct thumb pressure toward the eye on the other side for two minutes. Repeat both steps on the other side of the head.

When to get medical help
● You have repeated, unexplained headaches.

Get help right away if:
● You have a sudden, severe headache of a kind not previously experienced.
● You experience vomiting, a stiff neck, fever, rash, dislike of bright light, confusion, and/or vision problems (with a severe headache).

See also:
HANGOVER, MIGRAINE, STRESS

Hearing Loss

Deterioration of hearing presents a challenge to effective communication and reduces the amount of useful information we receive from our environment. Luckily, hearing loss is rarely total. Several causes of this problem, such as wax blockage, are often easy to prevent, and some others are treatable with natural remedies and therapies.

There are two types of hearing loss: conductive and sensorineural. Conductive hearing loss occurs when sound waves from the outside world fail to reach the inner ear, usually as a result of a blockage in the outer ear canal or problems in the eardrum or middle ear. In sensorineural hearing loss, sounds reach the inner ear but fail to reach the brain because of damage to the inner ear or the acoustic nerve. The chief causes of such permanent hearing loss are the effects of age, arterial disease (which can reduce the blood supply to the acoustic nerve), and prolonged exposure to excessive noise levels (above 85 decibels). Sudden or prolonged noise—for example, from a loud workplace or rock concert—can damage the hairlike endings of the acoustic nerve. Researchers now believe that such damage may be partly caused by a surge of unstable oxygen molecules, known as free

What is Ménière's disease?

Attacks of vertigo, nausea, ear discomfort, and tinnitus (ringing and other noises in the ear), combined with progressive hearing loss in one ear, are usually symptoms of Ménière's disease. This results from fluid build-up in the inner ear, which puts pressure on the hearing nerve endings. Factors that may trigger Ménière's disease include poor circulation, premenstrual fluid retention, and, possibly, food sensitivity. One in three sufferers also has migraine.

radicals, that follows exposure to loud noise. Some prescribed drugs can also affect hearing.

Common causes of conductive hearing loss include inflammation of the middle ear, a boil in the outer ear, and impacted wax in the ear canal. Other causes include thick fluid remaining in the middle ear after an infection, Ménière's disease (see box), and aging. Temporary hearing loss experienced when flying occurs because of the inability to equalize air pressure in the middle ear and the throat during takeoff and landing. This is more likely if the eustachian tubes are blocked due to allergy or infection.

PREVENTION

Measures to prevent hearing loss include boosting resistance to infection and allergy, stabilizing

Inside the ear
The ear is divided into three areas: the outer ear, the middle ear, and the inner ear. Blockage of the outer or middle ear leads to conductive hearing loss, which is usually reversible. Damage to the inner ear can cause sensorineural hearing loss, which is more likely to be permanent.

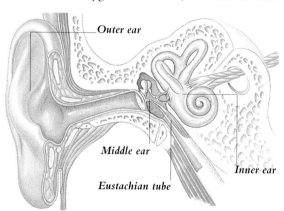

Outer ear

Middle ear

Inner ear

Eustachian tube

the body's fluid balance, combating arterial disease, and addressing the causes of premature aging. This means eating a healthy diet (see p. 9), with plenty of whole grains, fruits, and vegetables, and limiting your intake of sugar, refined carbohydrates, and salt. Get some exercise daily, and if you smoke, find a way to stop. If you have allergic rhinitis or Ménière's disease, try to identify and deal with any underlying triggers.

Avoid sudden or prolonged loud noise. Signs that the decibel level may be high enough to damage hearing include being unable to hear someone speaking directly to you and experiencing ringing in the ears during exposure and muffling of ordinary sounds afterward. If you cannot avoid loud noise, wear efficient earplugs or other protectors and take a supplement of antioxidants for a few days in advance. These nutrients will help neutralize any damaging effects of free radicals on the ear.

TREATMENT

Age-related hearing loss: Help slow down the progression of this condition by following a diet that preserves the health of the arteries and nerves supplying the ears (see "Prevention"). Take supplements of antioxidants and magnesium for two weeks after exposure to loud noise.

Nasal congestion: You can tackle hearing loss resulting from mucus congestion in several ways.
- Add a teaspoon of red sage tincture to half a cup of warm water. Use as a gargle.
- Drink plantain tea, which helps liquefy and loosen thick mucus.
- Drink a cup of tea made with one or more of

Removing earwax

To soften wax so that it will work its way out of the ear canal, place a few drops of warm olive, almond, or mullein oil in your ear, then lie on your side with that ear uppermost for 15 minutes. Repeat several times a day for two to three days. Caution: Don't put anything in your ear if you have a discharge or pain—your eardrum may be perforated.

the following herbs two or three times a day: chamomile, cleavers, echinacea, elderflower, goldenseal, and licorice.
- Put a few drops of eucalyptus or lemon oil on a tissue and inhale the vapor. Or add one or two drops of one of these oils to a teaspoon of cold-pressed vegetable oil and smooth over your throat and around your ears.
- Add lemon balm leaves to salads and soups.
Caution: For safety concerns, see pp. 34–37.

When to get medical help

- You have a severe earache or a discharge from the ear.
- You feel dizzy.
- Home treatment does not help within a few days.
- The hearing loss is sudden.

See also:
AGING, ALLERGIC RHINITIS, ARTERIAL DISEASE, COLDS, EARACHE, MIGRAINE, SORE THROAT

Hemorrhoids

About half the population in Western countries suffers at some time from hemorrhoids, which are swollen or twisted veins in the walls of the anus. Otherwise known as piles (from the Latin pilae, *meaning "balls"), these varicose anal veins can often be prevented by eating the right foods and, unless severe, they can usually be alleviated through natural therapies.*

Hemorrhoids may be internal—that is, within the anal canal—or external, when they may be felt as little knobs or balls around the anal opening. Prolapsed hemorrhoids protrude outside the anus. Symptoms may include painful defecation, itching, and rectal bleeding. Pain may be severe if a large hemorrhoid is inside the anus. Hemorrhoids are usually caused by constipation, when straining to pass hard stools increases the pressure in the anal veins, making them dilate. Constipation also makes existing hemorrhoids worse, since passing hard stools abrades dilated veins and the strain of trying to have a bowel movement puts pressure on the anus. Hemorrhoids often occur during pregnancy and immediately after childbirth. They are more likely if you are overweight or inactive, or if you eat a diet low in fiber and high in refined foods.

PREVENTION

Lose any excess weight. Eat a well-balanced, high-fiber diet (see p. 9) to provide the nutrients needed to keep veins strong and healthy and to prevent constipation. Drink at least six extra glasses of water daily to help soften stools. Exercise regularly to ensure good circulation. Be careful about reading in the bathroom; sitting too long on the toilet seat increases pressure on the rectum.

Potent fruits
Berries and cherries are rich in vein-strengthening antioxidant flavonoids called proanthocyanidins.

TREATMENT

During flare-ups of pain, take daily breaks (see photograph, left). Don't stand still for long periods, and exercise vigorously for at least 20 minutes on most days to improve circulation.

Diet: Eat plenty of fresh fruits and vegetables, whole grains, nuts, and seeds. These contain fiber, which helps treat constipation, as well as vitamin C, silica, and flavonoid pigments that help make vein walls strong and flexible. Berries, cherries, and buckwheat contain especially beneficial flavonoids.

Rest position
When hemorrhoids are painful, rest for two half-hour periods every day by lying or sitting with the feet above hip level.

From the drugstore: Strengthen vein walls with supplements of vitamin C, proanthocyanidins, rutin, and silica.

Herbal remedies: Gently wash and dry the anal area, then apply one of the following to soothe and shrink swollen veins:

■ A cold, astringent solution made from a tablespoon of distilled witch hazel and four drops of marigold (calendula) tincture in a cup of water.

■ Cooled tea made by boiling a teaspoon of grated bistort root in a cup of water for 10 minutes in a covered pan.

■ Pilewort (lesser celandine) ointment. Apply in the morning, at bedtime, and after washing.

■ A preparation available from the health-food store containing extracts of horse chestnut and black haw. Or apply a paste made by mixing two teaspoons of one or both of these powdered herbs with one to two teaspoons of walnut oil at night; remove by spraying with cold water in the morning.

Caution: For safety concerns, see pp. 34–37.

Homeopathy

■ Apply homeopathic cream containing Aesculus and Hamamelis to soothe the affected area.

■ Sulfur and Nux vomica, alternated on a daily basis, can often be helpful.

Aromatherapy: To strengthen vein walls, add six drops of lemon, lavender, rosemary, cypress, or juniper berry essential oil to your bathwater. Avoid juniper berry oil throughout pregnancy and rosemary and cypress oils during the first 20 weeks of pregnancy.

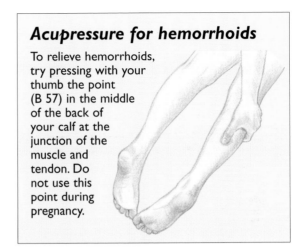

Acupressure for hemorrhoids

To relieve hemorrhoids, try pressing with your thumb the point (B 57) in the middle of the back of your calf at the junction of the muscle and tendon. Do not use this point during pregnancy.

Hydrotherapy

■ To ease itching, wash with unscented soap and water. Rinse the area with cold water.

■ Take alternate hot and cold sitz baths each day (see p. 49) to improve circulation.

■ If your hemorrhoids are very painful, apply crushed ice to the area for a few seconds or spray with iced water.

When to get medical help

● You notice fecal blood or rectal bleeding.
● You experience unexplained diarrhea or constipation for more than two weeks.
● Symptoms fail to improve with treatment.
● You feel ill or lose weight.
● You have protracted rectal pain or excessive discomfort during bowel movements.

Get help right away if:
● Rectal bleeding is severe.

See also:
CONSTIPATION,
DIARRHEA,
OVERWEIGHT,
PREGNANCY
PROBLEMS,
VARICOSE VEINS

Hiccups

The involuntary intakes of air known as hiccups are provoked by repeated spasms of the diaphragm, the sheet of muscle separating the chest and abdomen. Most attacks of hiccups, which include making an uncontrollable noise with each intake, last only a few minutes. Although irritating, hiccups are not serious, but you can try a variety of home remedies to stop an attack.

Hiccups often begin after having a large hot drink or a large meal, when an overfull stomach presses on the diaphragm. They also frequently follow a prolonged bout of uncontrollable laughter. But there may be no obvious cause. Attacks of hiccups usually stop of their own accord, rarely lasting more than 20 minutes. If they persist or make you uncomfortable or embarrassed, any of several simple traditional remedies may be effective. In rare cases, continuing hiccups signify an underlying disorder.

PREVENTION
Get into the habit of eating and drinking slowly. Avoid ingesting too much at one time, always chew thoroughly, and avoid stress at mealtimes.

TREATMENT
The following two remedies work by raising the body's level of carbon dioxide, which seems to relax the diaphragm.
- Take a breath and hold it for a while, but exhale before you get light-headed or dizzy.
- Hold a paper bag—never use plastic—over your nose and mouth and breathe in and out several times (see photograph, p. 196).

Acupressure: Apply firm pressure with finger and thumb on the point (GB 20) on each side of the neck under the base of the skull (see p. 237) for two to three minutes while taking short, shallow breaths. This calms the nerve that controls contraction of the diaphragm.

Herbal remedies: The antispasmodic and relaxant effects of peppermint on the digestive tract may help relieve hiccups resulting from an overfull stomach. Have the tea after main meals. Caution: For safety concerns, see pp. 34–37.

Rhythmic drinking

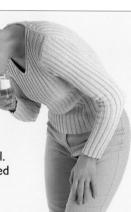

Slowly sipping a glass of cold water or sucking on an ice cube can sometimes stop a bout of hiccups. A variation is to bend your head forward over a glass of water and slowly sip from the other side of the rim.

These remedies may work, probably because most people breathe relatively little as they sip, thereby increasing their body's carbon dioxide level. The rhythmic contractions of the esophagus induced by slow sipping and swallowing also override the spasms of the diaphragm.

When to get medical help
- Your hiccups last longer than a day.
- You suffer from frequent attacks of hiccups.
- You also have difficulty breathing, chest pain, or light-headedness.

High Blood Pressure

A rise in pressure exerted by circulating blood on the artery walls is a normal response to stress and physical activity. However, if this pressure remains persistently high, it can overwork your heart and arteries, making arterial disease, heart attacks, and strokes more likely. Simple lifestyle changes can help reduce high blood pressure, or hypertension.

More men than women have hypertension, and the disorder is most common after middle age. No obvious cause for high blood pressure is found in about 90 percent of those affected; this type is called essential hypertension.

Because hypertension is usually symptomless, it is often discovered only during a medical examination. It must be taken seriously, because it increases your risk of a stroke, "mini-stroke" (transient ischemic attack, or TIA), heart attack, and other problems, such as kidney disease.

Causes

Smoking, a high alcohol intake, obesity, a sedentary lifestyle, and stress all increase the likelihood of hypertension. The stiffening and loss of elasticity of artery walls that accompany aging and certain forms of arterial disease can also elevate blood pressure. High blood pressure during pregnancy (preeclampsia) makes hypertension more likely later in life. Genetic factors can also underlie elevated blood pressure.

You may be at risk of high blood pressure if your mother did not eat a nutritious diet during pregnancy. This can adversely influence the long-term elasticity of the arteries, as well as encouraging low birth weight. Babies of low birth weight are more likely as adults to develop high blood pressure, along with obesity, elevated blood fats, and oversensitivity to insulin (which precedes diabetes). These symptoms are known collectively as the metabolic syndrome, or syndrome X.

Prevention

Help prevent high blood pressure by reducing all possible risk factors.

- Get regular, brisk exercise.
- Don't smoke.
- Eat a healthy diet (see p. 9).
- Avoid excessive alcohol intake (see p. 230).
- Keep off excess weight.

Losing weight is especially important if you are "apple-shaped," with excess fat carried around your middle, rather than your hips and thighs. A waist measuring more than 37 inches in a man, or 32 inches in a woman, slightly increases the risk of hypertension; more than 40 inches

How blood pressure is measured

Blood pressure is recorded as two values, the systolic (the pressure of the blood as it enters the aorta from the heart) and the diastolic (the pressure when the heart ventricles relax between beats). Normal blood pressure (BP) is usually defined as less than 140/90. However, a person's BP varies with age, and you can work out what your normal systolic pressure (the higher number of the two) should roughly be by adding 100 to your age in years (though this is not so accurate in later years). BP also varies with diet, weight, activity level, emotions, and degree of relaxation at the time of testing.

in a man, or 35 inches in a woman, increases it more significantly.

Because the epinephrine released by a high level of anger, anxiety, or other stressful emotion encourages high blood pressure, learn stress-management techniques to keep you calm. Conversely, feeling happy and relaxed tends to reduce high blood pressure.

TREATMENT

High blood pressure requires monitoring and, often, medical treatment. If you have only mild hypertension, you and your doctor may find that lifestyle changes and, perhaps, natural supplements will reduce your blood pressure sufficiently so that you have no need for prescription drugs. In other cases where medication is required, many of the following natural remedies can work to support that treatment.

Diet: Recent research has identified the benefits of certain minerals in the treatment of high blood pressure. The following tips will help you maintain your intake of the nutrients you need to keep your blood vessels in good condition while also helping you control your weight.

- Eat at least five daily servings of vegetables (not including potatoes) and fruits. These supply nutrients—such as vitamins B_6 and C, magnesium, and potassium—necessary for healthy arteries and heart function. Vegetables and fruits also supply fiber and natural salicylates, which may—like their relative, aspirin (acetyl salicylic acid)—reduce the risk of a heart attack resulting from hypertension.

Dietary helpers
Potassium can work to lower blood pressure. The richest sources of this mineral include bananas, tomatoes, and peas.

- If you need to lose weight, follow a sound weight-control diet (see p. 303), combined with daily exercise.
- Boost fiber intake by choosing whole-grain breads and cereals rather than refined products.
- Eat oily fish three times weekly; their omega-3 fatty acids may lower blood pressure.
- Reduce your overall intake of fat, especially saturated fat, but eat enough foods containing essential fatty acids (oily fish, nuts, seeds, and cold-pressed olive or sunflower oil).
- Eat more calcium-rich foods, such as dairy products. Choose low-fat types.
- Keep your sodium intake low. Don't add salt (sodium chloride) to food or eat commercially processed foods containing added salt. Between 70 and 80 percent of our salt intake comes from such processed products as breads, breakfast cereals, potato chips, and other snacks.

Testing for salt sensitivity

Salt encourages hypertension only in certain "salt-sensitive" people, but until a test to detect salt sensitivity becomes available, the only way you can detect it is to eat a low-salt diet for a month and have your blood pressure checked before and afterward.

- Cut down on sodium from foods containing sodium bicarbonate, fish or meat cured with sodium nitrite, and foods containing the flavor enhancer monosodium glutamate, or MSG.
- Use a salt substitute from the supermarket or drugstore. Such products are high in potassium and magnesium (which may help lower blood pressure), but low in sodium.
- Minimize your intake of caffeine-containing drinks, since caffeine may contribute to raised blood pressure.
- Keep your alcohol intake low.
- Have some garlic (raw or as capsules or tablets) every day. A substance, called allicin, in garlic dilates blood vessels.

From the drugstore: Supplements are sometimes used along with or instead of prescription drugs for very mild hypertension. However, consult your doctor before trying any of them to make sure they are safe for you and to find out the proper amounts and combinations. Also keep in mind that high blood pressure requires careful monitoring. Supplements that may be recommended include:

- Calcium, magnesium, and/or potassium
- The herb hawthorn
- The amino acids arginine and taurine

Herbal remedies: To help reduce mild high blood pressure, use remedies containing hawthorn or calcium elenolate (derived from a bitter antioxidant flavonoid called oleuropein in olive leaves). Drink a cup of tea or take a few drops of tincture made from one or more of these remedies once or twice daily for up to two

---

Progessive muscular relaxation

Relaxation exercises are among the most effective natural means of combating high blood pressure. Try the following method every day:

1 Lie down on your back with your legs slightly apart and your hands palms upward at your sides. Breathe deeply and steadily throughout the exercise.

2 Starting at your toes and slowly working up to your face, tighten and then consciously relax the muscles of each part of the body in turn.

3 When you have worked on all your muscles, lie still and enjoy the feeling of relaxation for about five minutes.

---

months. Do not use these remedies in addition to the supplements described in "From the Drugstore" (left). Consult your doctor first if you're already taking prescribed medication.
Caution: For safety concerns, see pp. 34–37.

Stress management: Reduce the demands of work and home when you can. For the unavoidable stress in your life, find ways to cope (see p. 347), if necessary by working with a counselor.
- Relax at regular intervals, using meditation and/or progressive muscular relaxation (see box). Consider also visualization (p. 47).

Exercise: Get daily aerobic exercise, such as brisk walking or cycling. The combination of

Aromatherapy massage for relaxation

The calming actions of some essential oils add to the relaxing and therefore blood-pressure-lowering benefits of massage. Ask a friend to follow these instructions to give you a peaceful, soothing, whole-body massage to reduce stress-induced hypertension. Make a massage oil from three drops each of ylang ylang, lavender, and marjoram oils, and one tablespoon of jojoba oil. Warm the oil to body temperature in a container of hot water.

1 Sitting as shown, oil your hands and rest them gently on the center of the upper back. Leaning forward from the hips, slide your hands down along each side of the spine, circling back up the sides. Repeat several times.

2 Glide one hand across the upper back, away from the direction your partner is facing. Follow with a stroke of the other hand. Repeat, alternating strokes of each hand. Then ask your partner to face the other way and work in the other direction.

3 Place your thumbs on one side of the neck. Glide your thumbs outward along the shoulder between the top of the shoulder blade and the shoulder muscle. Repeat, gradually moving a little farther toward the top of the shoulder. Work on the other shoulder in the same way.

4 Facing your partner's head, place your oiled hands on the lower back. Make counterclockwise circles with your right hand and clockwise circles with the left. Increase the pressure a little as you move toward the center of the back.

5 Place both hands on the back of the leg below the calf. Glide slowly up to the top of the thigh. Move your hands apart, allowing one to circle the hip and the other to move to the inner thigh, avoiding the genitals. Slide both hands back to the ankle and down the foot. Repeat several times on each leg.

this and weight loss lowers blood pressure more than either alone. However, avoid lifting heavy weights. This type of physical exertion causes a rise in blood pressure that might burst a blood vessel, leading to a nosebleed or bleeding in the retina or the brain (a stroke). Gentle forms of exercise, such as yoga (see below), promote relaxation, which helps lower blood pressure.

Yoga: Many studies have shown that the regular practice of certain yoga postures and breathing exercises can have a marked effect on hypertension, partly by teaching you how to keep calm.
- Practice the corpse pose with breathing exercises (see p. 54) for 30 to 60 minutes daily.
- Don't do any exercise that involves holding your breath, and avoid the shoulder-stand and other inverted postures. The half shoulder-stand can bring high blood pressure down, but should be done only under the supervision of an experienced yoga teacher.

Aromatherapy: Soak in a warm bathtub to which you have added a total of five to six drops of bergamot, German or Roman chamomile, or frankincense oil.

Light therapy: Exposure to the ultraviolet light of the sun may help reduce blood pressure. It elevates levels of vitamin D, which alters the

Soothing herb
Lime tree flowers aid relaxation of mind and muscles, and so have beneficial effects on high blood pressure caused by nervous tension. Drink a cup of this tea once or twice a day.

body's use of calcium and relaxes tense arteries, and which may in turn encourage a healthy blood pressure. Indeed, hypertension appears to be less common in areas that have more daylight. Expose your skin to daylight every day for 15 to 20 minutes, but stay out of the strong midday sun (10 A.M. to 3 P.M.) to avoid the risk of skin cancer.

Hydrotherapy: Alternate hot and cold footbaths are said to be useful for hypertension.
- Fill one bowl with hot water and another with cold. Put your feet in the hot water for three minutes, then in the cold for one minute. Repeat this process three or four times.

Other therapies: Studies suggest that acupuncture and autogenic training can reduce high blood pressure. A biofeedback teacher or counselor can teach you how to lower blood pressure elevated by stress-induced muscle tension.

When to get medical help
- You haven't had your blood pressure checked in the past 12 months.

Get help right away if:
- You have high blood pressure and feel poorly for any reason.
- You experience dizziness, faintness, unusual fatigue, or unusual headaches.
- You have shortness of breath, confusion, or chest or arm pain.
- You notice a sudden change in strength or feeling in a limb.

See also:
ARTERIAL
DISEASE,
DIABETES,
OVERWEIGHT,
STRESS

Hives

This type of itchy rash, also known as urticaria or nettle rash, is usually caused by an allergic reaction to something you have touched, such as a plant, or eaten, such as strawberries. About 20 percent of the population develops hives at some time. Women are more prone to the condition than men, but the reason for this is unclear.

Common culprits
Among the most prevalent dietary causes of hives are eggs, milk, nuts, shellfish, and strawberries. Skin contact with nettles can produce similar symptoms.

When an allergic reaction causes certain skin cells to release histamine, local small blood vessels dilate and their walls become permeable. Clear fluid called serum then leaks into the surrounding tissues and causes the characteristic inflammation and itchy, raised lumps of hives. Hives develop within minutes of eating or coming into contact with the offending substance. The lumps vary considerably in size, and larger ones may merge to form irregular patches known as weals. Initially a weal is red; later it becomes white at the center, leaving a red rim. It lasts for about a day, and then disappears.

Hives often result from an allergy to a food, stinging plant (such as nettle or poison ivy), medication (such as aspirin or penicillin), or insect bite. Sun exposure, temperature extremes, and stress may also cause hives.

PREVENTION

You can prevent a recurrence of hives if you are able to identify and avoid the cause. Sometimes it is easy to relate the symptom to a particular food, but more often the link is not obvious. To pin it down, keep a diary in which you list everything that enters your mouth—not only food and drink, but also supplements, medications (including over-the-counter drugs), toothpaste, and mouthwash.

If your symptoms reappear, you may be able to determine a connection between something you have ingested and your hives. If this is unsuccessful, try an exclusion diet, eliminating one or two foods at a time for a period of three weeks each (see illustration, left). If you have no further symptoms during this period, reintroduce the foods into your diet one at a time, every three weeks. If the hives recur, the most recently reintroduced food is probably causing the symptoms.

To lower your risk of allergic reactions to food, avoid highly refined foods, which can reduce the efficiency of the immune system, and eat

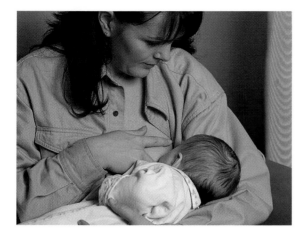

Protecting your baby
Breast-feeding a baby helps prevent allergies, which can cause hives, in later life. If possible, breast-feed your baby for at least a year.

more immunity-boosting foods, such as those rich in essential fatty acids and vitamins A and C (see p. 12). Vitamin C also has powerful antihistamine properties. Be aware that certain factors may weaken your immune system and make it react unusually to a normally harmless food. These include infection, stress, a lack of sleep, digestive problems, air filled with tobacco smoke or other pollutants, certain drugs, and pesticides and other chemicals in foods.

If you have had a baby, reduce his or her risk of developing a food allergy or other sensitivity by breast-feeding exclusively for a minimum of four months. While you are pregnant or breast-feeding, eat a wide range of foods to reduce your child's risk of developing allergies.

TREATMENT
Herbal remedies
- For hives induced by anxiety or stress, drink a cup of valerian or chamomile tea twice daily.
- Apply aloe vera gel to soothe the rash.
- Wash with tea made from chamomile, chickweed, or elderflowers.
- Drink a cup of tea made from nettles, burdock,

echinacea, myrrh, and/or marshmallow twice a day for their antihistamine action.
- Apply cream made from calendula, chickweed, comfrey, elderflowers, or plantain.

Caution: For safety concerns, see pp. 34–37.

Kitchen cabinet remedies
- Relieve itching by adding three tablespoons of baking soda to a warm bath and soaking for 10 to 15 minutes. Or add five tablespoons of coarse (colloidal) oatmeal to the water.
- Add nine cups of vinegar to your bathwater, or add a teaspoon of vinegar to a tablespoon of lukewarm water and apply with a cotton ball to the affected area. Vinegar helps prevent itching by acidifying the skin.
- Apply extracted cucumber juice to the affected area, or lay cucumber slices over it.

From the drugstore: Take 500 milligrams of vitamin C with flavonoids twice a day.

Homeopathy
- Urtica: if hives are very itchy.
- Rhus toxicodendron: if the rash is itchy, red, and sore, and you feel very restless.

When to get medical help
- The rash persists longer than a day or recurs.

Get help right away if:
- Your mouth and throat are affected.
- You experience faintness, shortness of breath, or a rapid pulse.
- The hives occur after taking medication.

See also:
FOOD SENSITIVITY,
INSECT BITES AND
STINGS, ITCHING,
SUNBURN

Incontinence

*U*rinary incontinence, the involuntary passing of urine, is often a result of injury or disease of the urinary tract. This loss of bladder control may be frustrating and potentially embarrassing, but in many cases the problem can be improved significantly with Kegel exercises, devised to strengthen pelvic-floor muscles, and various changes in routine.

In women, who are mainly affected, incontinence usually results from weakness of the bladder-neck muscle (urethral sphincter) around the top of the urethra, which helps close the bladder, or from weakness of the pelvic-floor muscles—the muscles that support the bladder and uterus and also help close the bladder. Weakness of these muscles may accompany aging, any disorder (such as a stroke) affecting the nerves supplying these muscles, or injury to the muscles or their nerves. Other causes of incontinence include irritation of the bladder lining and over-sensitivity of the bladder-wall (detrusor) muscle, making it contract unexpectedly. In men, incontinence may stem from prostate problems.

TYPES OF INCONTINENCE

Stress incontinence: The most common result of weakness of the bladder-neck and pelvic-floor muscles, stress incontinence is leakage of urine that occurs because of raised pressure in the abdomen, often caused by laughing, coughing, lifting, or jumping. The condition is widespread among women, especially during pregnancy, when the growing uterus puts pressure on the bladder neck and pelvic floor, and after childbirth, when the bladder neck and pelvic floor may be stretched or damaged. Standing or straining may provoke stress incontinence in men with an enlarged prostate or other prostate disorder. People of either sex may suffer from this problem if they are very overweight.

Urge incontinence: This sudden, irresistible urge to empty the bladder is often triggered by a change in position, for example, from sitting to standing. It may also occur during the night. One cause—often responsible for incontinence in older people—is overactivity of the bladder-wall muscle. This may happen as a result of stress, a full bladder, certain drugs (including diuretics, antidepressants, tranquilizers, and high blood pressure medication), or for no apparent reason. Other causes of urge incontinence include irritation of the bladder lining by a urinary-tract infection, over-concentrated urine from low fluid intake, nicotine, certain food colorings, sugar (with untreated diabetes), caffeine, and alcohol. Some researchers believe that fluoride-containing toothpaste is a possible cause.

Overflow incontinence: This occurs as a result of chronic urinary retention, when the bladder is unable to empty and is always full, leading to constant dribbling of urine. Possible causes

What are the pelvic floor muscles?
Located within the pelvis, these vital muscles provide a supporting web for the female reproductive and urinary organs and their outlets.

Spinal column

Anus

Pelvis — Vagina — Urethra

include an enlarged prostate, a prolapsed uterus, and certain medications.

PREVENTION

Performing Kegel exercises, especially during pregnancy and after childbirth, strengthens and tones the pelvic floor, and helps prevent stress incontinence. If you have done these exercises regularly, you will more easily be able to adjust the speed and ease of the baby's descent down the vagina in the second stage of labor. A controlled descent helps prevent subsequent urinary incontinence caused by overstretching of the

Bladder irritants
Restrict foods containing oxalate (such as strawberries, rhubarb, and spinach), which increase the frequency of urination in the morning.

pelvic-floor muscles. These exercises are also beneficial for men and older women.

TREATMENT

If you have stress incontinence:
- Do Kegel exercises every day.
- Women can also try vaginal muscle "weight-training." Cone-shaped vaginal weights of various sizes to insert and hold in the vagina are available from some drugstores.
- Lose any excess weight, since fat deposits put pressure on the bladder and pelvic floor.

If incontinence results from bladder irritation:
- Keep the genital area clean and dry to avoid irritation of the urethra from infection.
- Avoid caffeine-containing drinks and alcohol in the evening; these increase urine output and may irritate the bladder lining.
- Cut out artifically colored foods, as some food colorings may irritate the bladder lining.
- Stop smoking.

Kegel exercises

To recognize the pelvic-floor muscles, try to stop your urine flow midstream. Then, at least five times daily, sit or lie with your knees slightly apart, and tighten these same muscles for two seconds at a time, relaxing for two seconds in between. Repeat the cycle up to 10 times. Gradually work up to 10-second muscle tensing. Practice anywhere, standing or sitting. Check your progress each week by trying to stop your urine flow midstream.

When to get medical help

- Lack of bladder control is preventing you from undertaking normal activities.
- Urination is painful.
- You think a prescribed medication may be responsible.

Get help right away if:
- You suddenly lose bladder control.

See also:
PROSTATE PROBLEMS, URINARY-TRACT INFECTIONS, URINARY DIFFICULTIES

Indigestion

The term "indigestion" covers a range of symptoms that may arise after eating. These symptoms, which include discomfort, pain, and a feeling of fullness in the upper abdomen, are usually brought on by eating too quickly or too much, or by certain foods. Changes in your eating habits may prevent the problem. Otherwise, a variety of natural remedies can help.

If you regularly suffer from indigestion, it is important to exclude an underlying problem, such as a peptic ulcer, gastritis (inflammation of the stomach lining), esophagitis (inflammation of the esophagal lining), irritable bowel syndrome, inflammatory bowel disease, and stomach cancer.

Indigestion may stem from minor irritation of the esophagus, stomach, or intestines, which then cease or slow their contractions. The stomach or intestines consequently become distended with gas, partially digested food, and digestive juices (which include stomach acid, enzymes, and mucus made in the digestive tract, liver, and pancreas). Symptoms include belching, abdominal pain, nausea, bloating, and heartburn—a burning sensation behind the breastbone (sternum), perhaps with surges of acid stomach contents into the mouth (acid reflux).

CAUSES

The most common causes of indigestion are:

- Eating too fast. This can reduce the flow of digestive juices. You are also unlikely to chew well enough to break up the food and mix it with the digestive enzymes in saliva.
- Eating too much. An overfull stomach empties more slowly and encourages acid reflux.
- Eating certain foods, such as wheat flour or milk, to which you may be sensitive. Wheat and other carbohydrates and fibers can also cause discomfort simply by swelling as they absorb fluid. This can lead to bloating.
- Producing excess gas. This can occur if you eat fruit after a fatty meal. Fats need more time in

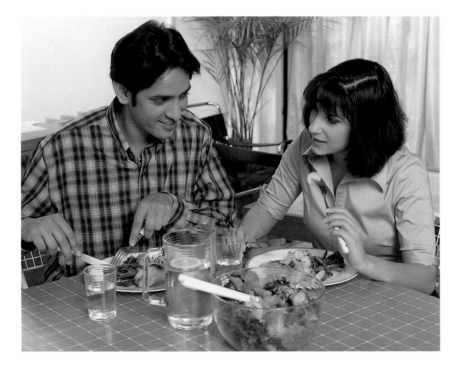

Enjoy your meal
Sit down for meals. Take your time, chew well, and relax as much as possible. If you can, remain seated for half an hour after finishing your food.

the stomach than do fruits, so eating fruit after fat means that the fruit remains in the stomach so long that it begins to ferment. Gas is also caused by an imbalance of intestinal micro-organisms and by inadequate stomach acid (see box).

■ Eating unripe fruit.

■ Having certain drinks. Sugar and carbonation in drinks can promote bloating and flatulence. Caffeine-containing drinks can elevate stomach acid levels, irritate any inflamed areas, and raise the levels of stress hormones (see next item). Alcohol can also increase acid production and irritate already inflamed areas.

■ Feeling stressed. This impairs digestion because stress hormones—for example, epinephrine (adrenaline) and cortisone—divert blood from

Bon appetit!
Stimulate the flow of digestive juices before a meal by eating a bitter food, such as olives, or by drinking tonic water or a tea made from bitter herbs.

the digestive system to the muscles, trigger contraction of the stomach muscles (which makes the stomach fill faster), and may increase stomach acid production. Stress also makes you more likely to swallow air while you eat.

■ Exercising too soon after a meal. Physical activity diverts blood from the digestive system to the muscles.

■ Taking nonsteroidal anti-inflammatory drugs, such as aspirin or ibuprofen, which may irritate the stomach lining.

■ Smoking. Chemicals in tobacco smoke may irritate the esophagus and weaken the valve-like mechanism between the esophagus and the stomach, encouraging acid reflux.

■ Having a hiatal hernia. In this condition part of the stomach protrudes through the diaphragm, leading to acid reflux. It is more common in smokers and those who are overweight.

■ Being pregnant. The growing uterus leaves increasingly less room for the stomach, thus encouraging acid reflux.

PREVENTION

To lower your risk of indigestion:

■ Don't overeat.

■ Don't let more than four hours elapse between meals, and always eat a good breakfast. Have your last meal of the day at least three hours before you go to bed.

■ Don't drink more than one average-sized glass of fluid during a meal.

■ Eat a balanced diet that includes foods rich in zinc and vitamins B and C (see p. 12).

■ If a food disagrees with you, stop eating it, or experiment to see whether you can tolerate a

---

Stomach acid: too much or too little?

Indigestion can be the result of either excessive or insufficient digestive acid being produced in the stomach.

Too much acid
This may result from a natural tendency to overproduction but may also be enouraged by eating fatty foods, which delay emptying of the stomach. Problems may also occur if the acid leaks up into the esophagus as a result of pressure on the stomach from pregnancy or a weakness of the valve that normally keeps the stomach closed. Excess stomach acid can also encourage the development of peptic ulcers.

Too little acid
Low acid production, or too dilute a concentration of stomach acid, may be the result of genetic factors, chronic stress, insufficient chewing, food sensitivity, drinking too much fluid with a meal, vitamin B deficiency, immune cell attack, or aging. Too little stomach acid leads to a failure to digest food, especially proteins, efficiently, and it may cause indigestion and other related problems.

smaller amount. You may find the problem clears up if you have it separately from other foods (see "Food Combining," facing page).

■ Deal with stress effectively (see p. 347).

■ If you are elderly, don't eat well, or have a food sensitivity, take a regular multiple vitamin and mineral supplement.

■ Before a meal, sip half a cup of tea made from parsley, chamomile, peppermint, dandelion, or burdock. If you feel stressed, add hops or lemon balm to the brew. For safety concerns about the use of herbs, see pp. 34–37.

■ Try avoiding particular combinations of foods (see "Food Combining," facing page).

■ Don't exercise for an hour after a meal.

■ After eating, chew cardamom, fennel, or caraway seeds.

■ If over-the-counter antacids do not relieve indigestion, you may have too little acid rather than too much. Before and during meals, sip water containing a teaspoon of apple-cider vinegar, or add vinegar to meat, fish, eggs, and cheese dishes. Or start meals with a supplement of digestive acid and enzymes (available from health-food stores).

■ Flavor food with rosemary, or incorporate chicory, watercress, or artichokes into some of your meals. These bitter foods make the digestive juices flow by stimulating the production of a hormone called gastrin.

■ Drink slippery elm gruel (see p. 172) before meals.

TREATMENT

Herbal remedies: If you sense the onset of indigestion after a meal, sip a cup of one of the following teas:

■ Meadowsweet with marshmallow

Enzyme action
Eat papaya, apples, dill, or ginger with meals. These foods contain enzymes that assist digestion.

Acupressure for indigestion

● Press with your thumb over the point (St 43) on the top of the foot in the furrow between your second and third toes, where the bones merge. Press firmly, moving your thumb in little circles, for two minutes.

● Use the same technique on the point (St 44) on the top of the foot in the web linking your second and third toes.

● Apply repeated pressure with your thumb on the point (HP 6) on the inside of the forearm two thumb-widths up from the wrist crease (see p. 282). Pressing the point St 36 may also provide relief (see p. 71).

- Two teaspoons of sage steeped in a cup of boiling water
- German chamomile with fennel or peppermint, or just rosemary
- Cloves, cinnamon, and ginger, in combination
Caution: For safety concerns, see pp. 34–37.

Kitchen cabinet remedies: Apples, cabbage, carrots, extra-virgin olive oil, eggs, and parsley all have antacid or demulcent (soothing) properties that can help prevent and treat indigestion and ulcers. Incorporate normal amounts of these foods into your meals on a regular basis. Raw potato juice has similar beneficial effects.

Other therapies: Consult a naturopathic doctor for detailed advice about possible changes in your lifestyle and diet that may improve your digestion and alleviate discomfort.

Food combining

Also known as the Hay Diet, this regimen is often said to improve digestion, although scientific evidence for its value is lacking. The theory is that because protein digestion occurs in an acid environment, and starch digestion in an alkaline one, you should not eat carbohydrates, such as potatoes, pasta, or bread, with proteins, such as meat, eggs, or fish. Food combiners also recommend eating fruit only between meals. However, some people with fruit-provoked indigestion can eat fruit at the beginning of a meal without experiencing discomfort afterward, and tropical fruits, such as pineapple, usually aid digestion.

Reflexology for indigestion

Working on certain reflex points thought to relate to the digestive system may help relieve discomfort.

Foot reflexology
Support your left foot with your right hand and press your left thumb across the central area of the sole in diagonal movements.

Hand reflexology
Press with creeping movements of the thumb across the central area of the left palm.

When to get medical help

- You have frequent attacks of indigestion.
- Your symptoms are severe.
- You have rapid and unexplained weight loss.
- You experience indigestion for the first time after the age of 40.
- You have little appetite, difficulty swallowing, or an unexplained cough along with symptoms of indigestion.
- You are taking painkilling medication or your symptoms begin after starting a new medication or supplement.
- You have discomfort after exercise and are not sure whether this is indigestion.
- Heartburn is present upon awakening.

See also:
ABDOMINAL PAIN, BAD BREATH, BLOATING, CANDIDA INFECTIONS, COLIC, DIVERTICULAR DISEASE, FLATULENCE, FOOD SENSITIVITY, GALLBLADDER PROBLEMS, HICCUPS, IRRITABLE BOWEL SYNDROME, NAUSEA AND VOMITING, OVERWEIGHT, STRESS

Influenza

Popularly known as flu, influenza is caused by a number of similar viruses. It occurs more often in winter and sometimes reaches epidemic proportions. It spreads quickly, especially in schools and institutions. Most otherwise healthy people recover quickly from flu without need for medical intervention, but those in poor health should see their doctor.

Keeping infection at bay
At the first sign of flu, gargle morning and night with two drops each of antiseptic tea tree and geranium oils in half a glass of warm water.

Flu usually starts suddenly with chills, fever, aching muscles, and sneezing. Soon you may develop a sore throat, a dry cough, sensitive skin, painful eyes, weakness, and a headache. You probably won't feel hungry. The fever accompanying flu generally lasts from three to five days. It is common to feel run-down for some weeks after these symptoms have passed.

PREVENTION

Try to improve your resistance to infection before the winter flu season gets underway. If you still get the flu, it may be a milder case.

■ Eat a healthy diet (see p. 9).
■ Get some aerobic exercise each day.
   ■ Take a daily multiple vitamin and mineral supplement (including beta-carotene, vitamins C and E, flavonoids, and the minerals selenium and zinc).
      ■ Try not to get too tired or stressed.
   ■ Don't expose yourself to crowds when there's flu around.
      ■ Take echinacea tea, tincture, or tablets two or three times a week in winter. Take a dose every day if you are in close contact with someone who has the flu.
         ■ Eat garlic or take garlic tablets daily.
         ■ Every three weeks throughout the winter take flu nosode, a preventive homeopathic remedy.

Cold or flu?

Both colds and flu can cause a sore throat, cough, and runny nose. Although there's usually no mistaking flu because of the severity of symptoms, the only sure way of distinguishing a bad cold from flu is for your doctor to send nose and throat swabs to a lab. However, this is rarely necessary.

TREATMENT

Treat flu carefully because it can cause serious complications. Stay at home so that you don't spread infection, and stay in bed because you need your strength to fight the flu viruses. Follow the recommendations for reducing fever on pages 206–207. Be wary of over-the-counter medicines that may mask unpleasant symptoms and make you think you can be up and about when you're actually still sick. Stay home for at least one day after your temperature has returned to normal.

Diet

■ Drink plenty of nonalcoholic, caffeine-free fluids, including water, fruit juice, barley water (see illustration, p. 358), and herbal teas (see facing page). Sipping black currant tea may soothe your sore throat even as it provides extra vitamin C, which helps fight infection.

Herbal remedies

- Drink echinacea tea three times a day, or take 200 milligrams of the supplement five times a day.
- A tea made from elderflower, peppermint, yarrow, and boneset may bring down a fever and reduce aches and pains.
- Elderberry extract may help stop flu viruses from multiplying.

Caution: For safety concerns, see pp. 34–37.

Aromatherapy

- Cajuput oil helps reduce fever and ease aching muscles. Add two drops of this essential oil to a tablespoon of jojoba oil and smooth behind the ears, over the forehead, on each side of your nose, and on your chest four times a day. Or add six to eight drops of cajuput oil to a warm (not hot) bath. Do not use this oil if you are in the first 20 weeks of pregnancy.
- Soothe congestion with steam inhalations, scented with a few drops of tea tree or eucalyptus oil (see p. 141).

Nature's medicine chest
The elder tree provides many remedies. The flowers and berries may ease colds and flu, the leaves may soothe bruises, and the inner green bark has been used as a purgative.

Homeopathy

- Aconite: if you suddenly become feverish, especially after catching a chill.
- Eupatorium: if the aching feels as though it is penetrating your bones.
- Gelsemium: if shivering and shaking are predominant symptoms.
- Oscillococcinum: as an overall remedy (take within the first 36 hours of the onset of your flulike symptoms).

Should you get a flu shot?

Immunization is especially recommended for people who are likely to become seriously ill with flu. These groups include:

- The elderly, particularly those with a history of frequent colds and/or flu.
- Those with long-term heart, lung, liver or kidney disease, diabetes, or sickle cell anemia.
- Those on corticosteroid or immuno-suppressant drugs.
- Those with no spleen.
- Those who live in residential care or nursing homes. Flu vaccine is also recommended for the staff in these homes and those who work in hospitals and clinics.

When to get medical help

- You are no better after a week or your symptoms worsen after three or four days.
- Symptoms remain after four weeks or recur.
- You cough up lots of green or yellow phlegm.
- You are among those for whom flu immunization is especially recommended.

Get help right away if:

- You experience chest pain or breathlessness.
- You have a stiff neck, a severe headache, an aversion to bright light, a rash, confusion, or severe joint pain.
- You cough up blood.

See also:
COLDS,
COUGHS,
FEVER,
HEADACHE,
SORE THROAT

Insect Bites and Stings

Blood-sucking insects, such as mosquitoes, inflict tiny puncture wounds when they bite. The stings from bees, wasps, and hornets contain venom. People vary in their reactions to bites and stings, but in most cases symptoms last only a day or two.

An allergic response to an insect's saliva or venom causes pain or itching, redness, and swelling at the site of a bite or sting. Some people experience a severe reaction to insect stings—a life-threatening swelling of the airways. Certain ticks transmit such diseases as Rocky Mountain spotted fever and Lyme disease, and mosquitoes cause malaria in some parts of the world.

PREVENTION

Keep your skin covered if you are in an area where insect bites are likely. Screen windows and doors. Repel insects by adding five drops of citronella oil to a cup of water and dabbing on exposed skin. Eat garlic and take a daily supplement of vitamin B_1 (thiamine) and zinc.

TREATMENT

General measures: Distilled witch hazel and calamine lotion are effective for soothing pain and itching from mosquito bites and other bites and stings. An ice cube, aloe vera gel, or onion juice are also good remedies.

Bee sting: Remove a bee stinger by pressing it out sideways with a thumbnail. Afterward, press out any poison.

Pain-relief paste
For a bee sting or ant bite, add baking soda or meat tenderizer to a little water and apply to the painful area.

Wasp sting: Apply lemon juice, vinegar, or cinnamon tea as soon as possible after being stung. Repeat if necessary.

Tick bite: If the tick is clinging to the skin, dislodge it by covering it with oil or petroleum jelly. Then gently twist it out with tweezers.

Homeopathy: Apply Hypercal cream and take Apis (if the bite is swollen and red), Arnica (if there is bruising and soreness), or Cantharis (if burning pain is predominant).

Aromatherapy: For any sting, apply one drop each of lavender and tea tree oils hourly.

When to get medical help

- With a suspected tick bite, you have localized redness or a circular rash, flulike symptoms, or joint pain.

Get help right way if:
- The wound is from a spider or scorpion.
- The bite or sting is on the face or in the mouth or throat, or you have hives, breathing difficulty, nausea, or vomiting.

See also:
ITCHING

258

Irritable Bowel Syndrome

*T*he most common of all intestinal disorders, irritable bowel syndrome may affect as many as one in three people in the Western world at some time. The condition tends to be recurrent, although symptoms can subside for long periods between attacks. Orthodox medicine offers no certain cure, but there are many natural ways of managing and easing symptoms.

Irritable bowel syndrome, or IBS, consists of a number of related symptoms, including intermittent abdominal pain and irregular bowel movements. The disorder is caused by a disturbance in the normal muscle movements of the wall of the large intestine. This creates problems in the way food moves through the digestive tract, which leads to diarrhea or constipation and/or pain from intestinal muscle spasms. The nerves in the intestinal wall may also overreact to painful stimuli, such as intestinal distension. IBS affects twice as many females as males. In some cases the disorder may result from too much or too little stomach acid or inadequate digestive enzymes (see "Indigestion," pp. 252–255, and "Food Sensitivity," pp. 212–215).

SYMPTOMS

Different individuals have different combinations of symptoms, which can also vary in severity from time to time in any one person. Most people who suffer from IBS have more than one of the following symptoms:

- Lower abdominal pain, eased temporarily by having a bowel movement or passing gas
- Bloating after a meal
- A rumbling stomach
- Excessive flatulence
- Diarrhea, especially early in the morning
- Constipation
- Alternating constipation and diarrhea
- A sense that the bowels are never completely empty, even after defecation
- Mucus in the feces

Headaches, fatigue, and depression are also common with IBS. Other associated symptoms include pain in the back or thighs, heavy or painful menstrual periods, pain during sexual intercourse for women, and a frequent or urgent need to urinate.

If you have IBS, your intestines may react adversely to one or more triggers. Possibilities include smoking, antibiotics, certain foods, a changing level of estrogen, excessive exercise, and anxiety, depression, and other forms of stress.

Several disorders produce symptoms that can easily be confused with those of IBS, including lactose intolerance, pelvic inflammatory disease, and endometriosis (a condition in which uterine lining cells stray into the abdomen, where they may cause pain, diarrhea, and other digestive symptoms by bleeding within the abdomen).

Many people find IBS much easier to live with once they have a diagnosis and realize that their symptoms are not the result of a serious underlying disease.

PREVENTION

This condition occurs less frequently in those who adhere to a high fiber diet. Therefore, a

valuable preventive measure is to consume natural, unprocessed foods, including a high proportion of vegetables and fruits. Regular moderate exercise seems to help regulate intestinal muscle action, and those who are physically active may be less susceptible to IBS. Dealing effectively with the stress in your life is a further key to preventing the disorder. If you smoke, stop or at least cut down. Smoking stimulates the release of epinephrine, a neurotransmitter that can interfere with the regular contraction of the intestines.

Time for yourself
IBS is closely linked to stress and tension. Try to find 20 minutes or so every day when you can relax on your own in a quiet place.

TREATMENT

Stress management: Because IBS is associated with emotional tension, learning to deal positively with the pressures in your life is essential. Practice meditation or another relaxation technique (see, for example, "Relaxation Through Yoga," p. 69). Anytime you're relaxing, focus your mind on a peaceful image, or on the air entering or leaving your body, to exclude intrusive and worrisome thoughts.

Yoga: Regular yoga practice can improve symptoms within a few weeks for some people. Follow a balanced program that emphasizes breathing exercises and deep relaxation.

Diet: Food is a significant factor in IBS, but no single diet helps everyone. Unless you are knowledgeable about nutrition, get advice from a doctor, naturopathic physician, or dietitian before making radical changes in your eating habits.

- If constipation is a problem, gradually introducing more fiber-rich foods (whole grains, fruits, and vegetables) may help. However, insoluble fiber (in rice, nuts, bread and other foods containing wheat or rye, and the skins and seeds of fruit) may make symptoms worse. In this case, boost fiber intake with foods containing only soluble fiber (peeled fruits and vegetables, peas and beans, rice bran, and oatmeal and other oat-containing foods). This type of fiber soothes the digestive tract, as well as producing bulkier stools.
- If you suspect food sensitivity, identify the foods that may be responsible (such as milk and other dairy products, wheat, and animal fat). You may have a food allergy or an inability to digest such foods properly—for example, if you produce too little of certain digestive enzymes.
- Limit your intake of alcohol and spicy foods.
- You may benefit from replacing animal fats with vegetable oils, especially those that are

cold-pressed. Try canola, olive, safflower, sunflower, and walnut oils.

■ Eat smaller, more frequent meals.

Supplements: IBS is sometimes associated with an unbalanced population of microorganisms in the intestine, perhaps following gastroenteritis or a course of antibiotics. If this is the case, take a preparation containing *Lactobacillus acidophilus* bacteria daily, or eat yogurt with live cultures.

Exercise: Regular exercise can soothe abnormal contractions of the intestine and thereby help reduce the symptoms of IBS. Get a half hour of moderate exercise, such as brisk walking, every day.

Herbal remedies

■ Peppermint helps relax the muscle of the intestinal wall. It is especially good for soothing abdominal pain accompanied by flatulence. Drink it as a tea (one or two cups daily), add fresh leaves to salads or cooked dishes, or take enteric-coated oil capsules (one capsule three times a day, between meals).

■ To relax the intestines and soothe inflammation, drink teas or tinctures made from a combination of wild yam, chamomile, peppermint, agrimony, marshmallow, and goldenseal, up to six times daily. When you are especially tense, add hops and extra chamomile.

■ Cinnamon and ginger may help relieve

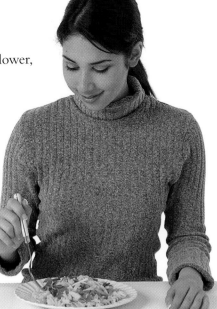

Relaxing mealtimes
Eat slowly and calmly, concentrating on chewing well and tasting and enjoying your food. Don't force yourself to eat when you are not hungry, and stop when you have had enough.

abdominal pain and expel gas. Add a good pinch of one of these powdered spices to slippery elm gruel (see p. 172), or add grated fresh ginger to one of the teas described above.

■ To help prevent constipation, take aloe vera juice or capsules (not to be confused with aloe latex) each day. As an alternative, try plantain seed gel, made by soaking two teaspoons of seeds in half a cup of water. Leave for 30 minutes before drinking the concoction.

Caution: For safety concerns, see pp. 34–37.

Aromatherapy

■ If stress makes your IBS symptoms worse, have an occasional relaxing soak in a warm bath. Add to the water three drops each of geranium and juniper berry oils and two of peppermint oil. Omit juniper berry oil if you are or might be pregnant.

■ To relieve diarrhea, add three drops each of tea tree and peppermint oils, and two each of geranium and sandalwood oils, to one fluid ounce of grapeseed or sweet almond oil. Use this to massage the lower abdomen with gentle circling movements, or ask a friend to give you a lower back massage.

Homeopathy

■ Colocynthis: for abdominal pain that comes in waves and makes you want to double up; is worse after eating, moving, or being touched; and is better with warmth.

■ Argentum: for diarrhea and gas that are worse if you have nervous tension or eat sugar.

➤ *continued, p. 262*

261

Reflexology for IBS

Hand reflexology is very convenient for self-treatment. The following technique may ease pain resulting from muscle spasms in the intestines. For the foot reflexology sequence (right), you'll need a partner.

1 Holding your right hand palm-upward, press with your left thumb on a point two finger-widths above the wrist crease, below the center of the little finger.

2 Move your thumb to the edge of your hand, and make tiny, creeping movements down the outer edge of the palm in a straight line until you reach the heel of the hand.

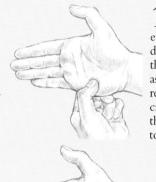

1 On the right foot, starting on the inside edge, press down and draw your thumb along the line above the heel, as shown. When you reach the outside edge, crook your thumb back toward you.

2 Still working on the right foot, use your left thumb to work the area between the ball of the foot and the heel, moving from the inner to the outer edge of the foot.

3 Work on the area described in the previous step on the left foot. There is no need to reverse hands.

■ Podophyllum: for painless diarrhea.
■ Sulfur: a general tonic for the intestines, but especially if you have a sensation of heat or burning and gas or bloating.

Other therapies: Hypnotherapy has one of the best success rates for IBS of any therapy. Initially, have treatment from a trained practitioner. Then ask the practitioner to demonstrate self-hypnosis techniques to use at home. Biofeedback is another useful therapy, which, once learned, can be practiced at home. Acupuncture, chiropractic, and osteopathy may also be effective.

When to get medical help

- You have recurring symptoms of IBS (see p. 259) and have not had an expert diagnosis.
- You notice black feces.

Get help right away if:
- You notice blood in the feces.
- Mild fever or abdominal pain or swelling suddenly becomes severe, or you develop severe diarrhea or constipation.

See also:
ABDOMINAL PAIN,
ANXIETY, BLOATING,
CONSTIPATION,
DEPRESSION, DIARRHEA,
DIVERTICULAR DISEASE,
FATIGUE, FLATULENCE,
FOOD SENSITIVITY,
INDIGESTION, STRESS

Itching

The intense, annoying, tickling sensation of itching may be felt over the entire body or in one area. There are a number of different causes of itching, including allergy, dry skin, and irritation from household or industrial chemicals. Some people, including many pregnant women and elderly folks, have especially sensitive skin.

Cooling inflammation
When you feel an urge to scratch, instead apply a wet, cold compress to the affected area.

Itching is often caused by excessive washing or bathing, harsh soaps, bath products and detergents, and rough clothing. In rare cases, generalized itching may arise from an underlying untreated condition, such as diabetes, a thyroid problem, or jaundice. It can also be a side effect of certain medications, or it may indicate a food sensitivity or other allergic reaction. Itching is a symptom of many skin conditions, including eczema, psoriasis, and wound healing, but often the reason for it remains unknown.

PREVENTION

If you are aware of an external cause for your itching, avoid it or at least minimize your contact. Don't use anything that dries out the skin, such as talcum powder and scented bath products. Use soaps and other toiletries formulated for sensitive skin. Soften dry, scaly skin with moisturizer or an emollient cream.

TREATMENT
General advice

- Try not to scratch, since this aggravates the irritation. It may also break or damage the skin and lead to infection.
- Avoid long, hot baths, which dry out the skin and may increase irritation.
- Use a mild, non-soap cleanser, or wash only with water.

Herbal remedies: The anti-inflammatory herbs marigold (calendula), chamomile, and chickweed are ideal for soothing itchy skin.

- Make a cold compress with marigold or chickweed tea and apply to the affected area.
- Add strong chickweed tea to your bath. Pour three cups of boiling water over 10 teaspoons of dried chickweed. Leave to steep for 15 minutes, then add to the bathwater and soak in it.
- Apply chamomile or calendula ointment.

Kitchen cabinet remedies: Add two tablespoons of cider vinegar or two cups of coarse (colloidal) oatmeal (from the drugstore) to warm bathwater. Relax in the tub for up to 15 minutes.

When to get medical help

- Itching continues even with treatment.
- Your skin becomes inflamed or infected.
- You suspect an underlying condition.
- You are pregnant and have persistent itching.

See also:
DERMATITIS, DIABETES, DRY SKIN, FUNGAL SKIN INFECTIONS, HAIR AND SCALP PROBLEMS, HEAD LICE, HIVES, INSECT BITES AND STINGS, PINWORMS, SKIN PROBLEMS

Jet Lag and In-flight Health

Flying through different time zones either shortens (going east) or lengthens (going west) a traveler's day. This disrupts the normal sleep-wake cycle and disturbs the body's usual hormonal rhythms, leading to jet lag. Flying can also have other ill effects on your well-being as a result of fluid depletion and long periods of immobility.

Throughout the 24-hour day, our bodily functions, such as alertness, temperature, sexual interest, and sleepiness, vary according to predictable rhythms. This happens in response to environmental factors, including time, temperature, and light levels. The hormonal activity responsible for these "biorhythms" is orchestrated by the hypothalamus and the pituitary and pineal glands in the brain. The pineal gland, for example, responds to the level of ambient light by producing a hormone called melatonin. Production rises as light falls in the evening, continues during the hours of darkness, and ceases as day dawns. Your body's melatonin level influences whether or not you are ready for sleep.

All these biorhythms are disrupted by a long-haul flight, producing the symptoms of jet lag. The symptoms, similar to those of a hangover, include fatigue, a desire to sleep during the day, and difficulty in sleeping during your new night-time. Memory and concentration may also be impaired. An eastward flight tends to produce more severe jet lag than a westward journey.

Flying entails other health threats besides jet lag. Breathing dry, recycled air on long flights can lead to dehydration, dry skin, and headaches. Sitting still for long periods can cause swollen feet and ankles and an increased risk of developing a potentially serious blood clot in a vein deep in the leg. Some people also suffer from stress as a result of a fear of flying.

PREVENTION
Before you go
- Have several good nights' sleep before traveling, so you don't start your flight already tired.
- When traveling east, begin to accustom yourself to what will be your new bedtime by going to bed an hour or two earlier for several nights.
- When traveling west, begin to accustom yourself to what will be your new bedtime by going to bed an hour or two later for several nights.

Gaining and losing hours
When traveling east to west, you lengthen your day. For example, after a five-hour flight from New York to San Francisco the local time of your arrival is only two hours later, so you "gain" three hours. When traveling west to east, you shorten your day. After a seven-hour flight from New York to Rome, the local time of your arrival is 13 hours later, so you "lose" six hours.

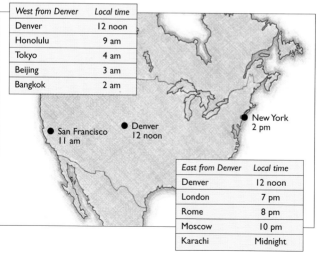

West from Denver	Local time
Denver	12 noon
Honolulu	9 am
Tokyo	4 am
Beijing	3 am
Bangkok	2 am

East from Denver	Local time
Denver	12 noon
London	7 pm
Rome	8 pm
Moscow	10 pm
Karachi	Midnight

San Francisco 11 am • Denver 12 noon • New York 2 pm

During the flight

- Set your watch to your destination's local time as soon as you board. Then, on the flight, begin to adjust your sleep-wake cycle to this time to reduce the adjustment your body has to make when you arrive.
- Prevent dehydration by drinking plenty of water or soft drinks. Avoid alcohol and caffeine, which can encourage fluid loss, and carbonated drinks, which may cause bloating.
- What you eat may also affect how you feel after flying. Avoid having foods on the plane that you don't usually eat. Take some fruit with you for a healthy snack.
- Walk around for 5 to 10 minutes at least every two hours. This helps prevent your ankles and feet from swelling and makes a blood clot in the legs less likely. Massaging your ankles and calves, using upward strokes, is also helpful.
- Don't cross your legs while sitting, as this encourages ankle swelling.
- Promote sleep with breathing exercises (p. 87) and progressive muscular relaxation (p. 245).
- Counteract tension with a neck and shoulder massage or by sprinkling a tissue with a few drops of a relaxing essential oil (such as lavender or geranium) and inhaling the scent.

TREATMENT

On arrival during the day

- Go outdoors immediately, and stay there for at least an hour. Exposure to bright light helps the body clock readjust.
- Try to make yourself stay awake (or take only a very short nap). Go to bed at the local time.

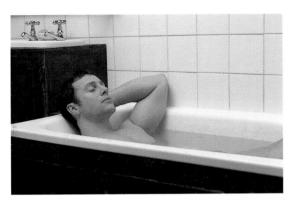

A wake-up bath
After you've been on a long flight, add a few drops of peppermint or eucalyptus oil to a bath. These oils are stimulating and will help revive you.

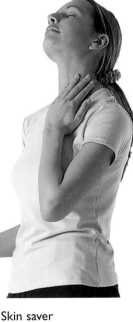

Skin saver
Apply moisturizer to your face and hands at regular intervals during the flight to counteract the drying effects of recirculated cabin air.

- Get some exercise—outdoors, if possible—to help you stay awake.

On arrival at night

- Go to bed at the normal hour, even if you don't feel sleepy. If you can't sleep, practice progressive muscular relaxation (see p. 245).
- To help you sleep, use a few drops of lavender or geranium oil in a bath.

Flower essences: Take Walnut to help your body adjust to the new time zone.

When to get medical help

- Severe jet lag lasts longer than a week.
- You have recurring, disruptive jet lag.

Get help right away if:
- On arrival, you experience a debilitating headache or any other type of internal pain.

See also:
SLEEPING DIFFICULTIES

265

Kidney Stones

When the urine is too rich in certain mineral salts, a stone may form in the kidney. This occurrence occasionally follows a urinary-tract infection. If the stone moves out of the kidney and lodges in the ureter, the duct to the bladder, it causes waves of intense pain, known as renal colic. Kidney stones affect men three times as often as they do women.

Most kidney stones result from excess oxalic acid, which produces stones composed of calcium oxalate. Less commonly, stones result from too much uric acid. Stones are less likely to develop if you drink plenty of water-based fluids to dilute the urine; limit your consumption of animal protein, fat, added sugar, and alcohol; and lose any excess weight. Don't smoke, since cadmium from smoke encourages stones.

TREATMENT
Diet
- Drink six to eight glasses of water a day.
- If you have calcium oxalate stones, eat fewer foods containing oxalates, such as beets, celery, cucumber, grapefruit, parsley, rhubarb, spinach, strawberries, sweet potatoes, nuts, chocolate, tea, and cola. Eat more foods rich in calcium, magnesium, potassium, and vitamin B_6 (see p. 12). You may want to consult a dietitian.
- If you have uric acid stones, cut down on foods containing purine—red meat, fish, shellfish, whole grains, beans, cauliflower, peas, spinach.

From the drugstore
- Daily supplements of vitamin B_6 (40 milligrams), magnesium (300 milligrams), and potassium citrate (150 milligrams) may help.

Herbal remedies: Drink two or three cups daily of corn silk, buchu, or couch grass tea. Caution: For safety concerns, see pp. 34–37.

The effect of calcium

Calcium in the diet may help prevent calcium oxalate stones—probably because calcium combines with oxalate in the intestine and so prevents the absorption of pure oxalate. Foods rich in calcium include milk, cheese, and yogurt (these can be low-fat), sardines, dark green leafy vegetables, nuts, seeds, and dried fruits. Taking calcium supplements during or just after meals may have a similar effect; however, taking them between meals can increase the risk of stones. You may want to ask your doctor about dosage and timing.

When to get medical help
- You have intense intermittent pain, probably starting in the back and moving to the groin.

Get help right away if:
- You have blood in your urine.

See also:
URINARY-TRACT INFECTIONS

Leg Cramps

Sudden muscle spasms can cause pain severe enough to make a person cry out. They usually strike the calf muscle but sometimes affect the foot, arm, or hand. For most people cramps are only an occasional nuisance, but for others they are a frequent occurrence. Home remedies can help, and simple lifestyle changes may prevent the problem from recurring.

Stretch for relief
When you have a cramp, lean forward against a wall, placing the affected leg out behind you with the foot flat.

The pain of a cramp results from excessive, prolonged, and unusual muscle contraction. Possible causes include a build-up of lactic acid in an overused muscle, nerve damage from repeated movement, sitting or lying in an awkward position, and poor circulation.

PREVENTION

- Eat fresh green vegetables (especially watercress and parsley), fresh fruits, whole grains, and low-fat dairy products to provide your muscles with the calcium, iron, magnesium, potassium, and zinc they need to function properly. Make sure you drink plenty of fluids.
- Get moderate daily exercise, but if this involves a repeated movement, such as when running or swimming, stretch and relax your muscles for five minutes every half hour.
- Take a warm bath before retiring and keep warm in bed.
- Avoid either too much or too little salt, since both extremes can cause cramps.
- Drink a cup of tea made from cramp bark, chamomile, and vervain before going to bed.

TREATMENT

Ease a cramp by stretching the contracted muscle (see photograph). Then knead and squeeze the muscle to disperse any remaining tension.

Acupressure

With your thumb, press the point (B 57) in the middle of the back of your calf where the muscle and the tendon meet. Begin with a brushing action, and build up to more force. Then press the point (B 54) in the middle of the crease at the back of your knee for a few seconds. Don't do this if you're pregnant.

Aromatherapy: Apply a hot compress made with lavender, marjoram, or ginger oil. Mix one or two drops of oil into a bowl of hot water. Lay a cloth on the surface of the water. Gently wring out and apply to the leg, oily side down.

Homeopathy: Apply Arnica cream to the affected muscle.

When to get medical help

- You suffer from frequent leg cramps.
- You experience leg cramps when walking.
- A leg cramp persists longer than an hour.
- A leg cramp is associated with circulation problems.

Memory Loss

We all experience forgetfulness from time to time, especially when preoccupied or under stress. Short-term memory loss also becomes more frequent during middle age. If you often forget where you've left something or have difficulty remembering people's names, you may need to learn ways to improve your memory. Simple lifestyle changes can make a big difference as well.

DID YOU KNOW?

There's some suspicion that microwave exposure from prolonged and repeated use of a cellular phone can impair short-term memory. Until the evidence is clearer, consider reserving your cell phone for occasional short conversations. Use a radiation-absorbing phone case or a hands-free adaptor.

The computer cannot compare with the miracle of the human brain, but there are some similarities. Both receive, store, and recall information, and each can fall prey to problems with these processes. Just as you can enhance a computer's memory, so too you can optimize your own.

Memory loss among older people may be the result of poor blood flow to the brain coupled with lack of mental stimulation. However, there are other causes of impaired memory—anemia, an underactive thyroid, depression, and chronic fatigue syndrome—that may need to be ruled out. A poor diet and excessive alcohol intake may also be factors. Alzheimer's disease is a less common cause of memory loss in the elderly.

PREVENTION

Reduce your risk of memory loss from poor circulation with a half hour's daily exercise, and by not smoking. Brain function is affected by nutrition, so be sure to eat a healthy diet (see p. 9). This is especially important as you get older, because you need fewer calories to meet your energy needs, and you absorb nutrients less efficiently.

Optimizing your memory

Try to present your brain with information in the way it prefers. Some people memorize best by seeing, others by hearing, and still others by the use of other senses. For example, if you learn best via your ears, record information on tape.

Jog your memory
- Use written memory aids, such as lists and diary entries.
- Mentally run through the alphabet when searching for a word.
- Refresh your long-term memory regularly with photographs, videos, letters, and other memorabilia.
- Use mnemonics—for example, "Every Good Boy Does Fine" for the notes on the lines of the music staff (E, G, B, D, F).

Train your brain
Use these memory-enhancing tricks:
- Keep repeating a new fact to yourself.
- Recall each day's events before falling asleep.
- Help to remember names by creating pictures from them. Mr. Lightfoot, for example, could be visualized as a lightbulb with a foot.

Stay interested
- Try to keep up with family, community, national, and world events.
- Keep your brain alert by reading, engaging in stimulating conversation, and doing crossword and other puzzles.
- Take up a new intellectual endeavor—for example, learning a foreign language.
- Make new friends and enjoy old relationships.

TREATMENT

Even if you have been absent-minded for some time, it is never too late to take steps to improve your memory or slow memory loss.

Diet

■ Eat frequent small meals to maintain a stable blood-sugar level, which is important for optimum mental function.

■ Eat plenty of whole grains, nuts, seeds, fruits, vegetables, and legumes. These foods contain high concentrations of beta-carotene, folic acid, calcium, copper, iron, iodine, magnesium, manganese, selenium, zinc, essential fatty acids, and vitamins B, C, and E. These nutrients are vital for maintaining the health of the brain and its blood supply.

■ Eat three servings of oily fish weekly. These are rich in brain-friendly omega-3 essential fatty acids, including DHA (docosahexaenoic acid) and phospholipids (important constituents of all membranes).

■ Don't drink too much alcohol.

From the drugstore: If you think your diet may be lacking in essential nutrients, consider taking the following supplements:

■ A multiple vitamin and mineral preparation.
■ Vitamin E.
■ Fish oil.

■ Phosphatidyl serine. The brain uses this phospholipid during memory recall, and supplements can slow age-related memory loss.

Breathing: The rapid, shallow breathing that accompanies anxiety reduces the brain's oxygen supply and, if prolonged, can interfere with memory. Use special strategies to handle the stress in your life (see p. 347). Yoga-based breathing exercises (p. 54), regular meditation, and/or other relaxation exercises may help improve memory.

Herbal helper
Ginkgo biloba may improve brain functioning and may prevent further short-term memory loss in people with Alzheimer's and other types of dementia. Take it as a tea or as a supplement.

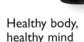

Healthy body, healthy mind
A half hour's daily vigorous exercise improves the brain's blood supply for more than 24 hours. It will also help you sleep soundly. Interrupted or inadequate sleep can contribute to forgetfulness.

When to get medical help

- You have severe or rapidly worsening memory loss.
- You are depressed.
- You have just started taking, or have increased the dose of, a prescribed drug.

Get help right away if:
- You suffer sudden memory loss following a head injury or loss of consciousness.

See also:
AGING, ANEMIA, ANXIETY, ARTERIAL DISEASE, CHRONIC FATIGUE SYNDROME, DEPRESSION, SLEEPING DIFFICULTIES, STRESS

Menopausal Problems

When menstruation ceases—usually between the ages of 45 and 55—a woman's natural capacity to bear children also ends. Menopause is the start of a new phase of life, which may bring exciting opportunities. However, this transition may also trigger physical and emotional problems, many of which respond to simple measures.

The timing of menopause is determined not only by genes, but also by medical conditions and by such lifestyle factors as smoking, diet, and stress levels. It is caused by reduced production of hormones by the ovaries, as the number of eggs in the ovaries dwindles. The supply of the hormone estrogen begins to fall before menopause, drops faster for a while afterward, then stabilizes. The same thing happens with progesterone, the other female sex hormone, but most experts think it is the reduced estrogen level that causes the majority of symptoms.

Especially if fertility has been at the heart of your sense of worth, you may experience a lowering of self-esteem at this time. Together with other possible major life changes—such as children leaving home, divorce, and elderly parents growing frail or ill—menopause can create a

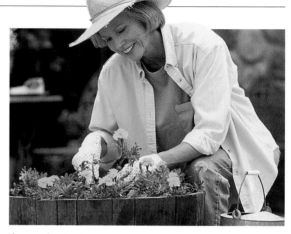

A new beginning
For many women, menopause signals the start of a time in life to concentrate on their own interests.

sense of multiple losses. If you are also dissatisfied with your life—struggling with a demanding job or other burdens—you may find this a hard time. On the other hand, you may welcome the release from menstruation and worries about contraception and the possibility of pregnancy. You may also enjoy increased freedom from responsibilities and discover a new zest for life.

SIGNS AND SYMPTOMS

Apart from the cessation of periods, the most common signs of menopause—experienced by four out of five women and sometimes predating the end of menstruation—are hot flashes and

Hormone replacement therapy

Many women are prescribed estrogen and progestogen supplements to counteract the adverse effects of menopause—not only such symptoms as hot flashes but also an increased risk of heart disease and osteoporosis. Such hormone replacement therapy (HRT) can be very effective, but it also carries possible long-term risks—in particular, that of breast cancer. Some evidence suggests that an HRT program involving treatment breaks may be the best option. Discuss the issues with your doctor, including whether natural therapies, such as consuming soy products, may offer a sound alternative to HRT in your case.

night sweats. These symptoms may continue for weeks, months, or even years. Many women find them to be little, if any, problem, but about 25 percent seek help because they interfere with sleep or are embarrassing or uncomfortable during the day. Vaginal dryness, leading to pain during intercourse, may occur. Other symptoms may include headaches, fatigue, insomnia, and depression. The skin may become thinner and drier.

Other body changes take place around this time as part of the natural aging process. The bones become less dense, and the risk of osteoporosis (weak, fragile bones prone to fracture) increases. Heart disease and strokes become more likely after menopause, largely because of the reduction in the protective effect of the female hormones.

Fit and active
Exercising regularly throughout menopause is one of the best ways to ease symptoms. There is evidence that aerobic exercise can boost estrogen levels.

PREVENTION

You will have a lower risk of osteoporosis if you have had plenty of calcium, magnesium, and other bone-building nutrients in your diet throughout your life. Regular weight-bearing exercise, such as walking or dancing, also boosts bone-mineral density. To protect against arterial disease, do an aerobic exercise, such as jogging or swimming, three times a week. Choosing the right foods can help ward

off heart attacks, strokes, and other forms of arterial disease (see pp. 92–95), as well as hot flashes and other menopausal symptoms.

Stress management is useful at any time, but after menopause it has the additional benefit of preventing a stress-induced fall in estrogen. This, along with regular sexual activity, reduces the risk of developing vaginal dryness.

TREATMENT

Diet: Foods that supply calcium, essential fatty acids, plant hormones, and vitamins C and E help maintain strong bones and the proper balance of various blood fats. They also help guard against hot flashes, night sweats, and vaginal dryness.

➤ continued, p. 272

A "Japanese" diet
For menopausal health, eat foods that contain plant hormones, including soy products, celery, fennel, rhubarb, alfalfa, fruits, whole grains, and flaxseeds. Essential fatty acids found in oily fish are also vital.

271

Women who eat a diet that includes soy products—such as tofu, tempeh, soy flour, and soybeans—have fewer hot flashes and night sweats. Research suggests that the plant hormones found in high concentrations in soy products mimic the action of human estrogen and thereby compensate for falling hormone levels. Most important, plant hormones can help block the action of estrogen when fluctuating hormone levels create an imbalance in the ratio of estrogen to progesterone.

Foods rich in essential fatty acids are critical for hormone production, as well as for healthy skin and nerves. Eat nuts, seeds, and whole grains; three helpings a week of oily fish (such as salmon, mackerel, tuna, and sardines); and cold-pressed vegetable oils.

Drink at least six glasses of water a day. If hot flashes are a problem, reduce your intake of hot drinks, especially tea and coffee, and avoid spicy foods and alcohol. Wean yourself off caffeinated drinks slowly by blending them with increasing amounts of decaffeinated coffee or tea. Stopping cold-turkey can lead to headaches.

Exercise: Regular exercise helps relieve depression, possibly by raising the level of endorphins, hormone-like substances that lift mood. It may also reduce hot flashes and, when combined with a healthy diet, make weight control easier and more permanent by raising your metabolic rate. Exercise also helps prevent or slow osteoporosis.

From the drugstore: Useful nutritional supplements include:

- Vitamin C and flavonoids: for hot flashes
- Vitamin E: for hot flashes and vaginal dryness
- A vitamin supplement designed for menopause, especially if you are not eating well
- Vitamin B complex and magnesium: for mild depression or anxiety
- Fish oil: for hormone production (if insufficient in your diet)

Herbal remedies: Many herbs rebalance hormone levels, often by acting as mild estrogens. For an all-round benefit, take red or purple sage and/or dong quai. You can also try flaxseed oil or evening primrose oil. For specific menopausal symptoms, try the following:

- Teas or supplements of chasteberry, black cohosh, or motherwort for hot flashes and/or night sweats.

Acupressure for symptoms

To alleviate hot flashes, night sweats, and anxiety, treat the points shown for two minutes each, every other day.

- Apply pressure with your thumb or fingertip, using a small, firm circling motion, on the point (H 6) half a thumb-width above the wrist crease, on the little-finger side of the forearm.

- Apply firm stationary pressure with thumb or fingertip to the point (K 6) a thumb-width below the tip of the inside ankle bone.

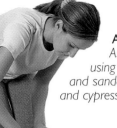

An aromatic relaxant
Ask a friend to give you a back massage using this mixture: two drops each of rose otto and sandalwood oils and three drops each of neroli and cypress oils in five teaspoons of sweet almond oil.

■ Peppermint, which has cooling qualities, is useful for treating hot flashes. Drink peppermint tea regularly, and carry a bottle of peppermint oil with you to relieve symptoms when they occur: sprinkle a few drops of the oil onto a tissue and inhale deeply.
■ St. John's wort for sleeping difficulties and depression.
■ Motherwort for anxiety.
■ Motherwort or dong quai for vaginal dryness.
Caution: For safety concerns, see pp. 34–37.

Herbal helpers
Peppermint, chasteberry, black cohosh, motherwort, St. John's wort, and dong quai may all alleviate menopausal symptoms. Yarrow may help regulate excessive menstrual flow in the months preceding cessation of menstruation, but avoid it if you have hot flashes.

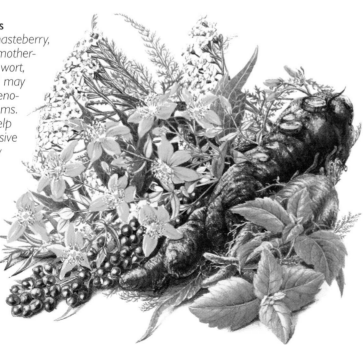

Aromatherapy: Essential oils that may help regulate hormone production include neroli, sandalwood, lavender, clary sage, rose otto, and geranium. To prevent a recurrence of hot flashes or other symptoms, add three drops of clary sage and two drops each of rose otto and geranium oils to a daily bath. A few drops of lavender oil in a vaporizer can help promote relaxation.

Flower essences
■ Larch: for lack of confidence.
■ Mustard: for depression with no apparent cause.
■ Scleranthus: for mood swings.
■ Walnut: to help you cope with change.

Homeopathy
■ Sepia: for hot flashes, anxiety, painful sex, and/or a decline in libido.
■ Lachesis: for hot flashes, heavy bleeding, night sweats, uterine cramps, and/or irritability.
■ Calendula ointment: for vaginal dryness.
■ Pulsatilla: for hot flashes, overwhelming emotions, or mood swings.

When to get medical help
● You have menopausal symptoms that are severe or suddenly change.

See also:
AGING, ANXIETY, ARTERIAL
DISEASE, DEPRESSION,
MENSTRUAL PROBLEMS,
OSTEOPOROSIS, SEX DRIVE
LOSS, STRESS, VAGINAL
PROBLEMS

Menstrual Problems

The delicate hormonal balance of the monthly menstrual cycle can be easily upset by such factors as stress, a change in weight or diet, and too little or too much exercise. Menstrual problems include painful or heavy periods, and irregular or infrequent periods. It is often possible to relieve symptoms by normalizing hormone levels naturally, without drugs.

Pain during a period (dysmenorrhea) is the most common menstrual problem, especially among teenage girls and young women. It often abates after the age of 25 and after childbirth. Symptoms, which usually start just before a period and last up to 12 hours, may be severe enough to interfere with everyday life.

Menstrual pain, felt as a cramping in the lower abdomen, often comes in waves and may be accompanied by low back pain and nausea. The cramps are caused by contractions of the uterus and are associated with high levels of hormone-like substances called prostaglandins. An unhealthy diet and a lack of exercise can make cramps worse.

If you start to experience such pain in your 40s or if it recurs after years of pain-free periods, it may be due to an underlying disorder, such as endometriosis, a condition in which patches of uterine-lining cells stray into the pelvic cavity and settle on other organs. Each month these cells swell and bleed, and they may inflame the underlying tissues.

Heavy periods are most likely soon after the onset of menstruation and in your late 30s and 40s. Possible causes include a hormonal imbalance from an unhealthy diet, stress, pelvic inflammatory disease, fibroids, or endometriosis.

Irregular or infrequent periods are common during the first few years after the start of menstruation, until regular ovulation is established. Periods may also be irregular in the few years before menopause. Disrupted periods and bleeding between periods may also be associated with difficulty in conceiving. The disruption may be caused by a hormonal imbalance due to stress or polycystic ovary syndrome, in which multiple cysts on the ovaries—often due to weight gain—disrupt hormone production.

Other causes of menstrual irregularity include uterine polyps and cancer of the cervix or uterus. Spotting of blood between menstrual periods may occur if you are taking contraceptive pills or undergoing hormone replacement therapy. Intensive exercise, weight loss, and eating disorders can also result in disruption of the normal pattern of menstruation.

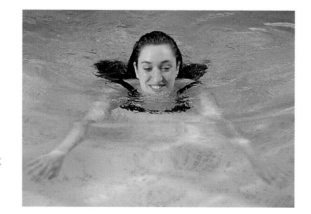

Exercise away pain
Swimming, as well as other activities that work muscles throughout the body, can help prevent menstrual cramps.

TREATING PAIN

Diet: In the week before you expect your period, take special care to eat a healthy diet; this helps prevent an imbalance of prostaglandins in the wall of the uterus. Choose foods rich in essential fatty acids, calcium, magnesium, zinc, and vitamins B, C, and E (see p. 12). Prevent constipation by drinking plenty of fluids and by eating vegetables, fruits, and whole grains daily. Avoid foods made with white flour, sugar, and saturated fats.

Massage: A daily massage of your abdomen and back in the week before your period helps prevent cramps by aiding muscle relaxation. Massage your abdomen yourself and ask someone else to massage your back (see photograph, below left). Use sunflower or sweet almond oil alone or with three drops of lavender oil added to each tablespoon.

Exercise: Get regular exercise that works your whole body. Try swimming, or join a yoga or

Sexual healing

Having an orgasm can help reduce menstrual pain and bring it to an end faster. It may be that the contractions of the uterus that occur during orgasm help prevent congestion of blood and tissue fluid as well as painful muscle spasms.

aerobics class. If you have cramps, kneel on all fours, then flex and stretch your lower back quickly and repeatedly. This pushes your hips up and down, which exercises the pelvis, boosts blood circulation to it, and helps prevent congestion in the uterine wall (see photograph, p. 312).

Heat: Take a warm bath, or rest in bed with a covered hot-water bottle over your lower abdomen or the small of your back. Alternatively, put a hot compress over your lower abdomen for two or three minutes, then replace it with a cold one for half a minute. Repeat two or three times. For severe pain, apply to your lower back and abdomen a compress soaked in hot water to which you have added four drops each of clary sage and sweet marjoram oils, and three of Roman chamomile oil.

Herbal remedies: For cramping pains combined with relatively light bleeding, drink tea made from prickly ash, cramp bark, blue cohosh, black cohosh (for intense pain), chasteberry,

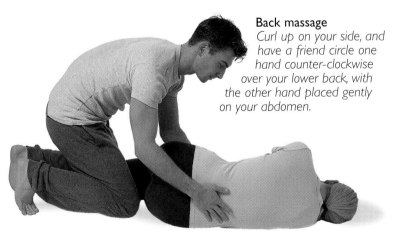

Back massage
Curl up on your side, and have a friend circle one hand counter-clockwise over your lower back, with the other hand placed gently on your abdomen.

Helpful hip-rocking
Lie on your back, and have a friend straddle your legs and use his or her hands to rock your hips rhythmically from side to side. Once the person has a rhythm going, a light touch is all that's needed.

275

chamomile, and ginger, taken singly or in combination. Drink a cup three times daily.
Caution: For safety concerns, see pp. 34–37.

Homeopathy: For persistent problems, consult a homeopathic practitioner. Otherwise, choose the remedy that most closely matches your case.

■ Belladonna: for violent pain along with bright red, clotted blood and a feeling of heat.

■ Colocynthis: for pain relieved by warmth or doubling up, and for irritability.

■ Lachesis: for menstrual cramps that start before the period, are worse on the left side, increase when pressure is applied, and improve when the flow starts.

■ Magnesia phosphorica: for shooting pain that improves with heat or gentle massage.

■ Nux vomica: for cramps, low back pain, irritability, and constipation.

■ Pulsatilla: for pain when you also feel extremely emotional, weepy, and needy.

■ Sepia: for pain accompanied by irritability and indifference to those close to you.

TREATING HEAVY PERIODS

Get medical advice if you have heavy bleeding. Your doctor may need to test for anemia and such disorders as fibroids and endometriosis.

Diet: Eat foods rich in vitamin C and flavonoids (see p. 12) to strengthen blood vessel walls, and those rich in iron to prevent and treat anemia that may result from excessive blood loss.

Aromatherapy: During menstruation, massage your abdomen each night with a blend of the following: two drops each of rose otto, Roman chamomile, and clary sage oils with four drops of sweet marjoram oil and two tablespoons of sweet-almond or olive oil.

Herbal remedies: Take a tea or tincture made from equal amounts of beth root, blue cohosh, agrimony, goldenseal, and raspberry leaves.

Acupressure for menstrual problems

● To dissipate pain that builds up just before a period and lasts for the first day or two, apply pressure first to the point (Liv 3) in the furrow between the first and second toes where the bones meet on the top of the foot.

Then try the point four finger-widths above your inner ankle bone, just behind the shin bone (Sp 6). Press each point firmly for two minutes, one at a time, with your thumb. Use small circular movements.

● Two points are useful for heavy periods: the point (Sp 1) on the outer corners of your big toenails, and the point (CV 4) four finger-widths below your navel. Press each

point firmly with your thumb or fingers in a downward direction for about two minutes.

Yoga for pain relief

Practicing yoga can help reduce cramps and other symptoms. The following exercise promotes healthy circulation in the pelvic region.

1 Sit with your back straight and knees bent, so that your soles touch and your heels are close to your body.

2 Hold your feet, then gently raise and lower your knees several times.

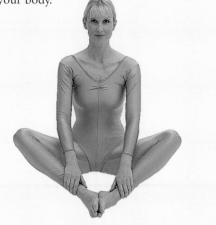

3 Next, lean forward slowly, bending from the hips and keeping your back straight. Hold this position for two minutes, feeling the stretch in your legs.

4 Relax and lean forward a little more as you exhale. Hold this position as you inhale. Repeat as necessary.

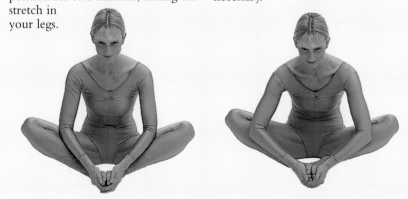

Dong quai and chasteberry are also effective. Take as tea or tincture three times each day. Caution: For safety concerns, see pp. 34–37.

TREATING IRREGULAR PERIODS

Diet: Try to maintain a normal weight for your height (see p. 302) and, most important, avoid crash diets and binge eating. Too low a body weight prevents ovulation, which may make periods irregular. Too high a weight can over-stimulate the ovaries, which may contribute to multiple ovarian cysts and disrupted periods. Get the professional help you need to lose excess weight and/or manage your eating disorder.

Exercise: Get regular exercise, but if your periods become irregular or stop, reduce your exercise time by 10 to 20 percent, and have one or two exercise-free days each week.

Other therapies: Acupuncture may be helpful in regulating hormonal imbalances.

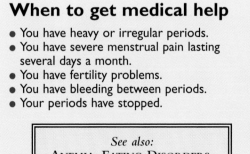

When to get medical help

- You have heavy or irregular periods.
- You have severe menstrual pain lasting several days a month.
- You have fertility problems.
- You have bleeding between periods.
- Your periods have stopped.

See also:
ANEMIA, EATING DISORDERS,
FERTILITY PROBLEMS, FIBROIDS,
PREMENSTRUAL SYNDROME

277

Migraine

A recurrent severe headache, usually accompanied by other disturbing symptoms, is known as migraine. It may last up to three days and be extremely disabling. The best way to manage a tendency toward migraine is to learn which factors trigger your attacks, so that you can try to avoid them. If a migraine does develop, various self-help measures may bring relief.

A clear head with yoga
Yoga can help relieve stress and reduce the frequency of migraines. Exercises that release tension in the upper back, shoulders, and neck may be especially beneficial. Ask a yoga teacher about suitable postures.

At least 10 percent of people suffer from migraine. The problem occurs three times more often in females than males, largely because of changing hormone levels before and during menstruation, pregnancy, and menopause (although for some women, menopause brings relief). A first attack of migraine usually occurs in the late teens or twenties; in some cases it happens at an even younger age. It is rare to have your first migraine over the age of 50. Attacks often become less frequent and severe as people get older: they are much less common in those over 65 years of age.

Migraine results from some sort of trigger (see box) making certain arteries in the brain first constrict, then dilate. Serotonin levels in the brain are low between attacks and high during them. Levels of other neurotransmitters may also be disrupted during attacks, as may calcium and magnesium levels.

Symptoms vary from one individual to another, but the common factor is a fierce, throbbing pain in one side of the head.

Migraine triggers

One or more of a large number of factors may set off a migraine. They include:
- Certain foods, especially cheese, chocolate, red wine, fried foods, and citrus fruits
- Low blood sugar, brought on by hunger or excessive intake of refined carbohydrates
- Dehydration
- Stress, shock, or worry
- Lack of sleep
- Bright light or certain colors of light
- Loud noise
- Weather or climate changes
- A dry atmosphere or a warm, dry wind
- Hormonal changes

You may experience one or more strange sensations—called an aura—that precede an attack and last up to an hour, such as flashing lights, zigzag lines, or a blind area in your field of vision. Once the headache begins, many people feel nauseated or vomit, and they may become sensitive to light and sound. Other possible symptoms are vertigo, tingling, and numbness.

PREVENTION

The simplest way to prevent attacks is to try, with experience and the help of a diary, to recognize your triggers, so that you can take steps to avoid them or minimize their effect. For example, if

both stress and premenstrual hormonal changes tend to bring about migraines, don't plan demanding events, such as a job interview, in the week before a period. If you know that motion sickness can precipitate a migraine, take steps to prevent the condition from arising, for instance by avoiding large meals before a long journey. A diary may reveal a cycle of regular attacks—for most sufferers, occurring every 10 to 40 days. Being aware of such a pattern helps you know when to be especially careful about staying away from triggers.

Diet: Prevent any nutrient shortage that might make migraine more likely by eating a well-balanced diet, including foods rich in vitamin B_2, or riboflavin, such as whole grains, egg yolks, milk, spinach, and lean meat. To avoid blood-sugar swings, eat smaller, more frequent meals, choosing slowly digested complex carbohydrates, such as whole grains and beans, rather than foods containing white flour or added sugar. Sugary, refined foods cause a rapid rise in blood-sugar level, followed by a steep fall (see p. 199). Such changes in blood-sugar level may provoke a migraine attack in susceptible people.

To help you discover whether any food triggers a migraine, keep a detailed food diary for several weeks. Some people are unable to tolerate foods containing tyramine, an amino acid that can cause migraine by affecting blood vessels in the brain. Tyramine-containing foods include chocolate,

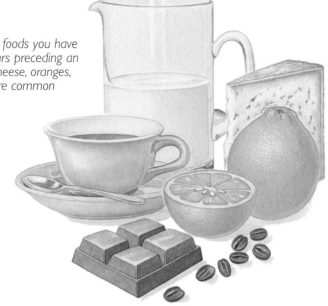

Culprit foods
Keep a diary of the foods you have eaten in the 24 hours preceding an attack. Chocolate, cheese, oranges, caffeine, and milk are common migraine triggers.

Protective foods
Eating oily fish, such as tuna and sardines, three times a week may protect against migraine because of their omega-3 fatty acids. Emphasizing whole grains over refined carbohydrates can also be beneficial.

cheese, beef, liver, eggs, beer, red wine and other fermented foods, and some fruits and vegetables (bananas, oranges, plums, broad beans, spinach, tomatoes).

Another possibility is a food allergy. Common culprits include wheat, milk, cheese, tomatoes, oranges, and potatoes. Some people develop a migraine after drinking tea, coffee, cola, or other caffeine-containing drinks.

However, there is one special difficulty in knowing whether any particular food is a migraine trigger. Before the headache itself begins, the already disrupted neurotransmitter levels may lead to a craving for certain foods. The foods commonly eaten before a migraine may not, therefore, actually cause the migraine, although symptoms tend to

occur after you eat them. The real trigger for your migraines may be another factor.

Light sensitivity: The glare from water, snow, and other surfaces can set off migraines in light-sensitive people. Wearing polarized sunglasses with good-quality lenses should help. If a very bright picture on a computer screen is a problem, adjust the contrast and brightness levels, and position the screen so as to avoid reflections. Ask your optometrist or ophthalmologist about trying tinted lenses to see if these help you. Certain blue or green tints may help prevent migraines in some people.

Air quality: Very dry air increases the proportion of positively charged ions in the atmosphere, which raises the body's level of serotonin, a neurotransmitter whose level increases during a migraine. Negative ions make the symptoms less severe and less long-lasting. Raise the concentration of negative ions in your home by opening windows and doors, having plenty of houseplants, and using a humidifier and/or an ionizer.

Stress: Stress is one of the most common triggers, so learning to handle it may reduce your migraine risk. Relaxation therapy can be very helpful, as can massage, yoga, meditation, and aromatherapy. Some people cope with stress while it lasts, but succumb to migraine afterward. If you recognize this pattern for your migraines, try to adjust your lifestyle so as to manage stress more effectively (see p. 347).

Supplements: There is evidence that the amino acid 5-HTP (5-hydroxytryptophan), a form of tryptophan, can help to prevent migraines. Take 100 milligrams three times a day. Some people experience nausea with this supplement. Seek medical advice first if you are taking antidepressant medication. Supplements of magnesium and calcium may also be beneficial. Take vitamin B$_2$ (riboflavin) if you find it hard to increase your dietary intake of this vitamin.

Herbal prevention: Substances in the bitter leaves of feverfew help combat inflammation and relax narrowed blood vessels. If you suspect that a migraine is starting, add two or three leaves of feverfew to a sandwich, which disguises the taste and helps prevent any possible irritant effect of the leaves on the mouth. If you prefer, take feverfew capsules or tablets. Feverfew can also be taken on a daily basis for the long-term prevention of migraines. Do not take feverfew if you

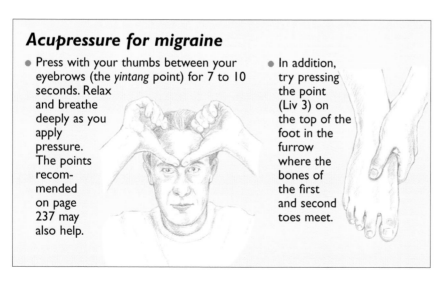

Acupressure for migraine

- Press with your thumbs between your eyebrows (the *yintang* point) for 7 to 10 seconds. Relax and breathe deeply as you apply pressure. The points recommended on page 237 may also help.

- In addition, try pressing the point (Liv 3) on the top of the foot in the furrow where the bones of the first and second toes meet.

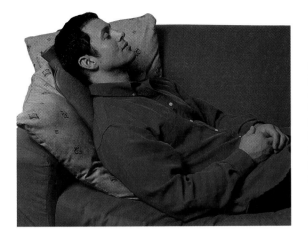

Cool relief
Rest your head against a hot-water bottle filled with cold water. Alternatives are putting your head under a shower of cold water, and pouring a basin of cold water over your head.

forehead and a hot one where your neck meets your skull, and switch them every two minutes. Repeat up to six times.

Other therapies: A cranial osteopath or practitioner of craniosacral therapy may be able to help with migraine. Utilizing biofeedback methods and the Alexander technique may also help reduce your susceptibility to this condition.

are pregnant or breast-feeding, or if contact with the plant gives you a rash.

TREATMENT

Rest and sleep: As soon as you feel you are about to get a migraine, lie down in a well-ventilated dark room. By doing this, you may cut short the attack or you may even succeed in staving it off completely.

Herbal remedies: Rosemary, lemon balm, and peppermint teas all have antispasmodic properties that may reduce the effects of a migraine.
Caution: For safety concerns, see pp. 34–37.

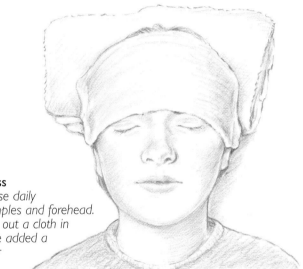

Aromatherapy compress
During stressful times, use daily compresses on your temples and forehead. Make these by wringing out a cloth in water to which you have added a few drops of lavender or marjoram oil.

Aromatherapy: If you feel an attack is imminent, add one drop each of peppermint and lavender oils to two teaspoons of sweet almond oil, and rub a little gently into your temples and the back of your neck.

Heat and cold

■ Place a cold compress against your forehead or neck. If this does not work, use hot and cold compresses. Start with a cold one on your

When to get medical help

- Migraines are more than an occasional problem or are severely disrupting your life.
- You are taking oral contraceptive pills.
- The pattern of migraines changes.

Get help right away if:
- You experience a debilitating headache for the first time.

See also:
HEADACHE, MOTION SICKNESS, NAUSEA AND VOMITING, STRESS

Motion Sickness

Some people experience nausea and/or vomiting when traveling by car, boat, train, or plane. This condition is especially common in children, whose balance mechanism is more sensitive than that of adults, and most people suffer less as they grow older. The sickness usually clears up quickly at the end of the journey.

Spicy relief
Take ginger for motion sickness two hours before departure and every four hours after that. Chew fresh ginger or drink ginger tea or a few drops of ginger tincture in warm water. You can also nibble crystallized ginger or a ginger cookie.

Motion sickness occurs when movement disturbs the semicircular canals, the balance mechanisms in your inner ear. Although your eyes adjust to the motion, your ears do not. In its mildest form, the condition causes slight discomfort or a headache; more severe cases produce nausea, sweating, and vomiting, which continue until the motion stops. A stuffy atmosphere, a full stomach, or the sight or smell of food makes the condition worse.

PREVENTION

Avoid large meals before traveling. Choose the front seat in a car or above the wing in a plane, and stay amidships on a boat. Get some fresh air—for example, by opening the car window. Look straight ahead at the road, or at the horizon if at sea. Avoid reading or any activity that involves focusing on nearby objects. Keep away from people who are smoking, since breathing the smoke may make you feel nauseated. If your child is prone to motion sickness, don't increase anxiety by talking about it before or during the journey, as this makes sickness more likely.

TREATMENT

Homeopathy: Take one dose of an appropriate remedy just before you set out, and then as necessary during the journey.

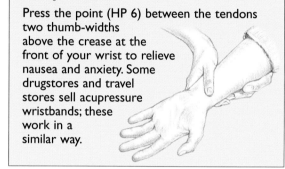

Acupressure

Press the point (HP 6) between the tendons two thumb-widths above the crease at the front of your wrist to relieve nausea and anxiety. Some drugstores and travel stores sell acupressure wristbands; these work in a similar way.

- Cocculus: for all symptoms of motion sickness.
- Tabacum: if the slightest movement brings on extreme nausea and vomiting, especially if you are pale or are sweating a lot.

When to get medical help

- You have a fever, severe headache, or feel faint or dizzy.
- Symptoms don't lessen within 24 hours.

Get help right away if:
- You have severe abdominal or chest pain.

See also:
DIZZINESS, NAUSEA AND VOMITING

Mouth Ulcers

Small white, gray, or yellow sores can occur singly or in clusters anywhere in the mouth, including the tongue. Often very painful, canker sores and other mouth ulcers affect about 20 percent of the population at any one time. They are most likely in people who have a poor diet or an underlying infection, or are under a lot of stress.

DID YOU KNOW?
You can speed the healing of canker sores by holding a cooled wet tea bag over them.

Saltwater mouthwash
Add one teaspoon of salt to a glass of warm water and rinse with this solution once or twice a day. This may cause stinging when the sore is new.

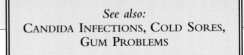

The many causes of the common mouth ulcers called aphthous ulcers include a vitamin deficiency, digestive upset, food sensitivity, infection, injury (such as biting the tongue or cheek), and poorly fitting dentures. They are more likely if you are exhausted or under stress. Occasionally ulcers are a sign of an underlying condition, such as tuberculosis, herpes simplex infection, celiac disease (intolerance of gluten, a cereal protein), Crohn's disease, anemia, or leukemia.

PREVENTION
Eat a healthy diet (see p. 9). Boost your resistance to infection by eating garlic, onions, foods rich in vitamin C and flavonoids (fruits and vegetables), and those containing zinc (nuts, seeds, root vegetables, shellfish), and by limiting your intake of refined carbohydrates.

TREATMENT
Kitchen cabinet remedies: Soothe mouth ulcers with a once or twice daily mouthwash or gargle of:
- Cold tea for its astringent effect.
- Sage tea for its antiseptic, healing, and astringent properties.

Aromatherapy: Antiseptic essential oils, such as geranium, lavender, lemon, myrrh, and tea tree, work well on ulcers caused by viral or bacterial infection. Avoid myrrh oil if you are in the first 20 weeks of pregnancy.
- Mix five drops of tea tree oil, three of lemon oil, and two of myrrh oil with two and a half teaspoons of grapeseed oil. Apply to the ulcers with your finger every two hours.
- Add one drop each of tea tree, geranium, and lavender oils to half a glass of water. Use as a mouthwash three or four times a day.
- Add a few drops of tea tree, geranium, or lavender oil to a cup of warm water and use as a mouthwash three times a day. You may apply tea tree or lavender oil undiluted, but it can cause stinging.

When to get medical help
- A mouth ulcer fails to heal within two weeks or increases in size over one week.
- The problem recurs frequently.
- You suspect the problem is caused by a tooth or dentures (see your dentist).
- You also have a cough, diarrhea, or a tendency to get recurrent infections elsewhere in your body.
- You are taking new medication.

See also:
CANDIDA INFECTIONS, COLD SORES, GUM PROBLEMS

Muscle Aches and Stiffness

Tender, stiff, aching muscles from too much exercise, heavy lifting, or other overuse—or from alterations in body chemistry—are a common complaint. The various remedies and therapies used to relieve them are a part of many people's healing repertoire, but these extra tips may provide relief the next time the problem arises.

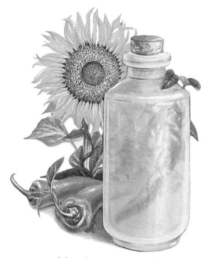

Muscle-warming oil
Dried chili infused in sunflower oil makes a warming massage oil, but test it on a small area first.

Stiffness and pain in the skeletal muscles (the muscles that control movement of the body) are frequent consequences of strains, cramps, and injuries. The affected muscles may go into a state of prolonged tension—or spasm—as a reflex to prevent further damage through movement.

Muscle tension may also be a response to injury or pain in an adjacent part of the body. If certain groups of fibers within a muscle become especially tense, they can be felt as taut, hard strands beneath the skin; these are most likely at the edges of the shoulder muscles. Sometimes tender lumps (fibrositic nodules) appear in strained muscles in the back, neck, and shoulders.

Muscle tension impedes local blood circulation, which inhibits the healing process in an injured muscle or other part. It also triggers the release of chemicals called cytokines and prostaglandins, which are responsible for the pain. If muscle tension is a response to pain from a compressed nerve (as in some back pain), the tension further compresses the nerve and increases pain.

One special type of muscle problem is described in the box below. Additional causes of aches and stiffness include:

- Stress, anxiety, or depression
- Exposure to cold air, as with a draft
- Insufficient nutrients, especially minerals
- Food sensitivity
- Cramps
- Chronic fatigue syndrome
- Tension headaches
- Repetitive strain injury
- Poor posture

Fibromyalgia: when you ache all over

Formerly called fibrositis or muscular rheumatism, this condition involves widespread muscle pain, morning stiffness, and tenderness over particular points where a muscle is attached to a bone. These are known as myofascial trigger points, or, in traditional Chinese medicine, "ah-shi" points, because when pressed, they tend to make a person cry out "ah shi!" (the equivalent of "ouch!"). It is thought that each skeletal muscle has a trigger point, and that this type of tenderness can result from any damage to that muscle or its protective coating of connective tissue. For a firm diagnosis of fibromyalgia, at least 11 out of 18 points must be tender.

People who suffer from fibromyalgia usually can't achieve deep sleep and are prone to depression, headaches, menstrual pain, restless legs, and Raynaud's syndrome. There is considerable overlap between the symptoms of fibromyalgia and those of chronic fatigue syndrome, but the cause of fibromyalgia is unclear.

PREVENTION

To protect muscles when doing physical work or exercising, follow some basic rules. Always warm up first, increasing the circulation to the muscles with some light whole-body exercise, because muscle aches and stiffness are more likely when muscles are cold. Once the body is warm, stretch each of the main groups of muscles. When you have finished your workout, cool down by gradually decreasing the intensity of the exercises, then stretch the muscles again.

Lifestyle factors can affect your susceptibility to muscle stiffness. Getting enough rest to balance the amount of exercise you get, and vice versa, helps prevent muscle problems and their sources, such as aching shoulders and back, fibromyalgia, cramps, restless legs, and tension headaches. Maintaining good posture so that no one group of muscles remains tense for too long is also important for preventing aches and stiffness. Two of the most important ways of doing this are keeping your head in line with your spine and not hunching your shoulders.

A healthy diet provides the nutrients your muscles need to perform well and to recover quickly from strain. Such nutrients include amino acids, calcium, magnesium, potassium, selenium, vitamins B and C, and flavonoids.

Warm-up stretches
To avoid stiff, aching muscles after your workout, start your routine with a program of stretches. Learn them from a fitness trainer or an exercise video that you know to be good.

Drinking enough fluids is important. Stress management (see p. 347) can help prevent stress-induced muscle tension and fibromyalgia.

TREATMENT

The most important aspect of treatment is to protect the muscles from further damage while healing the affected tissue. Relaxing the muscles helps alleviate symptoms and allows injured tissue to heal more quickly.

Rest: Rest stiff, aching muscles that result from overuse or strain, but resume normal activity after two or three days (long periods of inactivity are not advisable because this can result in shortening of the muscle fibers). Gradually resume normal exercise.

Exercise: After a few days' rest, start to gently stretch your stiff muscles. Exercise for a maximum of five minutes at first. Repeat several times daily, doing a little more activity every day, but stopping if you feel pain. After several days, weeks, or months—depending on the problem—you should be able to extend the muscle fully. Chronically stiff and aching shoulder and back muscles may take months to extend fully.

Aromatherapy: Having a massage or bathing with certain essential oils can provide pain relief.
- Mix 10 drops of rosemary oil, or two drops of German chamomile, with a tablespoon of sweet-almond or soybean oil, and rub gently over the sore area. Don't use rosemary oil in the first 20 weeks of pregnancy.
- Add three drops of lavender oil and three of

285

cypress to comfortably hot bathwater, and soak in it. Omit cypress oil if you are in the first 20 weeks of pregnancy.

■ Add three drops of a warming spice oil, such as ginger, to a hot compress and apply to the affected muscle.

Herbal remedies: Gently rubbing an herbal ointment over painful, stiff muscles three or four times daily may help.

■ Apply arnica ointment.

■ Make a warming oil to rub into aching muscles by infusing an ounce of dried chili in a pint of sunflower oil. Apply to a tiny area of skin first, since it makes some people blister. Alternatively, buy an ointment containing capsaicin (a chemical derived from capsicum peppers) from a drugstore or health-food store.

Caution: For safety concerns, see pp. 34–37.

Heat and cold: Stiff, aching muscles respond well to heat, whereas a torn or overstretched muscle generally feels better with a cold compress for the first 24 hours, then heat.

■ Warm stiff muscles with an infrared bulb placed at a distance of 20 to 30 inches for a half hour twice daily.

■ Place over a sore muscle a covered hot-water bottle, a gel-filled pack heated in the oven or microwave, or an electrically heated pad.

■ Have a long soak in warm (not hot) bathwater.

■ Apply a hot compress for three minutes, then a cold one for one minute, and repeat two or three times. Do this several times daily until you feel better. For added benefit, first soak the hot compress in half a pint of water containing

Massage away the aches

One of the best therapies for aching muscles is massage. Take a warm bath first, and have the massage in a warm room to encourage the muscles to relax. Ask a friend to follow the steps below.

1 Massage the sore muscles with gliding and kneading movements.

2 Encourage tense strands or points to relax with cross-fiber friction—moving your fingers across the muscle fibers without sliding on the skin.

3 Press tender points firmly with a fingertip.

two tablespoons of distilled witch hazel.

- Try an ice pack (such as a covered freezer pack or package of frozen peas) over painful muscles resulting from injury.

Diet

- Eat magnesium-rich foods (see illustration, right). Alternatively, take 300 milligrams of magnesium daily in the form of a supplement.
- Consider a calcium supplement (250 milligrams twice a day).
- Reduce your intake of animal protein (for example, meat, cheese, and eggs) and of foods containing white flour and added sugar.

Homeopathy

- Arnica: for muscle stiffness after overstrenuous or unaccustomed exercise; for muscles that feel bruised, as if from sleeping on too hard a bed, and more painful when you move, and for related restlessness and irritability.
- Bryonia: for aching muscles made worse by movement or by a dry, cold wind.
- Rhus toxicodendron: for muscle stiffness after overuse that improves with gentle movement.

Other therapies: If long-standing aching and stiffness result from poor posture, you may benefit from physiotherapy, Alexander technique lessons, or yoga classes. An osteopath, chiropractor, or shiatsu therapist may also be helpful.

Muscle-friendly magnesium
This mineral has marked muscle-relaxing properties. Include in your diet a variety of magnesium-rich foods, such as whole-grain cereals, nuts, and beans.

Acupressure for stiff muscles

To relax your muscles, treat the following points for two minutes at a time:

- Apply constant thumb pressure to the point (GB 34) in the depression below the outside of the knee joint at the top of the fibula (shinbone).

- Apply pressure with rotating movements of the thumb to the point (TH 5) two thumb-widths above the wrist crease on the back of the forearm.

When to get medical help

- Symptoms persist longer than a week.
- Symptoms worsen.
- Other symptoms, such as fever, headache, diarrhea, pain, bruising, and numbness, accompany muscle aches or spasms.

See also:
ANXIETY, BACK PAIN, CHRONIC FATIGUE SYNDROME, HEADACHE, LEG CRAMPS, NECK AND SHOULDER PROBLEMS, PAIN, REPETITIVE STRAIN INJURY, RESTLESS LEGS, STRAINS AND SPRAINS, STRESS

Nail Problems

*H*ealthy nails are smooth, evenly colored, and strong, with a pale pink or flesh-colored nail bed. A number of disorders may affect their appearance. Your nails can therefore be an indicator of your underlying state of health. There's much you can do at home through diet and externally applied treatments to improve the look of your nails.

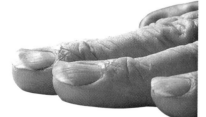

Tell-tale shape
Iron-deficiency anemia can cause the profile of each nail to become spoon-shaped.

The nails and surrounding skin can be infected by bacteria and such fungi as tinea and candida. These conditions can make the nails soft, discolored, thickened, and misshapen. Paronychia is a bacterial or fungal infection of the fold of skin at the side of the nail.

Certain skin diseases can also affect the nails, including psoriasis, which may cause thickening, pitting, or even separation of the nail from the nail bed. The patchy hair loss known as alopecia areata is sometimes associated with ridged, pitted, rough nails. Other, more serious conditions leading to nail problems include excessive production of the thyroid hormone (thyrotoxicosis), disorders of the blood-clotting process, and inflamed heart valves (endocarditis). Blueness of the nails may result from severe asthma, heart disease, emphysema, or bronchitis, while yellowing and excessive hardening of the nails may be a sign of bronchiectasis (damaged airways in the lung) or lymphedema (accumulation of lymphatic fluid in the tissues). Nail discoloration can also result from smoking or regular use of nail polish. Toenails may become ingrown—for example, because of the pressure from ill-fitting shoes.

Several nutritional deficiencies may also show up in the nails:
- Iron-deficiency anemia may cause the nails to appear pale and become thin, brittle, ridged, and easily cracked or broken.

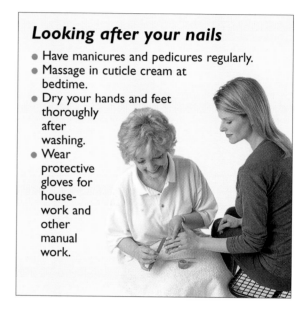

Looking after your nails

- Have manicures and pedicures regularly.
- Massage in cuticle cream at bedtime.
- Dry your hands and feet thoroughly after washing.
- Wear protective gloves for house-work and other manual work.

- Zinc deficiency leads to white spots and/or brittleness of nails.
- Severe protein deficiency makes the nail beds appear white.
- Lack of linoleic acid (an essential fatty acid) may cause the nails to split and flake.

TREATMENT
Diet: Adapt your diet according to your specific nail problem.
- For nail problems resulting from iron deficiency, follow the advice on pages 84–85.

288

Nutrition for nails

If your nails are brittle or flaking, give them a boost by increasing your intake of key nutrients, such as calcium (in milk), omega-3 fatty acids (in oily fish), vitamin C (in most fresh fruits and vegetables), and zinc (in seafood and poultry).

- For fungal or bacterial nail infections, boost immunity by eating garlic and onions, foods rich in zinc (nuts, root vegetables, shellfish), vitamin C and flavonoids (fruits and vegetables), and omega-3 fatty acids (nuts, seeds, dark green leafy vegetables, oily fish, canola oil).
- For splitting and breaking nails, increase your body's level of vitamin A by drinking carrot juice and eating more eggs, milk, and liver. Eat three servings of oily fish each week, and consider taking a fish oil supplement.
- For white spots in the nails, increase your intake of zinc and B vitamins by eating more poultry, seafood, and whole grains.
- For nail problems caused by psoriasis, eat more oily fish and other foods with essential fatty acids (whole grains, nuts, seeds).

Aromatherapy: Several essential oils are useful for nail infections.

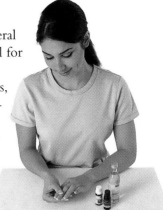

- For fungal infections, tea tree oil is particularly beneficial. Dab the oil directly onto the affected nail and cuticle, or mix five drops with the same amount of tagetes oil into two tablespoons of sweet almond oil, and massage into the nail.

Anti-infective oils
Keep your selected mix of essential oils in a dark bottle and use to massage around the nail bed three times daily while symptoms persist.

- For other infections, mix five drops each of eucalyptus and patchouli oils with 10 drops each of tea tree and tagetes oils, and two tablespoons of sweet almond oil.

Homeopathy

- Silica can often strengthen weak nails. Try one pill a day for a month.

When to get medical help

- Your nail problem continues to affect new nail growth in spite of treatment.
- You experience pain, swelling, inflammation, or pus around the nail.
- You suspect that your nail problem is a symptom of an underlying condition.

See also:
ANEMIA, FOOT PROBLEMS,
FUNGAL SKIN INFECTIONS,
HAIR AND SCALP
PROBLEMS, SKIN PROBLEMS

Nausea and Vomiting

Each of us is familiar with the unpleasant sensation of nausea, with its accompanying sweating, pallor, and faintness, and the feeling that we may vomit. In some cases, actual vomiting (the "throwing up" of stomach contents) soon follows these warning signs. Many simple natural remedies can help you feel better or stop you from feeling nauseated in the first place.

Nausea and vomiting most often result from a digestive upset caused by overeating, too much rich food, or food to which you are allergic, intolerant, or otherwise sensitive. Irritation of the stomach lining caused by too much alcohol or by infecting microorganisms or their toxins (food poisoning) may also produce these symptoms. Infection of the digestive tract may lead to diarrhea as well.

Other triggers of nausea and vomiting include anxiety, fear or shock, and migraine. Disturbance of the inner ear's balance mechanism that leads to dizziness—as with motion sickness, an inner-ear infection, and Ménière's disease—may also cause nausea and vomiting. Nausea, especially first thing in the morning ("morning sickness"), is a common occurrence in early pregnancy. Young children often vomit as a result of a feverish illness.

Vomiting can occasionally be a sign of an underlying disorder, such as a stomach ulcer, uncontrolled diabetes, jaundice, gallbladder disease, or cancer. Certain drugs, including some anticancer and anesthetic agents, may also cause nausea and vomiting.

PREVENTION
Always eat slowly and chew thoroughly to avoid nausea after meals. Avoid very large meals. You may suspect a food sensitivity if symptoms consistently occur after eating a particular type of food. In this case, avoiding the food is the simplest way of averting the problem.

Prevent digestive upsets from infection by paying careful attention to personal and kitchen hygiene (see p. 167). To help prevent sickness during pregnancy, eat frequent light meals, and have a ginger cookie or drink a small cup of ginger tea, sweetened with a little honey, as soon as you get up in the morning.

To avoid feeling nauseated when you are stressed or excited, practice breathing and other relaxation exercises so that you can more easily relax your mind and body when necessary.

TREATMENT
Maintain an adequate fluid intake if you are suffering from repeated vomiting, especially if it is accompanied by diarrhea.

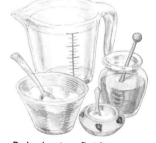

Rehydration fluid
Mix eight level teaspoons of sugar (or four heaping ones of honey) and one teaspoon of salt into one quart of water.

- Take frequent sips of water or fruit juice throughout the day.
- To replace salts and fluids lost through vomiting, make drinks using oral rehydration salts from the drugstore, or

make your own (see illustration, facing page).

■ Experiment to see whether warm drinks are easier to keep down than cold ones.

■ Avoid alcohol, as this boosts urine production and encourages dehydration. It also irritates the stomach and may therefore slow recovery.

Herbal remedies

■ Ginger counters nausea and vomiting. Chew a piece of fresh or crystallized ginger, take ginger tablets, or sip ginger tea.

■ To help settle nausea associated with anxiety, sip chamomile tea, which has a calming effect as well as digestive properties.
Caution: For safety concerns, see pp. 34–37.

Kitchen cabinet remedies: Warming spices, such as cloves, cinnamon, and cardamom, assist digestion and facilitate the elimination of toxins via the bowel. Use one or more of these spices to make a tea to sip when you feel nauseated. Do not use this remedy if you have a stomach ulcer.

Diet: After a bout of nausea and vomiting, give your system time to recover by returning to a normal diet gradually. Choose bland, easily digested foods at first, such as rice, clear soup, low-fat yogurt, whole-grain toast, and apple-sauce. Avoid coffee, tea, and fatty foods.

Homeopathy

■ Arsenicum: for acute gastrointestinal ailments, with diarrhea and burning stomach pains, exhaustion, and chilliness.

■ Ipecacuanha: for constant nausea. Other symptoms may accompany the nausea.

Acupressure

● Use the point (HP 6) described on page 282.
● Or if the risk of vomiting has passed, lie down and ask someone to press gradually and gently with the thumbs on the point (CV 12) four thumb-widths above your navel, using small circling movements, for up to two minutes.

■ Nux vomica: for nausea when you can't vomit but wish you could.

■ Sepia: for unrelieved nausea triggered even by the thought of food.

Flower essences: When nausea results from anxiety, try Mimulus if you know what you are anxious about or Aspen if you don't.

When to get medical help

● You have been suffering from bouts of unexplained nausea and vomiting for longer than 12 hours, or you have eaten undercooked food.
● A medication may be the cause.
● You have recently been to a tropical country.

Get help right away if:
● Vomit contains blood or black material resembling coffee grounds.
● You have a severe headache, dizziness, fever, severe abdominal pain, drowsiness, aversion to bright light, or chest pain.
● A young child or an elderly person is experiencing repeated vomiting.

See also:
ABDOMINAL PAIN, ANXIETY, ARTERIAL DISEASE, EATING DISORDERS, GALLBLADDER PROBLEMS, HANGOVER, INDIGESTION, MOTION SICKNESS, PREGNANCY PROBLEMS

Neck and Shoulder Problems

Pain and stiffness in the neck and shoulders can range from slight discomfort that hinders full movement to severe pain that prevents even minimal movement. Fortunately, the problem can often be prevented or relieved by reducing strain and tension in the muscles and joints.

DID YOU KNOW?
Neck and shoulder problems often occur during sleep, because we have little control over our positions. Some people find cervical braces or special pillows helpful.

In most cases, neck and shoulder pain is caused when the muscles go into spasm—that is, they contract and become rigid so that the joints are unable to move normally. This can result from the cumulative stresses of long periods of being in the same position, as when driving, sitting at a computer, or doing repetitive factory work.

"Whiplash" injuries sustained in automobile accidents and sports injuries (especially among those unaccustomed to strenuous activity) are common causes of shoulder pain. Before you try to treat any such injury, check the box on page 295 for danger signs. In addition, pain may recur at the site of an old injury.

Persistent pain and stiffness often result from arthritis, in which bony outgrowths from the vertebrae in the neck pinch nearby nerves and put pressure on the muscles and ligaments. There are many other causes of neck and/or shoulder pain that may require medical attention, including a herniated ("slipped") disk, tendinitis, bursitis, spinal disorders, and Lyme disease.

Muscular tension in the neck and shoulder area is a common physiological manifestation of psychological and emotional stress. In this case, the underlying source of the problem needs to be identified and addressed.

PREVENTION

Avoid strain by paying attention to how you stand, sit, lift, and carry (see advice in "Back Pain," pp. 105–108). Learn to recognize the signs of stress, and offset any negative physical effects by dealing with it properly (see p. 347). Always warm up and stretch before exercise; the overuse of cold muscles can cause pain and stiffness.

TREATMENT

For pain from minor strain or tension, try the following natural remedies:
- Ask a friend to give you the shiatsu massage described on the facing page. Enhance its soothing effects by adding a few drops of a relaxing essential oil, such as lavender or geranium, to your basic massage oil or lotion.

➢ *continued, p. 294*

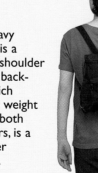

Carrying bags

Regularly carrying heavy shoulder bags (left) is a common cause of shoulder and neck pain. A backpack (right), which distributes the weight evenly on both shoulders, is a healthier option.

292

Shiatsu massage for painful neck and shoulders

This sequence will help relieve pain and stiffness when symptoms are not severe and do not include redness. The sufferer should sit on a chair, stool, or floor cushion. The instructions are for the person giving the treatment. Omit step one if the sufferer is pregnant.

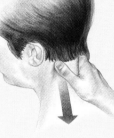

3 Apply firm but careful thumb pressure into the hollow between the neck muscles at the base of the skull. Work downward. Change sides and hands, repeating on the other side of the neck.

1 Stand behind the sufferer and lean straight down on the shoulders with open palms. Start with gentle pressure and gradually lean more heavily.

2 Move your hands so you can work on one side. Support the forehead with one hand and, with the other hand, squeeze the muscles at the back of the neck, working downward from the base of the skull.

4 Step back and place your hands, with arms extended, onto the shoulders. Apply slow and repeated pressure into the muscles on either side of the spine between the shoulder blades. Be guided by the person's response in judging the degree of pressure to exert.

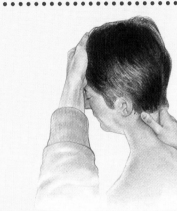

5 Finish by repeatedly squeezing and stroking the arms from the shoulders to the elbows in a series of quick movements to dispel any remaining tension.

293

■ Place a hot compress (see facing page) over the affected area. Or apply alternate hot and cold compresses for a total of 20 minutes. Leave each hot compress in place for three minutes and each cold one for one minute.

Posture: Much neck and shoulder pain results from muscle tension caused by poor posture, especially when driving or working at a desk.

■ Be sure your desk and chair at work are properly adjusted for your height (see p. 106).

■ Take care to adjust your car seat, especially before long journeys. Your back should be well supported along its length. It is especially important for shorter people to make sure that

A simple solution
If you are prone to neck pain or if you have to sit in the cold or a draft for more than a few minutes, prevent neck stiffness by wearing a scarf or a turtle-neck sweater, which will help keep the muscles warm and relaxed.

Neck-release exercises

Try the sequence of exercises described below to release tension in the neck and shoulders. Sit comfortably in an upright chair, and breathe slowly and evenly throughout. Repeat each exercise six times before going on to the next. Stop if you feel dizzy.

1 Allow your head to drop forward until your chin rests on your chest. Raise your head slowly.

2 Tilt your head to one side and then the other, while keeping your shoulders level.

3 Turn your head to face left and then turn slowly to face right.

4 Lift your shoulders up toward your ears and roll them forward and then backward.

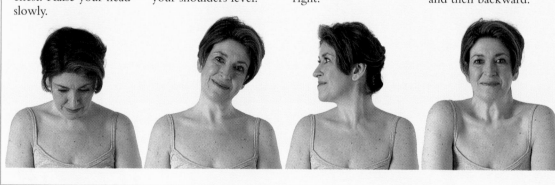

294

the seat is high enough to prevent the need to strain the neck to see clearly over the steering wheel. Use a cushion if your car seat is not fully adjustable.

Herbal remedies: Pain and stiffness in the neck and shoulders are often due to muscle tension resulting from emotional tension. Herbs with relaxing properties may help.
- Take a bath in warm water to which you have added tea made from rosemary or lavender. Avoid rosemary if you are in the first 20 weeks of pregnancy.
- Try chamomile, hops, passionflower, or valerian. Take as tea before bedtime.

Caution: For safety concerns, see pp. 34–37.

Homeopathy
- Arnica: for pain and stiffness arising from a recent injury. Take the remedy as tablets or apply it topically as ointment.
- Rhus toxicodendron: for long-standing pain and stiffness when symptoms are eased by gentle movement, warmth, and massage.

Other therapies: If you don't have any of the symptoms listed under "When to Get Medical Help" (right), seek advice from a qualified practitioner of a manipulative therapy, such as osteopathy or chiropractic. Acupuncture may also help. Long-standing neck and shoulder problems may benefit from improved posture achieved through the Alexander technique, the Feldenkrais method, or similar bodywork therapies. Practicing tai chi and yoga can also help prevent posture-related problems.

Making a neck compress

Applying a hot compress may relieve neck and shoulder problems resulting from muscle stiffness. Here's how to make one:

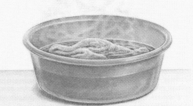

1 Soak a towel in hot (not boiling) water. Fold the towel and wring out well.

2 Unfold the towel and place over the back of the neck and shoulders. Cover with a dry towel. Leave in place for up to 10 minutes.

When to get medical help
- You also have a headache, a fever, dizziness, faintness, or sensitivity to bright light.
- You have swollen glands in the neck or difficulty swallowing.

Get help right away if:
- You also have difficulty in moving a limb, loss of bladder or bowel control, tingling or numbness in a limb, shortness of breath, chest pain, or shooting pains in one or both arms.
- The pain follows an injury.
- You have difficulty moving your neck.

See also:
ARTHRITIS, BACK PAIN,
MUSCLE ACHES AND STIFFNESS

Nosebleeds

Relatively common in childhood, when the tiny blood vessels of the nasal lining may be fragile, nosebleeds are usually insignificant. They occur less often in healthy adults but may become more frequent again during old age. You can easily treat most nosebleeds at home, using traditional techniques to stem bleeding and allow healing.

A nosebleed occurs when one or more blood vessels inside a nostril ruptures. This may happen after a blow to the nose or head, repeated sneezing, or picking or blowing the nose. An upper-respiratory infection also makes nasal blood vessels more fragile. Indoor heating can dry out the mucous membrane, affecting the vessels and causing a mild nosebleed. In rare cases, nosebleeds are a sign of an underlying disease, such as high blood pressure or a blood-clotting disorder.

PREVENTION

If you suffer from recurrent nosebleeds, eat more foods containing vitamin C and flavonoids (see p. 12) to strengthen capillary walls.

TREATMENT

Herbal remedies

- Apply to your nose and the back of your neck cold compresses soaked in dilute witch hazel.
- Hold a cotton ball soaked in marigold (calendula) tincture under your nose.

Aromatherapy: Cypress and helichrysum oils help stop blood loss. Put a few drops on a cotton ball and hold under your nose. Do not use cypress oil in the first 20 weeks of pregnancy.

Homeopathy

- Ferrum phosphoricum: use daily for a month if you are prone to nosebleeds.
- Phosphorus: for sudden heavy bleeding.

First aid for nosebleeds

- Sit up and lean slightly forward. Breathing through your mouth, pinch your nostrils together for 10 to 15 minutes.
- If you find it hard to maintain pressure, take two tongue depressors and place a rubber band around them (about one-third of the way down). Then position them over the nose so that a depressor is on either side (see illustration).
- Slowly release your nostrils.

If the bleeding has not stopped, pinch for 10 minutes more.
- Once the bleeding stops, gently clean away dried blood with lukewarm water.

When to get medical help

- Bleeding lasts longer than 30 minutes.
- Blood loss is severe.
- You suffer from frequent nosebleeds.
- You have high blood pressure.

Get help right away if:
- A nosebleed follows a head injury.
- You get a headache along with a nosebleed.

See also:
HIGH BLOOD PRESSURE

Osteoporosis

As people age, the density of their bones naturally decreases because of the gradual loss of minerals from the skeleton. Severe mineral loss, a condition called osteoporosis, causes the bones to become weak and increasingly susceptible to fractures. The disorder occurs most frequently in older women due to hormonal changes after menopause.

About 25 million Americans suffer from osteoporosis. Four out of five are women who have gone through menopause, though osteoporosis can also affect men and younger women. Each year in the United States an estimated 1.5 million fractures—primarily of the spine, hip, and wrist—result from this condition. By the age of 70, about 40 percent of American women have had at least one fracture caused by osteoporosis.

Osteoporosis often produces no symptoms until a fracture occurs after a fall. However, there may be back pain if the vertebrae (spinal bones) become weakened and collapse. Other indications of osteoporosis are loosening of the teeth, a loss of height, and kyphosis (an excessive curvature of the upper spine, also known as dowager's hump). A bone density scan can reveal the severity of suspected osteoporosis.

RISK FACTORS

Besides being postmenopausal, important risk factors in developing osteoporosis include being small-boned, underweight, and inactive. Excessive alcohol consumption, a poor diet, and smoking also increase the possibility. All these factors can make mature bones less dense and can prevent a young person's bone density from reaching its potential peak. If bone density does not

How osteoporosis develops

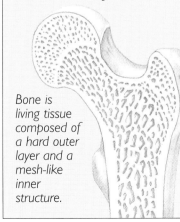

Bone is living tissue composed of a hard outer layer and a mesh-like inner structure.

Bone density increases throughout childhood and adolescence and for some years afterward. New bone cells are continually being produced and old ones broken down. The bones are usually at their most dense and resilient in the late 20s. Osteoporosis—which means "porous bones"—occurs when bone tissue breaks down faster than new bone is formed. As a woman nears menopause, more bone is destroyed than is produced, and her bones start to become less dense. The onset of osteoporosis may result from the naturally falling level of estrogen, which assists the body in absorbing calcium. After menopause the rate of bone tissue loss increases, and a woman's risk of osteoporosis begins to rise more steeply. In contrast, men's risk of osteoporosis is more gradual as they get older.

The amount of calcium available also plays a major role in determining the rates of bone formation and resorption. If insufficient calcium is provided by the diet and levels in the blood are inadequate for the needs of other vital body parts, such as the heart, nerves, and muscles, cells called osteoclasts ("bone cell destroyers") release calcium from bones. This results in more porous bones that become increasingly light and fragile.

develop fully, the natural demineralization that accompanies aging takes effect sooner and makes a person prone to osteoporosis at a younger age.

Osteoporosis may also have a genetic link. Experts suspect that a gene can interfere with the body's ability to use vitamin D, which is crucial for calcium absorption. People with small bones—such as, generally speaking, Caucasians and Asians—are particularly prone to osteoporosis. Other risk factors include diabetes, thyroid disease, and some prescribed drugs, notably corticosteroids and anticonvulsants.

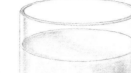

Estrogen boosters
Soybeans and soy products, such as tofu, miso, and soy milk, contain hormonelike substances that may mimic the bone-protecting properties of estrogen.

Calcium-rich foods

The following foods are good sources of calcium. The approximate amount of the mineral present in an average serving of a selection of foods is shown below.

Milk (8 ounces) ....250 mg
Hard cheese (2 ounces) ....300 mg
Yogurt (4 ounces) ....250 mg
Sardines (2 ounces, canned) ....250 mg
Green cabbage (4 ounces, raw) ....50 mg
Tofu (bean curd, 4 ounces) ....150 mg
Baked beans (4 ounces) ....50 mg

PREVENTION

You can do much to prevent osteoporosis from developing. It is never too early to begin. Encourage children to eat foods rich in calcium and other bone-building nutrients (see chart) to help ensure optimal bone density. Whatever their history, adults too can make their bones stronger or at least slow the rate of bone loss by improving their diet and making lifestyle changes.

■ Eat more fruits and vegetables, including soy products. When a man's or a woman's natural level of estrogen falls, plant hormones may take its place by locking onto cell receptors in the bone. This is thought to confer benefits similar to those of your own estrogen.

■ Eat a diet that will provide the minerals required to keep bones healthy. In addition to calcium, the most abundant mineral in bone, these include boron (for calcium absorption and retention), copper (for bone production), magnesium (for the efficient use of calcium), manganese (for strengthening connective tissue in bones), silicon (for bone resilience), and zinc (see facing page). Most experts recommend that an adult woman consume at least 1,000 milligrams of calcium daily.

■ Teenage, pregnant, breast-feeding, or post-menopausal women, as well as older men, need at least 1,200 milligrams of calcium a day. Sources include dairy products (milk, cheese, yogurt—choose low-fat varieties), dark green

leafy vegetables (kale, collards, broccoli), beans, carrots, almonds; and fish with edible bones (sardines, canned salmon, anchovies).

- If you are not eating well or have a high risk of osteoporosis, take a daily calcium supplement (with milk to increase absorption). Calcium supplementation can decrease bone loss by 40 percent after menopause.
- Increase intake of zinc-rich foods (shellfish, nuts, seeds, root vegetables). Zinc encourages the production of bone protein and gastric acid, which is needed for the optimal absorption of calcium. Reduce your intake of saturated fat and sugar, since both can reduce acid production. If you suspect that your acid production is low (for example, if you produce a

Strength from the sun
The body synthesizes vitamin D, a nutrient required for strong bones, in response to exposure to ultraviolet light. Being outdoors with bright light on your face for 15 minutes a day is usually sufficient. Avoid overexposure, which can cause skin cancer.

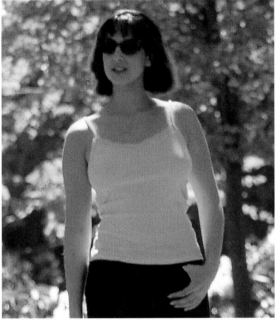

Feed your bones
Fruits, vegetables, dairy products, nuts, and oily fish contain many of the nutrients essential for healthy bones.

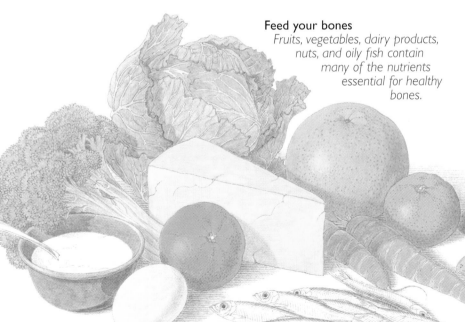

lot of gas and suffer from indigestion and a feeling of fullness for a long time after a meal), consider taking a product, such as betaine hydrochloride, that contains acid (from health-food stores) to enhance mineral absorption. Don't take it if you have an ulcer.

- Cut down on alcohol; drinking can accelerate the rate of loss of minerals from your bones.
- Limit your caffeine intake, because it can interfere with calcium absorption. However, some studies indicate that moderate caffeine consumption (defined as about two cups of average-strength coffee a day) has little or no effect. Adding

299

milk to tea and coffee helps replace the calcium being lost.

■ Cut salt intake, since salt may reduce bone density by increasing the amount of calcium that is lost in the urine.

■ Limit your intake of meat, which can promote calcium loss. Research shows that meat eaters are more likely to develop osteoporosis than those who follow a vegetarian diet.

■ Eat plenty of foods rich in vitamin A (dairy products, eggs, yellow and orange fruits and vegetables, green leafy vegetables) for bone protein production, and vitamin C (most fresh fruits—especially citrus—and vegetables) for the production of collagen, which helps keep bone's connective tissue strong.

■ Eat foods rich in vitamin D, such as oily fish and fortified dairy products.

■ Get some direct daylight—unfiltered by windows—on your skin every day. Take a daily vitamin D supplement if you do not get much sunlight, live in a region with little sunlight for much of the year, or don't eat a balanced diet. Most people need 400 IU a day. Be aware that vitamin D can be toxic in large doses, so do not exceed 600 IU a day.

■ Eat foods rich in vitamin K (leafy green vegetables); one in three people with osteoporosis has too little of this vitamin in the blood.

■ Stop smoking. Smoking increases the rate of bone resorption, probably because nicotine reduces calcium absorption in the intestines.

■ Exercise regularly. Weight-bearing exercise is especially good for bones.

■ Use stress-management techniques (see p. 347) when you feel emotionally overwhelmed. High levels of epinephrine and other hormones produced during periods of stress deplete the body of magnesium and other minerals necessary for strong bones.

TREATMENT

If you have osteoporosis, take the preventive measures above to minimize further bone loss. It is never too late. Take care with exercise, however: while regular exercise is important in treating the condition, seek medical advice first. Prolonged or strenuous exercise may make the problem worse or even cause a fracture.

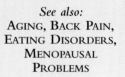

Building bone
Weight-bearing exercise increases bone density as well as muscle bulk, but you don't have to lift weights to gain this benefit. Forms of exercise in which you bear the weight of your body—such as walking, jogging, and dancing—also help build strong bones.

When to get medical help

● You have symptoms indicating osteoporosis, such as back or hip pain and loss of height.
● You have a condition or are taking a medication that increases your risk of developing osteoporosis.
● You are nearing menopause and have had many risk factors for much of your life.

See also:
AGING, BACK PAIN,
EATING DISORDERS,
MENOPAUSAL
PROBLEMS

Overweight

Carrying a lot more body fat than you should for your height and build increases the risk of health problems. Some people put on weight more easily than others, but with motivation and know-how, most overweight people can lose pounds and thereby improve their well-being. Scientists increasingly see regular aerobic exercise as one of the key factors to weight control.

DID YOU KNOW?
The old saying, "breakfast like a king, lunch like a lord, and dine like a pauper," has scientific backing. Your body burns calories more efficiently earlier in the day.

Approximately one adult in three in the United States is too fat. The problem affects more females than males and is more common in older people. Being overweight increases the risk of serious illness. Obesity—a body mass index of 30 or above (see p. 302)—makes more likely such disorders as arterial disease (heart disease, strokes, and high blood pressure), type II diabetes, osteoarthritis, digestive troubles (gallstones and constipation), certain cancers (for example, of the breast and uterus), infertility, pregnancy problems, varicose veins, and menstrual problems.

PREVENTION
Maintaining a healthy balance between energy expenditure and energy intake from an early age is the best insurance against excess weight gain. You need to get plenty of exercise (see p. 13) and to fuel your capacity for it by consuming all the nutrients you need for energy production and cell growth and renewal (see p. 9). Monitor your weight and adjust your exercise level and food intake to keep your weight within the optimum range for your height and build. Keep your calorie intake balanced: approximately 50 percent complex carbohydrates, 25 percent protein, 20–25 percent fats (with the emphasis on unsaturated fat).

TREATMENT
Whatever weight-loss program you use, aim to lose an average of no more than two pounds per week. If you lose any more than this, you are losing muscle, not fat. A dramatic drop in the first week usually results from fluid loss.

Diet: The only sure way of arriving at and maintaining a healthy weight is to change your eating habits permanently. Crash diets that promise rapid weight loss do not provide lasting results. On any one day in the United States, two in five women and one in six men are on a weight-loss diet. However, 98 percent regain their lost weight—or more—within five years.

➤ *continued, p. 303*

Causes of excess weight gain

Scientists are gradually learning why some people are especially prone to gaining weight. Proven factors include:
- The time of day at which food is eaten.
- How food is eaten.
- Genetic makeup—governing, for example, the levels of body chemicals that control appetite.
- Activity level.
- The body's metabolic rate—the rate at which it burns energy, which is influenced by genetic factors, activity level, types of food eaten, thyroid hormone levels, body weight, stress level, and food sensitivity.
- Increasing age. Many people also become less active as they get older, resulting in an even lower metabolic rate.

Are you carrying too much weight?

The most common way of judging if you are overweight is through the body mass index, which relates weight to height. Another useful indicator is your waist-to-hip ratio, since research now shows that those who accumulate fat in the abdominal area have a higher risk of health problems. A body fat percentage calculation distinguishes between those who are heavy owing to muscle bulk and those whose excess weight is the result of fat deposits.

Body mass index (BMI)

BMI is calculated by multiplying your weight in pounds by 700, then dividing the result by the square of your height in inches.
A BMI of:
- Under 20 suggests you are underweight.
- 20–24 is healthy.
- 25–29 means that you are overweight, but the risk to your health is low.
- 30 or more means you are obese, and your weight may be harming your health.

Use the chart (right) as a quick guide to your BMI.

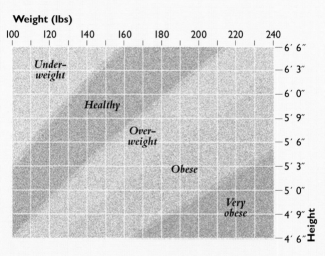

Waist-to-hip ratio

Measure your waist, with your stomach relaxed, and divide this number by your widest hip measurement. If the result is 0.85 or more (women) or 0.95 or more (men), you have an increased risk of health problems. The chart (right) provides a quick reference guide.

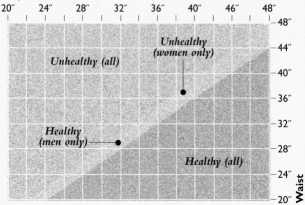

Body fat percentage

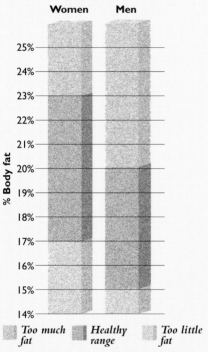

Too much fat   Healthy range   Too little fat

This measure of fat deposits needs expert assessment. Ask your doctor or fitness adviser to test you. Or you can measure it yourself on a special weighing scale that has this facility. It's natural for women to carry more body fat than men. The healthy range is 15 to 20 percent body fat for men and 17 to 23 percent for women.

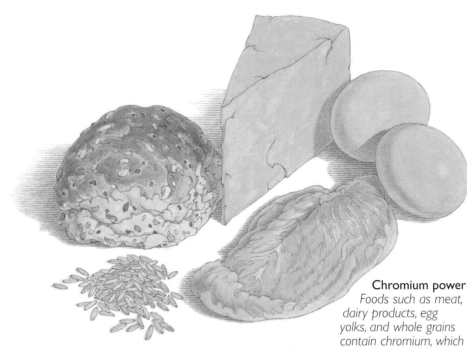

Chromium power
Foods such as meat, dairy products, egg yolks, and whole grains contain chromium, which assists weight loss because it helps regulate the release of energy from body cells.

To not only lose weight but also keep it off, follow these suggestions:

■ Eat a healthy diet with enough nutritious foods. If you choose a high proportion of refined foods (those made from white flour and sugar) and foods containing a lot of saturated fats but devoid of essential fatty acids, you are wasting a good part of your caloric intake, and your body may not get enough nutrients.

■ Choose high-fiber foods, such as brown rice, nuts, legumes, seeds, fruits, vegetables, whole-grain bread, cereals, and pasta. Fiber fills you up, prevents excessive blood-sugar swings, and converts to fat much more slowly.

■ Eat foods rich in essential fatty acids—oily fish, nuts, seeds, and whole grains. These help raise your metabolic rate.

■ Eat five or six small meals daily, rather than only one or two large ones. When you are hungry, your metabolic rate slows and you burn fewer calories to conserve energy, since your body expects famine. Eating small amounts frequently helps prevent this.

■ Have fresh foods whenever possible, because many processed foods have had their essential fatty acids destroyed to increase shelf life. They also tend to contain high levels of sugar and salt.

■ Cut down on fatty foods. These include butter, margarine, whole milk, cream, cheese, and foods made with these ingredients, as well as fatty cuts of meat. Instead, choose fish, poultry, lean cuts of meat (trim off any visible fat); buy low-fat (one percent, not two) or skim milk; and avoid fried foods.

■ Have a snack, such as a piece of fruit, about 90 minutes before a meal to prevent hunger from making you overeat during the meal.

■ Eat peppers and other spicy foods occasionally. These increase the metabolic rate for three or four hours afterward.

■ Drink green tea: studies suggest it can promote weight loss.

■ Eat less food with added sugar, such as cakes, candy, cookies, many canned vegetables and fruits, many canned or bottled drinks, and sweetened breakfast cereals. Take special care to avoid foods containing high levels of both sugar and fat, since eating sugar encourages your body to store fat.

■ Keep your alcohol intake low. Alcohol contains a lot of calories, and drinking alcohol before a meal is a well-known appetite stimulant.

■ If you suspect that food sensitivity is behind your weight problem, try an elimination diet (see p. 214). A food sensitivity can lead to fluid

retention because once the offending food proteins are captured by antibodies, they irritate the blood-vessel walls, which allows clear fluid to seep from the blood into the tissues. It can also trigger a craving for sweet, starchy food, and, perhaps, slow the metabolic rate. Wheat, milk, and potatoes are common causes of food sensitivity reactions.

From the drugstore

■ The antioxidants in multiple vitamin and mineral supplements help reduce the health risks arising from an increase in the level of fat in the blood, which is apt to occur when fat stores are utilized while you are losing weight.

■ Evidence suggests that taking a chromium supplement helps obese people with a high risk of diabetes to lose weight. Foods rich in chromium may not always provide enough of this mineral. Chromium supplements may also help prevent blood-sugar fluctuations, which can encourage binge eating. Consult your doctor before taking this mineral if you are receiving insulin treatment.

Yoga for regulating weight

Practicing yoga can help to restore and maintain healthy body weight by toning muscles and enhancing body awareness and willpower. The following exercises also help prevent or reduce a distended belly.

1 Lie flat on the floor with your legs together and your arms down by your sides. Inhale, raising both legs as high as possible. Then exhale, bringing your legs down again. Repeat this up to 10 times. If your abdominal or back muscles are weak, press your palms down as you lift your legs, and slightly bend your knees. Or try raising one leg at a time, but only as far as is comfortable. Your lower back should remain flat on the floor. Avoid this posture if you have lower back pain.

2 Stand with knees bent, your legs wide apart, and your hands on your thighs. Exhale completely, then, without inhaling, pull the abdomen in and up, expanding the chest at the same time. Then relax your stomach. Suck in the abdomen again, and pump it in and out (aim for 10 to 18 times) until you need to inhale. Take a normal breath, then exhale and repeat.

Exercise: Physical activity is vital to any weight-loss program, for a variety of reasons. Most important, it burns calories that would otherwise be stored as fat. An hour-long workout burns 200 to 400 calories and speeds up your metabolic rate for 24 to 48 hours afterward. Exercising with weights builds muscles, and muscle cells burn more energy, even when you are inactive, than fat cells. Strenuous physical activity also enhances your sense of well-being, partly by raising the level of mood-lifting chemicals, such as endorphins, and so helps you avoid eating too much to make yourself feel better.

Get your doctor's approval before starting an exercise program, especially if you are new to exercise, have a health problem, or are considerably overweight.

- Exercise four or five times weekly for about 30 minutes each session. Include aerobic exercise, such as brisk walking, swimming, cycling, or aerobics classes.
- Put your exercise sessions on your schedule to make sure you save time for them.
- Experiment with different sports and classes, such as tennis lessons, salsa dancing, and roller-blading, to find types of exercise that you enjoy.
- Ask a friend to join you. You will benefit from the stimulus of having company, and you'll be less likely to drop out if you know this will disappoint someone.
- Take every opportunity to be more active throughout the day. For instance, climb stairs instead of using the elevator, and walk to the store instead of taking the car. The extra calories you burn will soon add up.

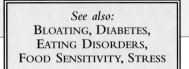

Walk away pounds
You don't have to do a vigorous workout to start burning fat. A regular brisk walk will help you lose weight.

Stress management: If food is your main source of comfort or security, you may find that you undermine your desire to lose weight at stressful or anxious times by overeating. Make a list of alternative, enjoyable activities to take the place of eating when times are tough. You might include having a scented bath, phoning a friend, and taking a walk (which is also good exercise).

Aromatherapy: Massage with essential oils helps to keep the skin smooth and supple during and after weight loss. Useful oils include celery, fennel, juniper berry, lavender, lemon, orange, oregano, and rosemary. Avoid rosemary oil in the first 20 weeks of pregnancy, and fennel, juniper berry, and oregano oils throughout pregnancy.

- Add six drops of your chosen essential oil to a warm bath.
- Alternatively, massage your feet, legs, and abdomen—or ask a friend to give you a massage—using four drops of your chosen oils in a tablespoon of sweet-almond or grapeseed oil.

When to get medical help

- You have a body mass index of 30 or above.
- The weight-reduction strategies suggested here do not work for you.
- Carrying excess weight is or may be creating health problems for you.
- You have sudden, unexplained weight gain.

See also:
BLOATING, DIABETES,
EATING DISORDERS,
FOOD SENSITIVITY, STRESS

Pain

*N*ever *ignore pain; it is a sign that something is harming you. The cause may be an external injury, such as a burn, or internal damage or disease. Once you know the source of the pain, you can often use natural remedies to ease the discomfort, while seeking medical advice, if necessary, to address the underlying cause.*

DID YOU KNOW?

There is a scientific reason why the pain goes away when Mom or Dad rubs a child's "boo-boo." The pain signals from the injured area are blocked by the pressure signals produced by massage.

Without pain to warn us about dangerous situations, human beings would probably not survive for long. For example, as children we need to learn that the pain from a wound is a sign that in the future we need to avoid the situation that caused it. Similarly, the discomfort from a sprain helps us understand that we need to rest the injured part. We therefore learn to prevent pain by protecting ourselves from its sources.

THE PERCEPTION OF PAIN

Everyone's pain threshold—the point at which a stimulus becomes painful—is the same, but each person's tolerance of pain varies. What seems a minor discomfort to one individual may be experienced as troublesome, or even agonizing, by another. People's responses also vary: someone brought up to suffer in silence will probably admit to less pain than someone from a background in which expressing feelings freely is accepted behavior.

You may also perceive the same level of pain differently at different times. A toothache that seems unbearable in the middle of the night may be unnoticed while you are enjoying a movie or cheering your football team. This may be either because your mind is occupied or because your enjoyment or excitement raises your body's levels of natural painkillers called endorphins (see "Natural Painkillers," facing page). Similarly, if you are in a car accident, you may not notice any pain from your injuries until later, when you are clear of the crash scene. The brain can suppress the sensation of pain until a crisis has passed and you are better able to cope.

TREATMENT

Addressing the underlying cause is the key to alleviating pain, so it is important to seek your doctor's advice about your symptoms. However, with many conditions it may take time for any type of treatment to begin to have an effect on your symptoms. In such cases, as with conditions that have no reliable cure, self-help measures can ease discomfort, help alleviate the mental stress associated with pain, and promote healing.

➤ *continued, p. 308*

Stress and pain

Whereas acute stress resulting from trauma may temporarily block pain (see "Natural Painkillers," opposite), chronic physical or emotional stress can cause pain and also affect your ability to cope with it. By heightening your response and lowering your tolerance to pain, stress makes existing discomfort worse. For example, if you are worried that pain results from a serious disease, it may be hard to bear, but once you know that this is not the case, you may find the pain much more tolerable. Long-term stress also causes physical tension, which makes you prone to headaches and minor injuries, such as strained muscles.

Pain pathways

The mechanisms enabling us to sense pain are complex. What you feel depends on many factors, including how active you are and whether or not you are already feeling stressed.

Painful messages

Skin receptors report a painful stimulus by sending electrical messages along sensory nerve fibers to the spinal cord. From there they travel to the brain, where the signals are interpreted as the sensation of pain. Sometimes you can feel pain in one part of the body even though the area affected is actually elsewhere. This is called referred pain, and one example is angina—pain originating from oxygen starvation of the heart muscle but felt in the upper arm, shoulder, and neck.

Pain message registers in the brain

Pain signal passes between nerve cells along nerve fibers

Natural painkillers

At times of acute stress, the brain produces chemicals, called endorphins, that block the action of the chemical messengers that transmit pain signals between nerve cells. This reduces the perception of pain.

Endorphin blocks pain signal in brain

The "gate control" theory

Pain may be partly or completely blocked by a process known as "gate control." Nerve messages carrying information from the skin about other sensations can sometimes bar the transmission of pain messages. This happens when nerve fibers carrying "non-pain" messages prevent nerve fibers carrying pain messages from relaying these signals up the spinal cord. It explains why therapies involving touch, pressure, heat, and cold can relieve pain.

Normal pain signal passing through "pain gate" in spinal cord

Pain signal blocked by other sensations

307

Relaxation: Counter the muscle tension that can exacerbate chronic pain by learning some relaxation techniques. Relaxation classes and cassettes, breathing exercises, yoga, meditation, visualization, and self-hypnosis can all help. Massage and aromatherapy are good for relaxing tense muscles; if you can't consult a professional, ask a friend or relative if he or she would be willing to learn the basic techniques.

Exercise

- A daily half hour of brisk exercise raises your body's levels of endorphins (natural painkillers in the blood) for several hours. To spread the effects of a raised endorphin level over a longer time, exercise for 20 minutes in the morning and another 20 minutes in the late afternoon.
- To lessen localized pain, exercise the affected part to increase local circulation. For example, gently bending and stretching a knee that is painful because of arthritis can assist the removal of inflammation-producing chemicals in the bloodstream.

Diet

- Limit your intake of animal proteins, which can increase the production of pain-promoting prostaglandins (hormonelike substances).
- Eat more foods containing salicylates, the family of natural painkillers from which aspirin was first made. These include most fruits (preferably unpeeled) and many vegetables, spices, nuts, and seeds. Some people are sensitive to salicylates, so seek medical advice if you notice unusual symptoms following a change in diet.

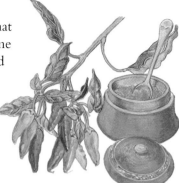

Pain-relieving pepper
A topical preparation containing capsaicin, a substance in cayenne pepper, can relieve arthritis or nerve pain. When first applied to the skin, it burns—an indication that it's working. Check with your doctor before using.

Healing touch
The contact of caring hands—for example, a friend giving you a massage or holding your hand—can be comforting if you are in pain.

Naturopathy

- Injuries to muscles, ligaments, or other soft tissues—such as a sprained ankle—can be improved by applying a cold compress to reduce swelling and inflammation and ease pain. Make a compress by wringing out a small towel or cloth in cold water. Lay this over the painful area and bind it in place with a bandage. Leave the compress in place for a half hour at a time. During the first two days after an injury, repeat as often as necessary to relieve pain.
- Some other types of pain, including menstrual cramps, may respond better to heat. A hot pack improves blood flow to the affected area, which helps clear away the inflammatory chemicals that contribute to pain. You can buy

a pack to heat in the oven or microwave, or use a towel wrung out in hot water or a hot-water bottle wrapped in a towel.

Herbal remedies: Drink one or two cups daily of the following herbal teas, according to your symptoms:

■ Black cohosh, wild yam, or meadowsweet: for pain from muscle tension.
■ Chamomile: for relaxation and relief of pain caused by tension.
■ Passionflower and St. John's wort: for backache resulting from tension.
■ Peppermint tea: for pain arising from muscle spasm.
■ Yarrow, wild yam, and meadowsweet: for pain arising from inflammation.

Caution: For safety concerns, see pp. 34–37.

Homeopathy

■ Arnica: for bruises, sprains, and aching muscles.
■ Belladonna: for throbbing pains, especially in the head, and when the area looks red.
■ Bryonia: for pain that worsens with the slightest movement and for pain on coughing.
■ Hypericum: for nerve injuries, especially when there are shooting pains.
■ Magnesia phosphorica: for neuralgia and abdominal pains, such as cramps, that are better with warmth and gentle rubbing.
■ Rhus toxicodendron: for sprains and strains with stiffness that eases after gentle movement.

Flower essences: Long-term pain can have a depressing effect, and this can add to your difficulties. Flower essences may help relieve emo-

A natural analgesic
Meadowsweet has pain-relieving properties similar to those of aspirin. However, whereas aspirin can irritate the stomach, meadowsweet has a soothing effect.

tional distress. Choose the essence according to your precise state of mind. For example:

■ Olive: for those who feel drained by a long period of illness.
■ Sweet chestnut: for those in despair, who are at the limits of their endurance.
  ■ Willow: for those who feel bitter or resentful about their illness.

Other therapies: Acupuncture, reflexology, biofeedback, meditation, yoga, and such healing therapies as reiki, can help those with chronic pain, as can counseling for stress. Some types of pain, such as lower-back, respond well to osteopathy and chiropractic.

When to get medical help

● You do not know the cause of pain.
● Pain continues despite home treatment.
● You have swelling or redness at the site of the pain, breathlessness, fever, or difficulty moving the affected part.

Get help right away if:
● You have severe pain of any kind.
● The pain is associated with numbness, tingling, or muscle weakness.

See also:
ABDOMINAL PAIN, ARTHRITIS, BACK PAIN, FACIAL PAIN, HEADACHE, MENSTRUAL PROBLEMS, MUSCLE ACHES AND STIFFNESS, NECK AND SHOULDER PAIN, RAYNAUD'S SYNDROME, SORE THROAT, STRAINS AND SPRAINS, TOOTHACHE

Palpitations

The sensation of your heart pounding, beating fast, missing a beat, or being out of rhythm can be alarming. Because it can indicate a serious heart disorder, the symptom always needs to be brought to your doctor's attention, but there is often a simple cause. Once your doctor has eliminated an underlying disorder, using appropriate natural remedies can help control palpitations.

Most of the time we are unaware of our heartbeat. However, when the heart works harder than normal, its pumping action becomes readily apparent. During and after exercise it beats faster to pump more blood around the body; this provides more oxygen and nutrients to the working muscles and removes carbon dioxide and other waste substances. Anxiety also increases heart rate, because high levels of epinephrine prepare the body for a possible "flight or fight" response to assumed danger.

Other causes of a racing heart with a regular beat include fever, caffeine-containing drinks (which raise epinephrine levels), and food allergy. Certain drugs (for example, those used for allergic rhinitis), an overactive thyroid gland, or arterial disease may also be responsible. Only in rare cases is a rapid heartbeat a sign of a heart disorder that may be life-threatening.

One type of very irregular heartbeat, atrial fibrillation, affects one in 50 people over the age of 65. It may be caused by thyroid disease or arterial disease and can be triggered by alcohol. This condition is a medical emergency. Another less serious cause of irregular heartbeat is an incompetent (prolapsed) mitral valve in the heart. This condition is present in up to one person in 20, and most commonly affects women. It requires expert assessment, but no specific treatment is usually needed.

PREVENTION

To diminish the risk of palpitations and at the same time reduce the likelihood of heart disease, keep fit with regular exercise, don't smoke, use stress-management strategies (see p. 347), eat a well-balanced diet, and maintain a proper body weight for your height (see p. 302).

TREATMENT

Palpitations manifested as an occasional rapid pulse or skipped beat usually need no treatment, unless they indicate underlying disease or are accompanied by dizziness or certain other symptoms (see box, facing page). But in all cases, it is important to get a medical opinion promptly.

Exercise: Aerobic exercise that provokes an uncomfortably rapid heartbeat indicates that your heart and lungs cannot supply your body with enough oxygenated, nutrient-enriched blood. An appropriate, graduated program of aerobic exercise over a period of months should boost lung capacity and heart strength. Be sure to consult your physician before intensifying your exercise level, especially if you have any cardiovascular risk factors, such as being overweight or a smoker.

Stress management: If you are suffering from stress-related palpitations, make time for regular relaxation and massage. Using stress-management

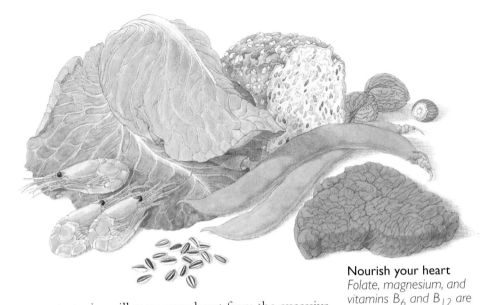

Nourish your heart
Folate, magnesium, and vitamins B_6 and B_{12} are essential for healthy heart rhythm. A diet that includes meat, shellfish, beans, peas, dark green leafy vegetables, and whole grains will supply these nutrients.

strategies will spare your heart from the excessive stimulation of a constantly high epinephrine level in the blood (see p. 347).

Diet

- Eat foods rich in folate, magnesium, and vitamins B_6 and B_{12} (see illustration).
- Lose excess weight. If you reduce the amount of body tissue the heart has to supply with blood, your heart will have to work less.
- If you suspect food sensitivity, take steps to identify the culprit food so that you can omit it from your diet (see p. 214).
- If caffeine makes your heart race and prevents you from sleeping, drink decaffeinated coffee and tea. Chamomile tea is a calming, caffeine-free, alternative beverage.
- If alcohol causes palpitations, cut your intake.

Herbal remedies: Do not take herbal remedies for palpitations except on the advice of a doctor experienced in the use of herbs. One remedy that he or she might recommend is hawthorn, which improves the pumping ability of the heart.
Caution: For safety concerns, see pp. 34–37.

Aromatherapy: Use calming oils, such as lavender, sweet marjoram, bitter orange, or neroli oils. Sprinkle a few drops onto a handkerchief and inhale, or use in a vaporizer. Rub two drops of bitter orange oil on your chest.

Other therapies: A qualified fitness instructor will work out a progressive exercise program to increase your cardiovascular tolerance to exertion, if lack of fitness is at the root of your problem. Biofeedback can help you manage your physical responses to stress, if anxiety is the cause. Regular yoga practice, with deep breathing and relaxation exercises, or meditation may also help regulate the action of the heart.

When to get medical help

- You have unexplained palpitations.
- You want to begin an exercise program and have a history of palpitations.
- You intend to use herbal remedies for palpitations.

Get help right away if:
- You have chest pain, a feeling of faintness, dizziness, a sudden change in vision, nausea, shortness of breath, or confusion.
- Your palpitations are very irregular, change in some way, or are associated with a pulse faster than 140 beats per minute.

See also:
ANXIETY,
ARTERIAL
DISEASE, STRESS

Pelvic Inflammatory Disease

This disorder, also known as PID, is a potentially serious infection of the internal female reproductive organs and the most common cause of female infertility in the United States. However, there is much you can do to prevent it and, if you have the disease, to increase the effectiveness of the treatment prescribed by your doctor.

Pelvic inflammatory disease may involve the cervix, uterine lining, fallopian tubes, ovaries, or the tissues surrounding the uterus, bladder, and bowel. Many kinds of bacteria, including chlamydiae and gonococci, can cause the disease. PID may develop after sexual intercourse with an infected partner, or, less frequently, after childbirth, miscarriage, or abortion. Those who use intrauterine devices (IUDs) have a higher than average risk of PID, as do young, sexually active women, especially those with multiple partners. Sometimes the cause cannot be found. Without adequate treatment, the infection can produce recurrent pain and can block the fallopian tubes—leading to an increased risk of infertility, ectopic pregnancy, or premature birth.

SYMPTOMS

The infected areas are sometimes tender and inflamed, but symptoms may be nonexistent, minimal, or vague. You may have painful, heavy, or irregular periods, bleeding between periods, an abnormal vaginal discharge, backache, fever, or nausea. You may also experience lower abdominal pain or a dull ache, whether intermittent or steady. Sexual intercourse may be painful.

PREVENTION

You can reduce the chances of catching any sexually transmitted disease by having an exclusive sexual relationship with one healthy partner. There is no risk if you were both previously celibate. Otherwise, you can reduce your risk of infection by always using a condom in addition to any other contraceptive method. This is especially important if you have recently had a miscarriage or an abortion. If you do not use condoms, arrange an annual test for chlamydia and gonorrhea (as well as HIV). If you have an IUD, you may want to consider an alternative method of contraception.

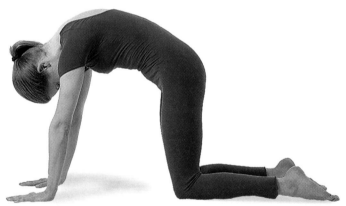

Back arching
Based on a yoga posture, this exercise alleviates back pain, tones the pelvic region, and strengthens the uterus. Arch your back upward, as shown, for a count of five, then inhale and slowly drop your back down, with your head stretched back. Repeat several times. Do not do this exercise if you have back pain from spine, muscle, or joint problems.

TREATMENT

Both you and your sexual partner should seek medical treatment and should abstain from unprotected intercourse until you are both free from infection. Use the following natural remedies alongside any prescribed treatment.

Heat: If you experience abdominal pain, rest until symptoms subside. Hold a covered hot-water bottle or an electrically heated pad against your abdomen to boost the circulation of blood and lymph and thus ease pelvic congestion of blood, lymph, and tissue fluid. Alternatively, take a warm bath to which you've added six to eight drops of rosemary, cypress, or peppermint oil. Later, when you feel better, try sitting in a warm bath, then a cold bath, and then a warm bath for 10 minutes each time.

Herbal remedies: Both echinacea and astragalus enhance the functioning of the immune system. Take either one as a tea, tincture, or tablet. Chamomile and hyssop teas may have relaxing and pain-relieving effects.
Caution: For safety concerns, see pp. 34–37.

Diet: Increase your resistance to infection with a healthy diet that includes foods rich in zinc, folic acid, flavonoids, and vitamins A, B_6, D, and E (see p. 12). Avoid refined foods, and if your consumption of alcohol and caffeine is high, cut down, since both substances can depress your immune system and your levels of B vitamins and zinc. If you are taking antibiotics, eat yogurt with live cultures daily to help prevent adverse effects on the digestive system.

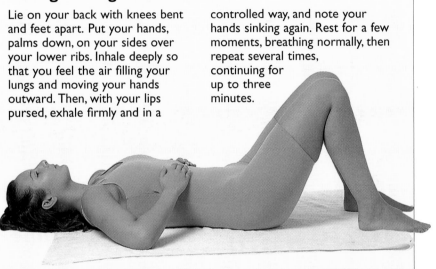

Strengthening the abdomen

Lie on your back with knees bent and feet apart. Put your hands, palms down, on your sides over your lower ribs. Inhale deeply so that you feel the air filling your lungs and moving your hands outward. Then, with your lips pursed, exhale firmly and in a controlled way, and note your hands sinking again. Rest for a few moments, breathing normally, then repeat several times, continuing for up to three minutes.

Exercise: If you feel well enough, do aerobic exercise regularly to help strengthen the immune system and stimulate the pelvic circulation, which allows more infection-fighting cells to reach the infected areas. Exercises for the abdomen (see box, above) and back help reduce congestion in the pelvis. "Crunches" are effective, as are yoga exercises.

When to get medical help

- In all cases in which symptoms suggest pelvic inflammatory disease.

See also:
ABDOMINAL PAIN, FERTILITY
PROBLEMS, MENSTRUAL PROBLEMS

Pinworms

Infestation of the intestines by these tiny worms is a common cause of anal irritation among children. Although the idea of having these parasites is unpleasant and, perhaps, embarrassing, pinworms pose little risk to health. Since the infestation is easily transmitted, all members of the family should be treated at the same time.

Testing for pinworms

You can often diagnose the condition by using the transparent tape method: Secure a piece of tape sticky-side up just outside the anus at bedtime. In the morning you may see the tiny white pinworms stuck to the tape.

Pinworms look like half-inch lengths of white cotton thread. The females emerge to lay their eggs at night, and their movements cause the characteristic nighttime itching. The eggs are too small to see with the naked eye, but if affected children scratch, they pick up eggs under their fingernails. If they later put their fingers to their mouths, the eggs readily travel from there to the intestines, where they mature, hatch, and start the cycle again. Dislodged eggs can live for some time away from the body, in bedding and on floors or other surfaces.

TREATMENT

General hygiene: Take these measures to prevent reinfestation if you have a case, and see that other affected household members do so as well.
- Wear cotton gloves in bed. If you scratch while half-asleep, the gloves will keep you from picking up eggs under your nails.
- Keep the nails clipped short.
- Wash your hands and scrub your nails after using the bathroom and before meals.
- Wash nightclothes, gloves, and bed linens daily, at as high a temperature as possible.

Eliminating infestation: Make a pint of herbal tea using one part of balmony, one part of peppermint, and one part of aniseed. Sweeten with honey, molasses, or fruit juice. Drink a cup of this mixture before breakfast, then another cup two or three times during the day, before meals. Use the treatment for a week, then repeat after a hiatus of two weeks.
Caution: For safety concerns, see pp. 34–37.

Dietary measures
- Grate a carrot and eat it mixed with a tablespoon of ground pumpkin seeds for breakfast.
- Eat raw onions, apples, and coconut, or add cayenne pepper and fresh or dried thyme to your meals to help kill worms.
- Add one or two cloves of crushed garlic to a little warm milk or a teaspoon of honey, and eat half an hour before breakfast.

Symptomatic relief: Apply a salve to the anal area at bedtime. Use calendula (marigold) ointment. Or mix two drops of lavender, eucalyptus, sweet thyme, or tea tree oil with two ounces of warmed petroleum jelly, and allow to cool.

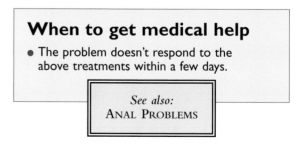

When to get medical help
- The problem doesn't respond to the above treatments within a few days.

See also:
ANAL PROBLEMS

Pregnancy Problems

*M*ost women remain healthy throughout pregnancy, but the enormous changes taking place in the body are capable of causing numerous problems and discomforts. Natural approaches, in addition to your regular prenatal care, are especially useful at this time, when only essential medications advised by your doctor should be taken.

The nine months of pregnancy have profound effects on a woman's body that can sometimes cause problems. The enlarging uterus may press on other internal organs, possibly leading to such disorders as heartburn, constipation, hemorrhoids, varicose veins, and stress incontinence. The growing weight of the baby, placenta, amniotic fluid, increased blood volume, and extra fat stores can mean fatigue and back pain. The baby's requirement for iron, calcium, and other minerals can result in maternal anemia and an increased risk of dental problems.

In addition, the body's changing metabolic, hormonal, and immunological states make diabetes, candida infection, fainting, itching, nausea and vomiting, gum problems, and leg cramps more likely.

A serious condition called preeclampsia may cause elevated blood pressure, migraines, fluid retention (which results in puffiness of the hands, face, and ankles), and protein leakage into the urine. If untreated, it can affect the supply of oxygen and nutrients to the baby and may cause miscarriage.

PREVENTION

Many minor problems of pregnancy can be averted or minimized by ensuring that you and

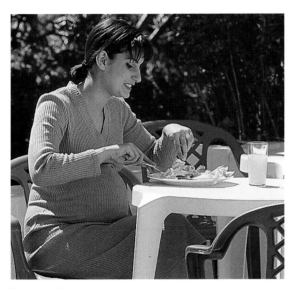

Pampered pregnancy
When you are expecting, focusing on your health is not self-indulgence but necessity. Getting enough rest and gentle exercise and eating a nutritious diet are among the most important ways of giving your baby a good start in life.

your partner are in optimum health before you conceive. Follow the advice on pages 202–205 for improving your health at this time. Once you know you are pregnant, adhere to the following guidelines for a naturally healthy pregnancy.

Diet: Continue to eat a healthy diet, with plenty of foods rich in folic acid, calcium, iron,

Essential prenatal care

It is important to have regular checkups by an obstetrician or other appropriate specialist so that any problems with you or your baby can be identified and treated as early as possible.

315

essential fatty acids, and vitamins B$_1$, B$_2$, C, and D. The average woman needs about 200 extra calories per day—roughly equivalent to a small tomato sandwich. Well-balanced meals and snacks will increase the chances of your baby having a normal birth weight, and, research suggests, will reduce the likelihood of the child suffering from diabetes, obesity, high blood pressure, and arterial disease as an adult. A good diet will also help protect you from deficiency of essential nutrients.

- Eat at least five servings daily of fruits and vegetables. Many of these contain natural salicylates, which are chemically similar to aspirin and make the blood less likely to clot. It's thought that a high intake of salicylates might reduce your risk of preeclampsia and miscarriage. Some studies already suggest that a daily dose of aspirin (which should be pre-scribed by a physician) lessens the risk of miscarriage in a few women at risk of preeclampsia and in women with Antiphos-pholipid Syndrome (APS), an immune-system disorder that interrupts the baby's blood supply by causing blood clots to form in the blood vessels of the placenta.
- Avoid or limit consumption of liver, liver prod-ucts, and vitamin-A-enriched foods. Too much vitamin A may cause birth defects.

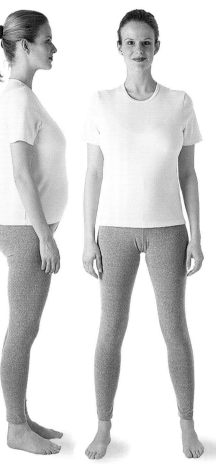

Avoiding back trouble
To reduce the risk of back strain and other aches and pains when standing, keep your feet shoulder-width apart, your shoulders relaxed, and your buttocks tucked in.

Abdominal pain

Mild tightening of the abdomen commonly occurs from about the fifth month of pregnancy onward. However, this should not cause more than slight discomfort. Abdominal pain at any stage of pregnancy should be taken seriously, especially if accompanied by vaginal bleeding. It may indicate a problem requiring urgent medical attention.

- Don't eat any food you are sensitive to. Also avoid having a large amount of any protein food at one time, as this might increase a baby's risk of developing an allergy to that food.

From the drugstore
Protect your nutrient stores from becoming depleted by taking a multiple vitamin and miner-al supplement designed for pregnancy. Ask your doctor for specific recommendations.

Exercise: Exercise moderately every day.
- If you have already had a miscarriage or pre-mature baby, or are at risk this time, don't play contact sports or engage in other jarring exer-cises, such as high-impact aerobics and jogging.
- Do Kegel exercises (see p. 251) several times daily. These make urine leaks less likely, give you more control of the baby's descent through the vagina during the second stage of labor, and lower the risk of postnatal stress incontinence.

Rest: Get sufficient rest, and take maternity leave sooner rather than later. Research indicates that women who remain at work during most of their

Yoga-based exercise program

Specially modified yoga exercises help reduce the normal aches and pains of pregnancy and prepare your body for childbirth. If you have back pain, check with your doctor before trying them.

Pelvic tuck-in

This exercise releases tension in the lower back.

1 Kneel on all fours with your knees and shoulders about 12 inches apart.

2 Drop your head and tuck in your buttocks, allowing your back to arch. Hold for a few seconds and relax. Repeat 5 to 10 times a day.

Pelvic release

This exercise releases stiffness in the pelvic area and helps widen the pelvic outlet.

1 Sit on your heels with your knees apart and toes pointing inward. Keeping your shoulders relaxed, raise your arms above your head. Breathe steadily.

2 Bend forward from your hips and rest your forearms on the floor or on a large pillow. Keep your buttocks as close to your heels as possible. Hold for 30 seconds.

Inner thigh stretch

This exercise releases tension in the inner thighs and helps reduce ankle swelling.

1 Lie down so that your buttocks are touching a wall and your legs are up against the wall. Breathe deeply and allow your legs to drop apart and your lower back to relax toward the floor. Bring your arms over your head and rest them on the floor. Relax and breathe deeply.

2 Bend your knees and bring your heels together as close to your body as you can without strain. Press your knees gently toward the wall. Hold for 30 seconds, then slowly roll onto your side to come up.

317

pregnancy have a higher risk of premature labor. Try to avoid exerting yourself and standing for long periods, since both can induce miscarriage.

Light: Exposure to bright sunshine boosts the body's production of vitamin D (which protects the bones) and serotonin (a "feel-good" neurotransmitter that helps you cope with stress). Go outside for 10 minutes at midday—longer at other times—to get sunlight on your skin, but take care not to burn.

Smoking: Stop smoking, or at least cut down. Chemicals in tobacco diminish the flow of blood to the placenta and reduce the supply of oxygen and vital nutrients to the baby. The more you smoke, the more likely your baby is to be born prematurely and the higher the risk of sudden infant death syndrome (SIDS, also called crib death). Be aware that low-tar cigarettes produce higher levels of carbon monoxide, which further reduce a baby's oxygen supply.

Tooth and gum problems: Both are more likely during pregnancy, so take extra care to protect yourself with good oral hygiene (brushing twice a day along with a session of flossing) and an adequate intake of calcium-rich foods.

Vaginal bleeding

Slight blood loss occurs in 1 out of 10 normal pregnancies without serious cause. However, vaginal bleeding can be a symptom of an impending miscarriage, an ectopic pregnancy, or a blood disorder. In all cases of bleeding, even spotting, notify your physician—immediately if you bleed heavily, have abdominal pain, or feel faint. If you have noticed bleeding of any kind, avoid physically strenuous activities, including lifting heavy weights, at least until a few days after the bleeding stops, and don't stand for long periods.

Avoiding infection: Do your best to ward off infections, which can harm the baby.

- Flu: Keep away from infected people and crowded places during an outbreak. Wash your hands often.
- Toxoplasmosis: Wear rubber gloves when gardening and handling raw meat. Wash fruits and vegetables well. Don't eat undercooked meat, and don't empty cat litter (have someone else disinfect the litter tray daily) or handle a sick cat.
- Listeria bacteria: Don't eat pâtés and deli meats, blue-veined and soft, mold-ripened cheese; feta cheese; soft ice cream; precooked poultry that's been kept warm for long periods; prepackaged salads (unless well washed); store-bought refrigerated meals (unless reheated thoroughly).

TREATMENT

Always consult your doctor about any troubling symptoms that you experience during pregnancy, and mention any home remedies that you are considering.

Nausea and vomiting: This is one of the most common problems in

Sound sleep
If you find it difficult to fall asleep because you can't get comfortable, try lying on your side with the upper knee resting on a pillow.

Semi-squatting

Whether or not you intend to use this position for labor, consider practicing semi-squatting regularly to open your pelvis and ease the baby's passage. Stand with your feet turned out, about 18 inches apart. Bend your knees to lower your body as far as is comfortable. If necessary, hold on to a chair or have your partner support you, as shown.

pregnancy. It typically diminishes after about 12 weeks, but these unpleasant symptoms continue longer for some women. Prevent attacks by eating smaller, more frequent meals and staying well rested. Avoid fatty foods and other foods or drinks that seem to provoke attacks. When nausea or vomiting occurs, try the following:

■ Eat a little bread or a cracker.

■ Sip some water.

■ Drink a cup of ginger or chamomile tea, sweetened with honey, or chew fresh ginger.

■ Press the acupressure point HP 6 (see p. 282).

Fatigue

■ Rest with your feet up for at least a half hour daily, or take a daily nap.

■ Get some whole-body exercise each day; lack of activity will make you more tired than a good balance of exercise and rest.

Carpal tunnel syndrome: This causes numbness and tingling in the middle three fingers, generally as a result of pressure on the nerves in the wrist resulting from fluid retention.

■ Don't dangle your bent wrist in an attempt to relieve discomfort. If you do this when asleep, put on a wrist splint before going to bed.

■ Take a five-minute break every half hour if your symptoms arise from working at a keyboard (see also the box on p. 325).

■ Every hour, exercise your arms and wrists for two minutes to increase the circulation of blood and lymph.

Other therapies: Seek advice on backache and other postural problems from an Alexander technique teacher.

When to get medical help

Ask your doctor about all unexplained symptoms. In particular, report the following:
● Severe nausea or repeated vomiting.
● Itching lasting more than a few days.
● Abnormal vaginal discharge.
● A bad cold, the flu, diarrhea, or a fever.

Get help right away if:
● You have abdominal pain, vaginal bleeding, or sudden and severe swelling of the hands, feet, or ankles.
● You have dizziness, severe headaches or shortness of breath, chest pain, or a sudden increase in frequency of urination.
● You have yellowing of the skin or the eyes.
● You have rubella, chicken pox, or a genital herpes infection.

See also:
ANEMIA, BACK PAIN, CANDIDA INFECTIONS, CHILDBIRTH, CONSTIPATION, FATIGUE, GUM PROBLEMS, HEMORRHOIDS, HIGH BLOOD PRESSURE, INCONTINENCE, INDIGESTION, LEG CRAMPS, MIGRAINE, NAUSEA AND VOMITING, SWOLLEN ANKLES, VARICOSE VEINS

Premenstrual Syndrome

During the second half of the menstrual cycle, many women experience a number of physical and/or emotional changes known collectively as premenstrual syndrome (PMS). Symptoms usually begin at or after ovulation (up to about 14 days before the next period) and gradually increase in severity until the onset of menstruation.

About 80 percent of ovulating women suffer from premenstrual syndrome, or PMS, at some time in their lives. It may be masked by taking contraceptive pills that contain both estrogen and progestogen, which override the body's normal hormonal cycle. Although the condition is extremely common, only one in 20 women is so severely affected that PMS greatly disrupts her life. As many as 100 symptoms have been ascribed to PMS. They fall into four categories:

- **Type A (for Anxiety):** anxiety, tension, irritability, and mood swings.
- **Type C (for Cravings):** cravings for foods containing sugar and other refined carbohydrates, increased appetite, faintness, dizziness, and headaches.
- **Type D (for Depression):** tearfulness, forgetfulness, insomnia, and confusion.
- **Type H (for Hydration):** fluid retention, with weight gain, swollen ankles and fingers, bloating, and breast tenderness.

PMS was long thought to result from an abnormal balance between estrogen and progesterone, but it now seems more likely that some women are simply oversensitive to the normal hormonal fluctuations of the menstrual cycle. Another possible cause of PMS is that premenstrual hormonal changes lead to an altered food intake, which results in nutritional deficiencies that trigger symptoms.

PREVENTION

Help even out mood swings by exercising daily and practicing relaxation techniques. Avoid or limit alcohol and caffeine-containing drinks, since they may worsen tension and depression. Also limit your intake of processed foods, animal fats, and sugar, but increase consumption of fruits, vegetables, and complex carbohydrates, such as whole-grain bread and pasta. Eat plenty of foods containing calcium, magnesium, and vitamins B_6 and E (see p. 12).

TREATMENT
Diet
- Eat more foods that contain helpful plant hormones (see illustration).
- Eat frequent small meals, based on whole grains, fruits, and vegetables, to help stabilize the blood-sugar level and reduce mood swings and cravings.
- Reduce your salt intake a few days before symptoms usually begin.

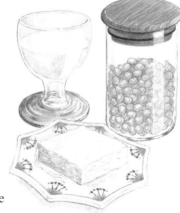

The soy factor
Soybeans and soy products, such as tofu and soy milk, contain plant isoflavones, which can help balance hormonal activity and ease PMS symptoms.

Supplements

- Two days before the onset of symptoms until the second day of your period, take supplements of vitamins B_6 and E, magnesium, and calcium, or a multiple vitamin and mineral formula specifically for PMS.
- Boost chromium intake (200 milligrams a day) to help regulate blood-sugar level and possibly control cravings for sweet foods.

Herbal remedies

- Chasteberry, along with dong quai and black cohosh, can help regulate hormone levels for all types of PMS. Take these herbs as tablets or tea. Supplements containing combinations of herbs for PMS are widely available.
- Teas made from herbs that help prevent a high level of estrogen by improving liver function, such as dandelion root or milk thistle, may also be helpful.
- Take evening primrose oil (1,000 milligrams twice a day) two days before the usual onset of symptoms until day two of your period, to help regulate any hormonal imbalance and relieve breast tenderness.
- For Type A, the calming herbs recommended for anxiety (see p. 89) may alleviate symptoms.
- For Type D, try St. John's wort tablets.
- For Type H, take horsetail and celery seed tea (two cups daily).

Caution: For safety concerns, see pp. 34–37.

Homeopathy

- Nux vomica: if you feel irritable.
- Pulsatilla: for tearfulness and a feeling of not being loved.
- Sepia: for moodiness, irritability, and a general feeling of exhaustion.
- Lachesis: if you feel jealous and quarrelsome.

Flower essences: These remedies may help dispel the emotional symptoms of PMS. Choose one or more remedies that match your symptoms and personality type (see p. 33).

Aromatherapy: Soak in a warm bath with three drops each of Roman chamomile (for its calming properties) and geranium oils and two drops of lavender oil (see illustration).

Light therapy: If depression is your main symptom, exposure to two hours of bright light in the late afternoon may help. In the winter months, a full-spectrum light box can provide an alternative to daylight (see p. 157).

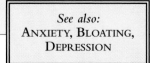

Soothing scents
Essential oils of geranium and lavender are said to help balance the emotions—a property that may enable them to curtail the mood swings often associated with PMS.

When to get medical help

- You are suffering from extreme depression.
- Your symptoms are so severe that they interfere with daily life and/or relationships.

See also:
ANXIETY, BLOATING, DEPRESSION

Prostate Problems

The prostate gland, which lies just below the bladder in men, is normally the size of a walnut. It secretes a fluid that is believed to enable the sperm to swim and reach the cervix at ejaculation. Problems arise if the prostate becomes enlarged or inflamed. The gland is also a common site for cancer in older men.

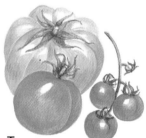

Tomato power
A high intake of lycopene, a flavonoid found in large amounts in cooked tomatoes, can help prevent cancer of the prostate.

The prostate gland begins to enlarge in most men around the age of 50. This condition, known as benign (that is, not inflamed or cancerous) prostatic hypertrophy, requires no treatment unless it produces symptoms. If the prostate swells enough to compress the urethra, which passes through it, it will obstruct urine flow. This can lead to a desire to urinate frequently, day and night, and the flow may become increasingly slow and hesitant. You may be unable to pass urine except in small amounts, yet you may suffer from incontinence.

Inflammation of the prostate is known as prostatitis. It may be a result of infection, usually transmitted sexually, or occur after jarring exercise (such as jogging) with a full bladder. Symptoms include a heavy feeling just behind the scrotum and pain in the lower back and abdomen. You may also experience pain while

Protect your prostate
The following are best avoided, especially if you have enlargement of the prostate:
- Delayed urination despite a full bladder
- Jarring exercise with a full bladder
- Constipation
- Smoking
- Unprotected sexual intercourse, unless in a long-standing, monogamous relationship

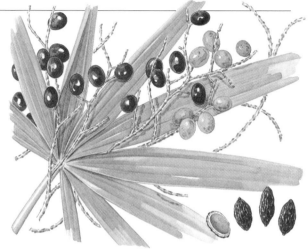

Science meets tradition
Saw palmetto is a remedy long used by Native Americans for prostate trouble. Research now shows that this plant contains substances that help block the production of hormones, especially testosterone, that stimulate prostate cell growth.

urinating. The urine may be cloudy, contain blood, and smell fishy, and you may have a fever.

Prostate cancer risk begins to rise in the early 40s. The cancer may be symptomless, so it's very important for men of this age and older to be medically tested (a PSA blood test).

PREVENTION
Eat foods rich in zinc, beta-carotene, flavonoids, and vitamins C and E (see p. 12). Eat more beans, nuts, and seeds, and have three servings of oily

Yoga for prostate health

The following exercise stimulates circulation to the prostate and nearby areas. It may also reduce any inflammation.

1 Lie on your back with your arms by your sides. Raise your knees and move your feet close to your buttocks.

2 Put the soles of your feet together —or, if you find this difficult, just let the inner edges of your soles touch. Relax your knees and allow them to sink toward the floor. Hold the position for about five minutes.

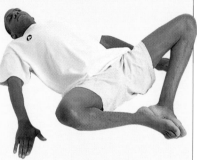

fish every week. Their omega-3 fatty acids boost immunity, thus guarding against infections and other causes of prostatitis. Daily exercise helps the prostate by stimulating pelvic circulation. Regular ejaculation is also good for the prostate.

TREATMENT

Prostatitis

This disorder generally requires prompt medical treatment. To promote healing, eat plenty of vegetables and fruits, as well as foods containing essential fatty acids, selenium, and zinc. Try to avoid physical and psychological stress.

Benign enlargement

Diet

- Reduce your consumption of dairy products and refined carbohydrates.
- Eat more foods containing zinc (including shellfish, root vegetables, and pumpkin seeds).
- Have more soy-based foods, such as tofu. Soybeans contain substances called isoflavones,

which may protect against prostate disease.

- Increase intake of foods containing beta-carotene, vitamins C and E, flavonoids (see "Tomato Power," facing page), magnesium, fiber, and essential fatty acids.
- Include lentils, nuts, and corn in your regular diet. These foods contain an amino acid called glutamic acid, which is thought to reduce prostate enlargement.
- Drink fewer caffeinated drinks.

Hydrotherapy: Take alternating hot and cold sitz baths (see p. 49) every day or two to stimulate circulation to the prostate gland.

Herbal remedies: Take the recommended daily dose of a remedy made from rye grass pollen, saw palmetto, or *Pygeum africanum*. Flaxseed oil (one tablespoon a day) contains essential fatty acids that may combat the symptoms of prostatitis and enlargement of the prostate.

Caution: For safety concerns, see pp. 34–37.

When to get medical help

- You need to urinate frequently and/or the stream is weak.
- You have pain when urinating.
- You have a fever, possibly with lower back and abdominal pain.
- You have a discharge from the urethra or blood in the urine.

Get help right away if:
- You are unable to urinate or have lower abdominal swelling or severe pain.

See also:
INCONTINENCE,
URINARY-TRACT
INFECTIONS

Raynaud's Syndrome

This disorder of the blood vessels causes the small arteries supplying the fingers and toes to contract suddenly, usually upon exposure to cold. The nose and ears may also be affected. The resulting reduction in blood circulation produces a succession of color changes in the skin, accompanied by pain, numbness, and tingling.

Maintaining circulation
When sitting still, keep the feet moving, and stimulate blood flow to the hands by repeatedly squeezing a small rubber ball.

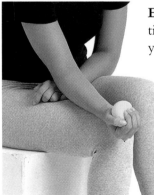

The symptoms of Raynaud's syndrome occur when the muscles surrounding the tiny blood vessels in the fingers and toes constrict, cutting down the blood supply to those areas. A cold environment, working with vibrating power tools, or certain drugs (including beta blockers) can cause an attack. The skin turns white from lack of blood, then blue as blood flow starts to return; finally, the skin reddens and may hurt. Raynaud's syndrome sometimes occurs with rheumatoid arthritis or arterial disease.

PREVENTION

Avoid known triggers. Smoking constricts the arteries, so quit or at least cut down. Keep hands and feet warm by wearing gloves and socks. Also wear several layers of clothing. Such fabrics as wool, silk, and polypropylene help conserve heat.

Exercise and massage: Improve your circulation by getting daily vigorous exercise that raises your heart rate. Regular massage may also help.

Diet: You may need extra magnesium, flavonoids, vitamins B and E, and essential fatty acids (see p. 12). Consider a daily multiple vitamin and mineral supplement. Limit your intake of alcohol and caffeine since these are triggers for some people.

Herbal remedies: Add such warming spices as cayenne, ginger, coriander seeds, cloves, and cinnamon to food, or drink one or two cups of tea made with one of these spices each day.
Caution: For safety concerns, see pp. 34–37.

TREATMENT

Heat: Warm yourself up, for example, by taking a comfortably warm, but not hot, bath. A mustard footbath (see p. 141) or hand bath may also be helpful during an attack.

Exercise: During an attack, hold your hands above your head for a minute, then whirl them around for half a minute to boost circulation. Rubbing your hands together for one to two minutes may also help alleviate symptoms.

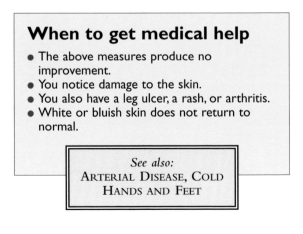

When to get medical help

- The above measures produce no improvement.
- You notice damage to the skin.
- You also have a leg ulcer, a rash, or arthritis.
- White or bluish skin does not return to normal.

See also:
ARTERIAL DISEASE, COLD
HANDS AND FEET

Repetitive Strain Injury

Injury to the muscles, ligaments, tendons, or nerves of the wrists, hands, arms, or shoulders that results from repeated movements is known as repetitive strain injury, or RSI. This includes such conditions as carpal tunnel syndrome, tenosynovitis, and tendinitis. In severe cases RSI can be painful and disabling, but there is much you can do to lessen the symptoms.

Repetitive strain injury—sometimes called work-related upper limb disorder—results from performing the same movement repeatedly throughout the day. This commonly occurs in the workplace, as when working on a computer keyboard for long hours or doing assembly-line production. Musicians are also susceptible to RSI. The damaging effects of the repeated action are encouraged by incorrect posture, poor working conditions, lack of rest breaks, and failure to perform muscle-stretching exercises.

SYMPTOMS

- Pain or aching in the hands, wrists, arms, or shoulders, aggravated by movement
- Restricted movement
- Swelling over the back of the hand or wrist
- Fatigue and weakness in the hands, wrists, arms, or shoulders
- Weak hand grip and/or lack of wrist strength
- Tingling and numbness in the fingers

PREVENTION

If your work involves small repeated movements for long periods of time, make sure that you take a regular five-minute break every hour. Use this break time to move around and stretch your hands, arms, and shoulders.

➤ continued, p. 326

Avoiding RSI at the computer

- Adjust the height of your desk and chair as described on page 106.
- Choose a chair with arms that support your elbows.
- Arrange your position so your forearms are parallel to the floor.
- Position the screen at a right angle to the window or strongest light to avoid glare.
- Make sure that your eyes are at the same height as the screen, which should be about 25 inches away from your eyes.
- Sit directly facing the keyboard and screen.
- Use soft but firm wrist supports, so you don't need to flex your wrists upward.
- Use a stand that holds documents at eye level to minimize neck bending while typing.

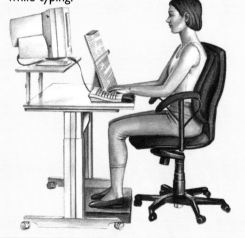

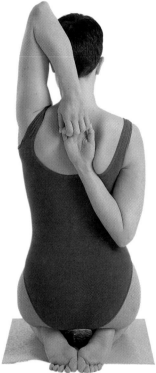

Stretch out
Yoga postures that release tension in the neck, shoulders, and upper back may help relieve symptoms of RSI.

TREATMENT

Self-help measures reduce the risk of a problem becoming chronic and causing serious and permanent damage.

- Rest the affected area as much as possible. If the condition is already serious, you may need to rest it completely for several weeks.
- Wear a splint to protect and support an affected wrist or arm. You may need to wear this while working to prevent the condition from becoming worse.
- Get regular upper body exercise to maintain mobility. Include stretching exercises, such as yoga postures (see photograph), to improve the range of motion of the affected part.

Diet: A deficiency of vitamin B_6 has been linked to carpal tunnel syndrome, a type of RSI in which swelling of the soft tissues in the wrist pinches the nerve that runs between the hand and the arm. Increase your intake of foods rich in this vitamin (lean meat, fish, whole grains, peanuts, beans, avocados, and bananas).

Hydrotherapy

- To reduce pain and swelling, apply either a cold compress (or ice pack) or a hot compress (or wrapped hot-water bottle), according to preference, to the affected area every half hour, as needed. Leave in place for as long as is comfortable—except for an ice pack, which should be applied for a maximum of three minutes.
- Avoid very hot baths. Although a soak in a hot tub may temporarily soothe aching muscles, too much heat may ultimately increase inflammation and therefore worsen RSI.

Herbal remedies: Comfrey is a traditional herbal remedy for inflammatory conditions. Apply comfrey ointment over a sore tendon or muscle. Do not use this herb if the skin is broken, and do not take it by mouth.

Aromatherapy: Some essential oils help reduce inflammation and muscle stiffness.

- Mix 10 drops each of peppermint, lavender, and eucalyptus oils with three tablespoons of sweet almond oil or a cold-pressed vegetable oil. Use this mixture to massage the affected area morning and evening.

Homeopathy

- Ruta: for most types of RSI, especially of the hand and wrist.
- Rhus toxicodendron: for pain relieved by gentle movement.
- Arnica: for any injury, when there is a sensation of bruising. Arnica cream may be massaged into the affected area.

When to get medical help

- Pain and/or stiffness is severe.
- Discomfort continues even during rest.
- Your range of movement is restricted.
- You notice wasting of muscle, especially near the thumb.
- You have numbness or tingling in the hand.

See also:
BACK PAIN, PAIN,
STRAINS AND SPRAINS

Restless Legs

This disorder is characterized by unpleasant aching, prickling, itching, or tickling sensations in the legs. The legs may twitch or feel tired, heavy, or tense, as if swollen. The most effective way to relieve the discomfort is by moving the legs. A few simple changes in your routine can reduce the frequency and/or the severity of symptoms.

Restless legs affect up to one in six people, and symptoms usually occur after prolonged sitting in the evening or while sleeping at night. The condition sometimes runs in families. It affects mainly middle-aged women but is also common toward the end of pregnancy. One in four people with rheumatoid arthritis develops the disorder, and it is also sometimes associated with iron-deficiency anemia, varicose veins, diabetes, and lung disease. The arms may also be involved.

The exact cause of restless legs is unknown, but possible triggers include smoking, fatigue, stress, alcohol, caffeine, and a lack of iron, folic acid, or vitamin E.

Cold comfort
Relieve affected muscles with a covered cold pack—a package of frozen peas or a picnic ice pack.

PREVENTION

- Eat more foods rich in iron, magnesium, vitamin E, and folic acid (see p. 12).
- Take a daily multiple vitamin and mineral supplement. Be aware, however, that most men and postmenopausal women do not need extra iron (contained in some daily supplements). Check with your doctor if you think lack of iron may be causing your restless legs.
  - Don't smoke.
  - Avoid alcohol in the evening.
  - Reduce your caffeine intake.
    - Get some moderately strenuous exercise every day.
    - Get enough rest and sleep.

TREATMENT

When symptoms appear, massage your calves with firm, kneading movements. If you can, take a walk and/or do some leg-stretching exercises.

Aromatherapy: Add 15 drops each of basil (avoid during first 20 weeks of pregnancy) and marjoram oils to three teaspoons of sweet almond oil and use this to massage your legs.

Hydrotherapy: Try the following therapies to see which works best for you.
- Apply a hot compress, such as a towel wrung out in hot water, for two minutes, and then a cold compress for one minute.
- Similarly, apply a hot-water bottle for two minutes and then a cold pack for one minute.
- Have a cool leg bath in a tub of shallow water.
- Alternate hot leg baths for two minutes with cold for one minute.

When to get medical help
- Your symptoms persist or worsen.
- Your sleep is seriously interrupted.

See also:
MUSCLE ACHES AND STIFFNESS,
SLEEPING DIFFICULTIES

Sex Drive Loss

The level of desire for sex, also termed libido, changes throughout life in response to both emotional and physical factors. These include fatigue, stress, illness, childbirth, and relationship difficulties. Understanding the reason behind any fluctuation is the first step in dealing with it. Natural therapies can help by boosting your general health so that you feel your best.

As is the case with most other aspects of human behavior, we all differ in our need for sex; there is no rule about what is "normal." A low sex drive is no cause for concern in itself, provided that you and your partner are content with the amount of sex in your relationship. However, reduced interest in sex can indicate an underlying problem. Depression and other psychological difficulties can lower libido, as can such physical illnesses as arthritis, diabetes, and arterial disease.

Several medications, including certain anti-depressants and blood-pressure lowering drugs, may reduce sex drive. Some older men have difficulty in becoming aroused or maintaining an erection. Women who are past menopause may not want to have intercourse because of discomfort resulting from vaginal dryness or other hormone-related changes.

TREATMENT

Aromatherapy: Ylang ylang and clary sage oils can encourage feelings of relaxation and sensuality. Rose otto oil is traditionally associated with a heightening of sexual desire, while sandalwood and geranium are said to help stimulate desire subdued by depression. Avoid clary sage in the first 20 weeks of pregnancy.

■ To restore calm and harmony—a prerequisite for resolving sexual difficulties—place a blend of four drops each of ylang ylang and clary sage

General help for loss of libido

- Share your concerns with your partner and involve him or her in your treatment plan.
- Try not to worry about your lack of sexual energy, as anxiety will only aggravate the problem.
- Practice stress-management strategies, including yoga, deep breathing, meditation, creative visualization, or other relaxation techniques.
- Exercise regularly to increase general, as well as sexual, energy. This will also help relieve anxiety and increase awareness of—and confidence in—your body.
- Get enough sleep. Fatigue is one of the major causes of a lack of interest in sex.

oils, or of sandalwood and geranium oils, in a vaporizer, or use eight drops of rose otto oil alone. Or sprinkle a few drops of selected oils on your bedsheets.

■ Add two drops each of ylang ylang and clary sage oils and three drops of geranium oil to two and a half teaspoons of sweet almond oil or other cold-pressed vegetable oil, and use this mixture to massage your partner's back, legs, and abdomen.

■ To boost energy levels, add two drops each of ylang ylang and clary sage oils and three drops of geranium oil to an evening bath.

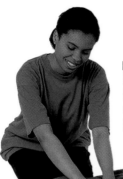

Easy closeness
Relieve anxiety and strengthen the bond between you and your partner by giving each other a gentle massage, perhaps with fragrant oils.

Herbal remedies: Certain herbal teas may be useful for countering a low sex drive.

- Women who are affected should drink a cup of tea in the evening made from raspberry leaves or take a few drops of a tincture made from this herb in half a cup of water. Tea or a few drops of tincture made from a combination of dong quai, licorice, nettles, prickly ash bark, and wild oats can increase vitality.
- To aid relaxation, men and women may benefit from a daily cup of tea made from a soothing herb, such as chamomile or vervain.
- Improve male libido with a cup of tea or a few

Specially for men
Damiana (Turnera diffusa) *has an ancient reputation as an aphrodisiac. Modern herbalism confirms its action as a tonic for the nerves and male hormonal system.*

drops of tincture made from damiana, saw palmetto, cinnamon, licorice, and ginger.
Caution: For safety concerns, see pp. 34–37.

Diet: A poor diet probably accounts for many people's low sex drive.

- Eat foods rich in vitamins A, B, and E, magnesium, manganese, zinc, essential fatty acids, and protein (see p. 12). These nutrients are important for sex hormone production and the maintenance of healthy reproductive organs.
- Eat raw fruits and vegetables every day to ensure maximum vitamin and mineral content.
- Avoid too much alcohol; it tends to impair sexual performance.

Other therapies: Marriage counseling can provide valuable help for those whose sex drive loss originates in a relationship problem or creates stress in the relationship. Psychotherapy may also be effective.

When to get medical help

- Your relationship with your partner is adversely affected.
- You suspect you have—or you are taking medication for—an underlying condition.
- You have other symptoms, such as pain during or after intercourse.
- You are depressed.
- The problem comes on suddenly.

See also:
ANXIETY, ARTERIAL DISEASE,
DEPRESSION, MENOPAUSAL
PROBLEMS, STRESS

329

Shock

Emotional shock is the mental distress that may occur after a sudden traumatic or upsetting event. Although it may require medical attention, it is quite different from clinical, or medical, shock, which follows serious injury or illness and always requires urgent attention. Natural remedies apply only to mild or moderate emotional shock.

Emotional shock may occur after such experiences as receiving news of bereavement or job loss or being physically attacked. The shock may be strong enough to affect the nerves that control blood pressure, leading to fainting (see p. 194).

Clinical shock is a potentially severe physical reaction to an injury or another medical emergency. It follows a sudden fall in the body's circulating blood volume, which leads to a reduction in the amount of oxygen reaching the brain and other vital organs. Untreated, it can damage these organs and may even be life-threatening. Causes of clinical shock include heart attack, serious accident, burns, severe allergic reaction (anaphylactic shock), acute pain, hypoglycemia, and internal or external bleeding. When this type of shock is suspected, seek emergency medical help.

After either type of shock, it is possible to develop a constellation of symptoms known as post-traumatic stress disorder. This may include flashbacks, sleep disturbance, depression, and relationship problems.

TREATMENT

The following treatments should be used only in cases of emotional shock that do not require emergency help.

Homeopathy

- Arnica: the primary remedy for emotional shock. Take doses of Arnica and Rescue Remedy (see "Flower Essences," facing page) every few minutes until you feel better.
- Aconite: if the shock is accompanied by feelings of terror and impending doom.
- Ignatia: if you feel faint or hysterical from an emotional upset.
- Gelsemium: if the shock is accompanied by weakness, trembling, diarrhea, or frequent urination, or occurs in anticipation of an event.
- Carbo vegetabilis: if the shock is accompanied by a feeling of icy coldness and the need for fresh air.

First aid for clinical shock

1 Call for medical assistance immediately.

2 If you are able, treat any obvious cause, such as bleeding.

3 Lay the person down and raise their legs higher than the heart.

4 Loosen tight clothing, and cover the victim with a blanket or extra clothing, to prevent heat loss.

5 Do not move a person in shock after a serious injury or if unconscious, except into the recovery position (see p. 195).

6 Do not give anything to eat or drink, though you can wet the person's lips with dabs of water.

Aromatherapy
- Massage your legs, arms, or face, or ask a friend to give you a massage. Mix a massage oil from one dro... nium, a... of swee... calming... and pal...
- If an em... lavende... scent fr...

Flower
four drop...
put four...
quarter o...

Herbal
- Sip tea...
- For lin... sip ging...
- For fee... of tea—...

Sym...
- Rapi...
- Pale,...
- Clam...
- Wea...
- Rapi...
- Faint...
- Anxi...
- Naus...
- Thir...
- Visu...

from lemon balm and chamomile. Do this four times daily.
- To help stimulate appetite...

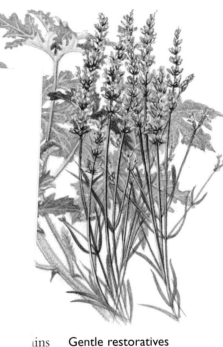

Gentle restoratives
Such essential oils as geranium and lavender can help induce a sense of calm in those who have experienced an emotional trauma.

in minutes!

or pesky health problems

Suffering from pollen allergies? **Turn to page 81** now and find out how some petroleum jelly could help.

Indigestion troubling you? **See page 254 and 255** to find out which delicious foods you can include with dinner tonight to help bring relief.

Feeling tired lately? See the collection of smart solutions on **page 200** for a natural pick-me-up.

For every ailment you look up, you'll discover a whole range of smart, natural remedies including: herbs, foods, acupressure, yoga, massage, meditation, aromatherapy, vitamins, and much more!

Plus, not only will your new book help you cure

Skin Problems

*T*he skin is your body's first line of defense against damage from infection, extremes of light and temperature, pollution, and physical injury. Its health can be affected by internal disorders as well as external factors. Look after your skin carefully—with natural therapies, when necessary—and it will continue to serve you well for a lifetime.

Essential skin protection
Contact with detergents can cause dryness, inflammation, and cracking of the skin. Protect your hands by wearing rubber gloves whenever possible.

The most common skin problems in adults include oily or dry skin, acne, psoriasis, and eczema and other forms of dermatitis. For skin to remain healthy, smooth, and supple, it needs an adequate production of sebum (the oily substance secreted by glands attached to the hair follicles); good hydration; a healthy circulation of blood and lymph; sufficient nutrients; the proper hormonal balance; the opportunity for repair and renewal; and the absence of irritation from detergents, ultraviolet sun rays, and other potentially damaging agents.

PREVENTION

Encourage sebum production by managing stress effectively, eating a healthy diet, maintaining a normal body weight, and avoiding temperature extremes, strong winds, and contact with harsh soaps and detergents. Apply a moisturizer each day, and hydrate the skin from within by drinking at least six glasses of water every day. Boost your circulation and help prevent fluid retention with regular brisk exercise and a sound diet. Protect your skin from wind and sun (use a sunscreen with an SPF of 15 or more). Wash your face and body with a mild soap containing vegetable extracts, such as palm kernel and coconut oil, or with a soapless cleansing bar containing synthetic ingredients to help maintain the skin's natural acidity. Encourage the repair and renewal of your skin cells by getting enough sleep and by not smoking (see box, below).

Diet: Prevent premature aging of skin by eating plenty of raw fruits and vegetables. Limit your intake of saturated fats, refined foods, and alcohol, all of which tend to speed skin aging. Only about 13 percent of your calories should come from animal protein foods, such as meat, eggs, and cheese. Try to lose excess weight: slim yet well-nourished people tend to age more slowly.

Vitamin C, flavonoids, and zinc help keep skin supple, so make sure your diet contains foods rich in these nutrients (see p. 12). You also need foods

Aging effects of smoking
- Toxins from inhaled smoke restrict the blood flow to the skin, thereby depriving it of oxygen. This reduces the ability to heal and regenerate new skin.
- After years of regular smoking, the skin may become much thinner than that of a nonsmoker, resulting in deeper wrinkles.
- Smoking reduces the collagen content of the skin so that wrinkles develop more quickly.

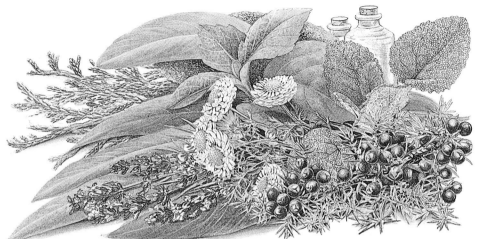

abundant in carotenoids; vitamins B (especially biotin) and E; and the minerals copper, manganese, and selenium. Include foods containing essential fatty acids, together with those that contain magnesium, zinc, and vitamin B_6, which are needed to metabolize them.

TREATMENT

Aromatherapy: The balancing, cleansing, and regenerative qualities of essential oils are excellent for improving the appearance and health of the skin. Used daily, they can improve skin texture, especially that of the face and hands—the areas most exposed to the elements.

Create your own range of aromatherapy skin products by mixing the oils in the items that follow with sweet-almond or jojoba oil or an unscented body lotion. Apply your mixtures to problem areas, or use for massage. You can also add diluted oils to your bathwater or mix them with water for a compress, but don't apply undiluted oils, other than tea tree and lavender, directly to the skin.

Fragrant skin care
Essential oils may help a wide variety of skin conditions. The plants from which some of the most effective are obtained are (clockwise from far left) eucalyptus, cypress, peppermint, clary sage, juniper berry, chamomile, and lavender.

- Clary sage is soothing and anti-inflammatory. It also helps preserve moisture in dry or mature skin. Do not use this oil during the first 20 weeks of pregnancy.
- Cypress, which is astringent and soothing, may help regulate the production of sebum in oily skin. Do not use this oil during the first 20 weeks of pregnancy.
- Eucalyptus is cooling and antiseptic. Use it to treat boils and pimples.
- Geranium has astringent and balancing properties. It helps cleanse and tone the skin, reduces inflammation, and can soothe acne, eczema, and minor wounds.
- Juniper berry is astringent and cleansing. It is beneficial for acne, oily skin, and oozing eczema. Do not use this oil at any time during pregnancy.
- Lavender is antiseptic and anti-inflammatory. It can soothe eczema, sunburn, and insect bites. It also helps promote cell growth and healing, thus possibly minimizing scarring.
- Peppermint oil cools and cleanses the skin. It can soothe itchy skin, though too much can make itching worse.
- Roman chamomile is soothing and antiseptic, and good for sensitive or dry skin. It helps heal acne and dermatitis and reduces other types of skin inflammation.
- Sandalwood helps soften dry, mature, or wrinkled skin. It may also reduce irritation from sunburn, hives, and other rashes.
- Tea tree oil has antiseptic, anti-inflammatory, and antifungal properties. It is good for boils and rashes, as well as countering skin infections of all kinds.

Food sensitivity: Such skin problems as rough-ness, hives, and eczema may result from food sensitivity. Sometimes it is easy to relate a skin problem to a particular food, but often the link is not obvious. Identifying a culprit food may be difficult if it is one that you eat frequently or if your symptoms are vague and long-standing.

You may want to try an exclusion diet, avoiding the suspected foods for three weeks. (Milk products, eggs, and wheat are among the most common culprits.) Then reintroduce these foods one at a time, with a gap of three weeks between each one, to help determine which, if any, are causing problems.

You may be able to boost your immunity and help heal any inflammation—thereby lowering your risk of food sensitivity—by avoiding refined foods and eating more foods rich in essential fatty acids, such as most cold-pressed vegetable oils, nuts, and seeds. Supplements of omega-3 fatty acids (found in fish oil) and evening primrose oil may be beneficial. Eating foods abundant in vitamins A and C may also be useful in preventing food sensitivity.

Herbal remedies: Many herbs are excellent for healing skin conditions. They can ward off infection, relieve pain, and reduce scarring. Use them either in a compress, made by soaking gauze in herbal tea and binding it to the damaged area, or in cream or ointment form.
- Aloe vera gel softens and nourishes dry skin and encourages skin regeneration after injury. It also helps prevent "barber's rash"—the crop of tiny pimples that may appear after shaving.
- Burdock seeds are cleansing. They're good for

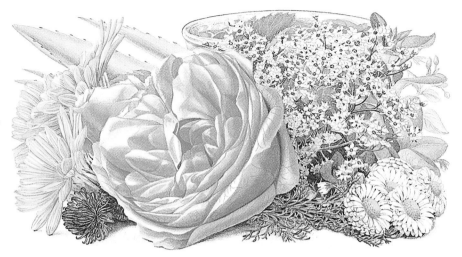

Help from the herb garden
Herbal teas and ointments are gentle treatments for skin conditions caused by infection, inflammation, or allergy. Many of these herbs have been used for centuries.

treating eczema, dermatitis, psoriasis, boils, abscesses, and acne.
- Chamomile's antiseptic oils have a soothing and anti-inflammatory effect. They help stimulate skin repair.
- Chickweed soothes such irritating skin conditions as eczema and psoriasis. It also softens the skin and alleviates itchy rashes and eruptions.
- Elderflower, an anti-inflammatory, is a traditional remedy for ulcers, burns, cuts, and wounds. Distilled elderflower water makes an excellent facial toner and cleanser.
- Marigold (calendula) is a good first-aid remedy for cuts, burns, and bruises, since it combats infection and reduces inflammation.
- Rosewater cleanses and tones the skin, smoothes wrinkles, and can help clear up acne. It cools the skin by acting as an astringent, aids skin repair, and reduces swelling and bruising.
- Witch hazel, widely available in drugstores, was traditionally used by Native Americans. It is strongly antiseptic and healing: its astringent tannins stop bleeding and lessen inflammation

and scarring. It is also effective for bruises and irritated varicose veins. Apply straight witch hazel to unbroken skin, but dilute with water for application to broken skin (any stinging will stop quickly).
Caution: For safety concerns, see pp. 34–37.

Kitchen cabinet remedies
- Baking soda applied to a poison ivy rash will help keep it dry.
- Beet and cabbage juices are good blood cleansers and helpful in cases of oily skin prone to acne. Drink half a glass of one of these juices once or twice a day for 10 days.
- Carrots are antiseptic and help speed wound healing. Apply cooled carrot broth to your skin to soothe chapping, roughness, and itching.
- Cucumber soothes inflamed, itchy rashes, such as eczema, and cucumber water also makes an ideal cleanser and toner for oily skin: cut a cucumber into cubes and boil in two pints of water for 15 minutes. Strain and press through a cloth or sieve.

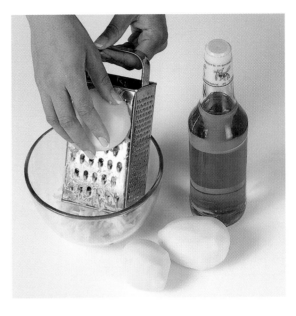

Versatile vegetable
Raw potato juice is a traditional remedy said to soothe inflammation and help heal dermatitis, wounds, and ulcers. To treat cracked skin, use grated potato mixed with olive oil.

- Flaxseeds are rich in omega-3 essential fatty acids, which aid skin health. Apply flaxseed tea to dry skin, or add it to bathwater to soften skin.
- Honey has antiseptic properties; smooth a little over infected skin.

When to get medical help
- A skin condition worsens or fails to clear up after home treatment.
- The problem is close to the eyes.
- A baby or young child is affected with a skin problem besides typical diaper rash or cradle cap.

Get help right away if:
- A rash occurs along with a raised temperature, a headache, drowsiness, a stiff neck, shortness of breath, or faintness.

See also:
ABSCESSES AND BOILS, ACNE, AGING, CANDIDA INFECTIONS, CHAPPED LIPS, COLD SORES, CUTS AND SCRAPES, DERMATITIS, DIAPER RASH, DRY SKIN, FOOD SENSITIVITY, FUNGAL SKIN INFECTIONS, HAIR AND SCALP PROBLEMS, HIVES, INSECT BITES AND STINGS, ITCHING, SUNBURN, WARTS

Sleeping Difficulties

A good night's sleep regenerates the body and refreshes the mind, but nearly everyone complains of difficulty sleeping at some time or another. Anxiety about your lack of sleep can make the situation worse, but using natural techniques (known collectively as sleep hygiene) may be all you need to start slumbering deeply once again.

The average American sleeps between six and seven hours a night, even though it's believed that most adults require about eight hours. Women report more problems with sleep than men, and sleeping difficulties become more common as we get older. If you do not sleep well, you may feel tired and generally unwell. Chronic lack of sleep reduces physical and mental performance during the day and may lead to anxiety, depression, or other problems.

PREVENTION

Sleep hygiene: This is a way of reorganizing your routine to create conditions that are conducive to sleep. Paying attention to sleep hygiene can help prevent problems with sleeping and can

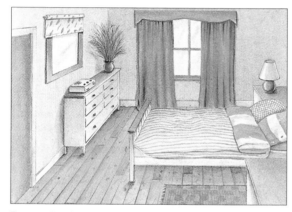

Dream land
Make your bedroom a peaceful, clutter-free space.

even help overcome established insomnia. You are unlikely to get a good night's sleep if you are uncomfortable, hungry, thirsty, or too hot or cold, so it is important to ensure that these factors do not interfere with your sleep.

■ Make sure that your bed is comfortable. If the mattress is more than 10 years old, you probably need to invest in a new one. Choose a mattress that is firm enough to provide support, but not so hard as to put pressure on your hips and shoulders.

■ Check that the temperature in your bedroom is neither too hot nor too cold—research indicates that a temperature of around 65°F is right for most people. Your bedroom should also be

---

Types of sleeping problems

● Difficulty getting to sleep often occurs because you're unable to stop thoughts and worries from whirling around in your mind. The cause is usually anxiety or a strong emotion, such as anger, that you have not dealt with during the day. Anticipatory excitement can also make it difficult to drop off. Physical reasons include indigestion, restless legs, and alcohol-induced agitation.

● Waking up early and being unable to get back to sleep may be a symptom of depression and/or anxiety. It can also occur if you have drunk too much alcohol or caffeine.
● Waking up frequently during the night and being unable to drop off again immediately is more common in older people and is sometimes linked to depression and/or anxiety.

dark and quiet. If it is not, consider using an eye mask and earplugs.

- Choose a restful decor, with warm, soft colors.
- In the hour or two before going to bed, do not smoke, eat large or indigestible meals containing animal fats and refined carbohydrates, drink alcohol or caffeine-containing drinks, watch exciting or disturbing TV programs, read stimulating articles or books, or do strenuous exercise. Have a warm bath just before bedtime.
- Eat a light, sleep-inducing snack (see "Treatment"). Hunger can keep you from getting to sleep or can make you wake up during the night or in the early morning.
- Ideally, your bedroom should be a peaceful haven associated with sleep. Do not use it for such activities as working and ironing.
- If you stay awake for more than half an hour after going to bed, get up, go to another room, and do something else, such as yoga or light reading, until you feel sleepy.
- Get into the habit of going to bed and getting up at the same times each day. Set your alarm to help you wake up, if necessary.
- Do not nap during the day.
- Exercise daily for at least 30 minutes.
- Try—unless you are on shift work—to take full advantage of the bright early-morning light by being awake then, rather than sleeping in a darkened room until mid-morning. The natural variation of light intensity throughout the 24-hour day has powerful effects on the brain's pineal gland, which helps regulate our daily rhythms. Sleeping when it is dark and staying awake when it is light can help reinforce a healthy pattern of sleep and waking.

TREATMENT

Soporific snacks: A light, easily digested snack before bedtime can often prevent hunger pangs from disturbing your sleep. Moreover, certain foods or food combinations can promote sleep. Such foods are high in carbohydrates and rich in vitamin B, calcium, magnesium, essential fatty acids, and the amino acid tryptophan, which is used by the brain to make sleep-inducing chemicals (see p. 86). This combination of nutrients allows the tryptophan to reach the brain and may help you feel sleepier within about half an hour. Snack suggestions include:

- A whole-grain bread and lettuce sandwich
- Boiled potato and cauliflower mashed with a little hazelnut or walnut oil
- Sliced banana with chopped dates
- Warm milk and cookies

If you suspect that certain foods disagree with you, cut them out of your diet for a couple of weeks to see if this improves your sleep. If you find that cheese causes nightmares, for example, eat it only early in the day.

Herbal remedies: Herbs are often a gentle alternative to prescription sleeping pills.

- Drink a cup of celery-seed tea before going to bed. Add two teaspoons of the crushed seeds to a cup of boiling water and steep.
- If your sleep problem is long-standing, opt for a cup of passionflower or valerian tea. Take this before bedtime. You can have another cup of this tea if you awaken

The sleep hormone

Melatonin, the body's sleep-inducing hormone, can be obtained in supplement form. Consult your doctor before taking this remedy.

Snooze foods
Eating snacks made from whole-grain bread, bananas, lettuce, cauliflower, and dates may be better than counting sheep.

during the course of the night and find it hard to fall asleep again.

■ Help yourself unwind by adding essential oils or herbal tea to your bathwater in the evening. Lime tree flower, lavender, Roman chamomile, frankincense, neroli, and rose oils are all suitable, as are teas made from lime tree flower, chamomile, catnip, lemon balm, and hops. St. John's wort tincture or tablets contain melatonin, which aids sleep.

■ Put a mixture of your favorite soothing and sleep-inducing herbs inside your pillowcase, or take a small fabric bag, stuff it with herbs, and put it near your head so you breathe in the

Yoga as sleep preparation

These simple yoga techniques can help if you have difficulty "switching off" at bedtime.

1 Stand with your arms straight out in front of you at shoulder height, and your palms facing each other, fingers stretched forward.

2 Move your arms out to each side as you inhale. Then return your arms to their original position as you exhale. Breathe in time with your arm movements. Repeat 10 times.

3 Stand with the palms of your hands on your chest and your fingers linked. As you inhale, move your arms out in front of you, at chest height, with palms outward and fingers stretched forward. Bring your hands back to their original position as you exhale. Do this three times. Then repeat, but this time lift your stretched arms to form an angle of 45 degrees to your body. Bring them back to your chest. Then repeat, this time raising your arms above your head. Do the entire exercise six times.

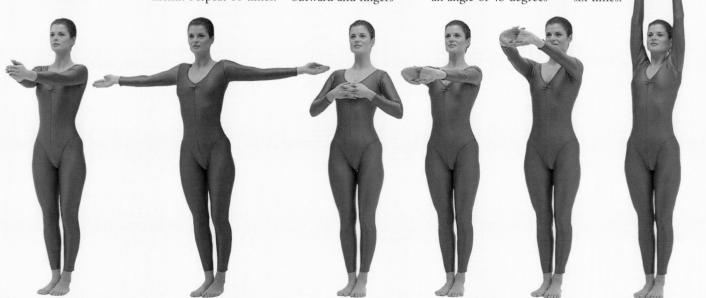

scent during the night. Suitable calming herbs include lavender, lime tree flower, chamomile, catnip, lemon balm, and hops.
Caution: For safety concerns, see pp. 34–37.

Homeopathy: Try the remedy that most closely matches your symptoms:
- Arsenicum: if anxiety is preventing you from sleeping.
- Coffea: for an overactive mind, crowded with unwanted thoughts.
- Passiflora: for uneasy sleep.

Herbs for sleep
Chamomile, passionflower, or hops can be used to make a soothing, caffeine-free bedtime drink.

Flower essences: These are gentle remedies designed to address emotional problems and are particularly appropriate for the treatment of sleep disorders. Choose a flower essence that seems to suit your emotional state—for example, Rock Rose for terror, Mimulus for fear, or Agrimony for worry (see p. 33). Add two drops each of your chosen remedies to a one-ounce, dark glass vial three-quarters full of spring water, and top off the bottle with brandy as a preservative. Use glycerin instead of brandy if consuming alcohol creates problems for you.

Take four drops of your mixture, either directly on the tongue from a dropper or added to spring water. Do this four times a day before a meal or snack. If this doesn't help after four weeks, add up to three more remedies to the mixture and continue taking as before.

Stress management: Lessening the stress in your life will probably improve your sleep. Some stress is unavoidable, but there are positive ways of handling it. Classes in relaxation, meditation, visualization, yoga, or assertiveness training may help you to manage stress. Self-hypnosis can also be effective. These techniques are especially good if you have been using food, cigarettes, or alcohol or other recreational drugs as a way of dealing with pressure. If you can't handle stress on your own, consult your doctor or a trained counselor.

Exercise: Regular exercise reduces anxiety, improves the circulation, and burns up the adrenaline and other stimulating hormones you make when you're feeling stressed. However, you should do serious exercise during the day rather than in the evening, or you may be too stimulated to sleep.

When to get medical help
- Your sleep problems last longer than a week or two.
- You fall asleep or cannot function properly during the day (especially important if your work requires you to be alert, physically strong, or well-coordinated).
- You fear that tiredness is affecting your family relationships.
- You suspect that an illness, such as depression or severe anxiety, underlies your sleep problem.
- You also have such symptoms as night sweats, fever, chills, abdominal pain, and neck ache.

See also:
ANXIETY, DEPRESSION, INDIGESTION, RESTLESS LEGS, STRESS

Snoring

People who snore are usually unaware of the noise they make, but the disorder can easily become the bane of their partner's life by seriously disturbing their sleep. There is no certain cure for snoring, but you can take several measures that may reduce or even prevent this annoying problem as well as improve your general health.

Sleep on your side
Sew a tennis ball into the back waistband of your pajamas to keep you from rolling onto your back and allowing the tongue and uvula to block the throat.

During waking hours, the activity of the throat muscles keeps the airway open. During sleep, these muscles relax and in certain people allow the airway to collapse. Their breathing then needs to deepen to force the airway open and allow air to enter the lungs. This deeper, more forceful breathing through the mouth causes a loud vibration and rattling of the soft palate and uvula (the small flap at the back of the soft palate), which produces the noise of snoring. Several factors may temporarily cause or increase snoring: a cold, allergic rhinitis, polyps in the nose, and enlarged adenoids. The following groups are most likely to snore:

■ Men—the problem affects three times as many men as women.
■ People of middle age and older.
■ Overweight people. Fat beneath the lining of the throat reduces the size of the airway and encourages breathing through the mouth. The larger you are, the more likely you are to snore.
■ Smokers. Smoke irritates the nose and throat and swells the lining of the passages. This constricts the airway and encourages breathing through the mouth.
 ■ Those who have consumed alcohol within the last few hours before bedtime. Alcohol relaxes the throat, face, and jaw muscles, encouraging breathing through the mouth.

TREATMENT
To prevent or reduce snoring:
■ Lose excess weight.
■ Don't smoke.
■ Reduce alcohol intake.
■ Eat your evening meal at least three hours before you go to bed.
■ Go to sleep and get up at about the same times every day.
■ Use books or blocks to elevate the head of your bed by three to four inches.
■ During a cold or an attack of allergic rhinitis, gargle before bedtime with one drop of peppermint oil in cold water. This remedy enlarges the airway by shrinking the swollen lining of the nose and throat.
■ Use nasal strips (from the drugstore) designed to help you breathe correctly.

When to get medical help
● The measures described don't help.
● You or your partner experiences daytime fatigue and sleepiness.
● Your partner reports that you sometimes stop breathing while snoring (sleep apnea).

See also:
OVERWEIGHT, SLEEPING DIFFICULTIES

Sore Throat

This common complaint may be caused by viral or bacterial infection, allergy, dry air, or by inhaling smoke and other airborne pollutants. A sore throat is often the first sign of a cold, the flu, laryngitis, or infectious mononucleosis ("mono"). Choose from a number of natural remedies to soothe your symptoms and fight infection.

A sore throat, which may look red, feels raw and rough, making it painful to swallow. It may be accompanied by a fever and congestion. In most cases, symptoms clear up quickly.

PREVENTION
- Keep warm.
- Drink at least six glasses of caffeine-free, non-alcoholic fluids daily.
- Don't smoke, and avoid polluted environments.
- Eat foods rich in folic acid and vitamins A, B, C, D, and E, as well as flavonoids, iron, magnesium, and zinc (see p. 12). Increase your intake of raw fruits and vegetables, and limit that of refined carbohydrates, caffeine, and alcohol.
- Include several cloves of crushed raw garlic in your food daily.

TREATMENT
Herbal remedies
- Gargle three to six times daily with tea made from thyme, goldenseal, or myrrh, or a few drops of tincture in a little water. Or use red sage tea with a teaspoon of apple-cider vinegar. These herbs are both antiseptic and soothing.
- To boost your immunity, drink every two hours a cup of tea made from echinacea, wild indigo, and sage. Add soothing mullein, marshmallow, or coltsfoot if your throat is very sore or you have a cough. If you have congestion or a fever, add elderflower, yarrow, and peppermint.
- The Chinese herbal supplements astragalus and reishi mushrooms have a powerful strengthening effect on the immune system. Add them to teas or use them in cooking.
Caution: For safety concerns, see pp. 34–37.

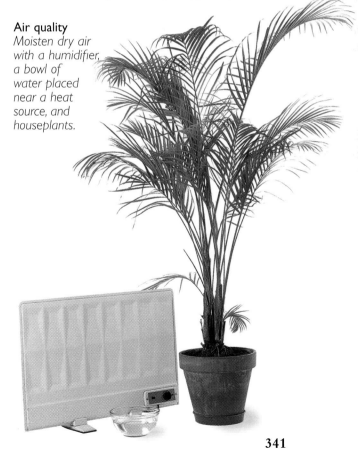

Air quality
Moisten dry air with a humidifier, a bowl of water placed near a heat source, and houseplants.

Aromatherapy: Sandalwood and lavender are soothing; lemon, geranium, pine, and tea tree help fight infection; and eucalyptus, peppermint, and Atlas cedarwood help clear congestion. Choose from these treatments:

■ Every two hours, gargle for several minutes with two drops each of sandalwood and lemon oils, or two drops each of Atlas cedarwood and eucalyptus oils, in a glass of warm water, then spit the water out.

■ Gargle with warm water to which you have added three drops of geranium or lemon oil.

■ Massage your face and chest with a blend made with three drops of sandalwood oil, two drops of eucalyptus oil, and one drop of peppermint oil in two and a half teaspoons of sweet almond oil or unscented lotion.

■ Inhale the steam from a bowl of very hot water containing two drops of eucalyptus or pine oil and two drops of peppermint oil. Do this for 5 to 10 minutes twice daily.

Homeopathy

■ Aconite: for soreness that begins suddenly, begins or worsens at night, and makes your throat hot and dry. Swallowing is difficult, although you are thirsty.

■ Apis: if your throat is red, stinging, and puffy, and cold drinks help.

■ Belladonna: if you have a sudden dry, burning, throbbing soreness, with bright red throat.

■ Hepar sulphuris: if your throat feels as if a fish bone were stuck in it. You feel bad-tempered

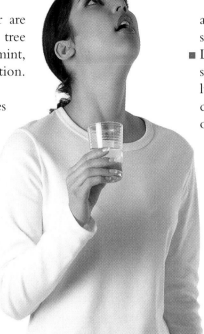

Acid action
A gargle made with a teaspoon of lemon juice or apple-cider vinegar in a glass of warm water is a traditional remedy for a sore throat. The acid in these ingredients is hostile to the bacteria and viruses that most often cause the problem.

and intolerant of cold, but your throat is soothed by warm drinks.

■ Lachesis: if swallowing solids is less painful than swallowing liquids. You feel as if you had a lump in your throat, and you cannot bear any constriction around the throat. The pain is often on the left side, or it begins on the left and moves to the right.

■ Lycopodium: if the right side of your throat feels worse or the pain moves from right to left. Warm drinks help, and you feel worse in the late afternoon or early evening.

■ Phytolacca: if your throat looks dark or bluish-red, and the pain is especially bad on swallowing. You feel as if you had a hot lump in your throat, and your body aches.

Kitchen cabinet remedy: Mix one teaspoon of salt with warm water. Gargle or use as a mouthwash up to six times daily.

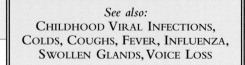

When to get medical help

● Your symptoms last longer than a few days, or if severe, a day.
● You have a high fever, a rash, dizziness, a severe headache, enlarged glands in the neck, or extreme difficulty swallowing.

Get help right away if:
● You have concurrent chest pain or palpitations.

See also:
CHILDHOOD VIRAL INFECTIONS,
COLDS, COUGHS, FEVER, INFLUENZA,
SWOLLEN GLANDS, VOICE LOSS

Splinters

A small splinter of wood, metal, glass, or other hard substance that becomes embedded in the skin can be surprisingly painful. If not removed, such a foreign body may cause inflammation and tenderness and may become infected. Splinters are often quick and easy to take out, however, using simple first-aid techniques.

The hands, feet, and knees are the areas most likely to come into contact with splintery materials. Although splinters may seem insignificant, don't ignore them. If left alone, they can be a source of infection that can spread to other parts of the body.

TREATMENT

Aromatherapy: Before and after removing a splinter, apply one drop of lavender, tea tree, or myrrh oil (avoid myrrh during first 20 weeks of pregnancy). These essential oils encourage healing and, because of their antibacterial properties, help prevent infection from taking hold.

Herbal remedy: To draw out a splinter, apply slippery elm ointment or a slippery elm poultice for 24 hours.

Kitchen cabinet remedies

- To help bring a deeply embedded splinter to the surface, apply a warm poultice (see p. 37) of bread or bran several times throughout the day. Then apply comfrey ointment and cover with a light bandage for 24 hours.
- Draw out a stubborn splinter by covering it overnight with an adhesive bandage spread with honey or kaolin (from a drugstore).

Homeopathy: Silica, taken orally, may help bring a small splinter to the skin surface.

Removing a splinter

- Clean the skin around the splinter with soap and warm water.
- If the splinter projects from the skin, use tweezers to grasp the end of it, as close to the skin as possible, and gently pull it out. If the splinter lies under the skin, sterilize the tip of a sewing needle by holding it in the clear part of a flame for a few seconds. Allow it to cool, then use it to ease the splinter out.
- When the splinter is out, squeeze the wound to encourage a little bleeding, apply a topical antiseptic, then cover with a dressing.

When to get medical help

- The splinter is large or cannot be removed.
- The splinter lies over a joint.
- The area surrounding the splinter is red, swollen, or hot.
- The wound around the splinter looks dirty.
- Pus has formed in the area of the splinter.
- You have not had a tetanus immunization within the past five years.

See also:
CUTS AND SCRAPES

Strains and Sprains

A strain is damage to a muscle and its tendon, and a sprain is damage to a ligament, which connects and supports the bones on either side of a joint and the fibrous capsule that encloses the joint. Both types of injury are caused by a sudden pulling or twisting of the affected part that overstretches or tears the tissues. They are a frequent consequence of falls and sports accidents.

The symptoms of strains and sprains are pain, swelling, and bruising. A strained muscle is most likely to occur with unaccustomed exertion or when exercising or lifting carelessly. An ankle sprain often happens after turning the ankle on uneven ground. The tissues around finger joints and facet joints of the spine (see p. 105) are other common sites of sprains.

To prevent sprains, watch your step, wear proper shoes for sports, and discard shoes that permit your ankles to turn easily. To prevent strains, warm up and stretch before exercising, and cool down and stretch afterward.

TREATMENT

- Apply a well-wrapped ice pack or a cold compress for 10 minutes several times daily for the first two days. After that, alternate a hot compress or heating pad with a cold compress. Apply an elastic bandage. If the skin becomes numb or blue, remove the source of cold. Get medical advice if normal sensation and color do not return within a few minutes.
- Elevate the injured part to reduce swelling.
- Rest the joint or muscle for at least 48 hours. Then gradually start moving the affected part.

Diet
- Add turmeric to your food. This spice is a potent anti-inflammatory agent.
- Eat pineapple. It contains bromelain, an enzyme that helps reduce inflammation.
- Eat foods rich in calcium and magnesium (see p. 12). These are key nutrients for muscles.

Herbal remedies
- To encourage healing, apply comfrey or arnica ointment over the injury before bandaging. Do not use either remedy on broken skin.
- To reduce inflammation, make a tea or take a supplement of the Indian herb boswellia.
Caution: For safety concerns, see pp. 34–37.

Homeopathy
- Arnica: for immediately after injury.
- Rhus toxicodendron: for severe strains, when the pain is eased by gentle motion.

RICE remedy
Treat sprains and strains with rest, ice (or a cold compress), compression, and elevation—a combination often abbreviated as RICE.

When to get medical help
- Your symptoms are severe or don't improve within two or three days.

Get help right away if:
- The part appears misshapen and/or you cannot move it.

See also:
BACK PAIN, MUSCLE ACHES AND STIFFNESS

Stress

People experience stress in response to various physical, mental, or emotional stimuli. Some stress in our lives can bring out the best in us, but if the level of tension is too high or lasts too long, we may lose our ability to cope and may even become ill. Everyone needs to learn effective ways of dealing with unavoidable stress.

The challenge of stress can be exciting, stimulating, or energizing. Some individuals thrive under continual stress, but most people find that they can cope for only so long before developing physical problems, or "distress."

Stress hormone levels normally fall once the stress is over and you can relax. The hormone levels may stay elevated if the stress continues or recurs frequently, or if you get into the habit of reacting to any stress, however minor, with distress. Research indicates that as much as 75 percent of disease is stress-related.

Stress-related illnesses include high blood pressure, heart attack, stroke, depression, anxiety, chronic fatigue syndrome, irritable bowel syndrome and other digestive disorders, obesity, migraine, and respiratory problems. Feeling continually stressed also disturbs the immune system, making you more likely to develop infections, cancer, and autoimmune disease, in which the

Causes of stress

Common causes of continual stress include:

- Loss or bereavement
- Poor relationships
- Money worries
- Unemployment
- Poor time-management
- Insufficient recreation and relaxation
- Boredom
- Ill health

immune system turns against the body's own cells. Examples of autoimmune disorders are rheumatoid arthritis, lupus, thyroid disease, and certain types of anemia and fertility problems. Smoking, overeating, and other common addictions are often stress-related.

PREVENTION

It is not always possible to prevent the events that cause stress, but you can modify your response to stimuli. Learn stress-management strategies (see p. 347) so that the next time you feel stressed, you can choose one that is appropriate for you. This will allow your stress hormone levels to fall and help you "flow" with whatever life brings. Many

Symptoms of stress

The prolonged presence of high levels of stress hormones may produce one or more of the following mental and physical symptoms:

Raised heart rate	Shaking	Headaches
Rapid, shallow breathing	Weight loss or gain	Difficulty concentrating
Dry mouth	Indigestion	Irritability
Sweating	Recurrent infections	Sleeping difficulties
	Tearfulness	

345

things influence your response to stress, including birth order, age, gender, education, experience, personality, expectations, and health.

TREATMENT

General measures: The first part of stress management is to take note of what or who makes you feel stressed, and how you react. The second is to reduce avoidable stresses in your life by, for example, leaving an unsuitable job, living within your means, and making your workplace more comfortable. The third element of stress management is to use various strategies to help you respond to unavoidable pressures in a constructive way (see facing page).

Diet: During periods of stress, the body uses up nutrients faster than usual. This may lead to deficiencies and consequent lowering of immunity unless the nutrients are replaced through the food you eat or by supplements.

- Eat regularly, and aim for relaxed mealtimes.
- Eat foods rich in vitamins A, B, C, and E, flavonoids, calcium, magnesium, selenium, and essential fatty acids (see p. 12).
- Reduce caffeine and alcohol intake.
- Eat more fruits, vegetables, and whole-grain cereals. Consume less animal protein and fewer refined foods made with white flour or added sugar, which tend to reduce immune function.
- Take a daily multiple vitamin and mineral supplement.

Aromatherapy: Use relaxing essential oils—for massage, in the bath, or for inhaling from a vaporizer or a tissue. Massage yourself or, even better,

---

Relax with acupressure

To reduce feelings of stress, use your thumb to press the following points firmly and repeatedly for two minutes each:

- The point (LI 4) in the web between the thumb and index finger on the back of your hand (see p. 88). Do not use this point during pregnancy.
- The point (Liv 3) in the furrow on the top of the foot between the first and second toes, where the bones merge (see p. 276).

---

ask someone else to do so. Use a massage oil made by mixing a total of eight drops of lavender, neroli, and/or ylang ylang oil into one tablespoon of sweet-almond or grapeseed oil. You can also use this oil for a shiatsu neck and shoulder massage (see p. 293), which may serve to relieve tension.

Meditation: The calming effects of meditation —feelings of being centered and at peace—can help you feel more detached about the causes of stress. You can learn basic meditation techniques by joining a class (see also pp. 46–47). Take time to practice meditation every day.

Herbal remedies: Teas made from calming herbs are helpful at especially stressful times. Drink a cup of chamomile, valerian, lime tree flower, or clover blossom tea once or twice daily. Caution: For safety concerns, see pp. 34–37.

➤ continued, p. 348

Exercise troubles away
A daily 30 minutes of brisk exercise reduces distress by "burning off" excess levels of stress hormones and by raising blood levels of mood-lifting chemicals called endorphins.

Stress-management strategies

Relaxation
The many forms of relaxing include:
- Taking regular work breaks.
- Going on vacations.
- Enjoying hobbies.
- Doing breathing exercises (see p. 87).
- Writing in a journal.
- Watching film comedies.
- Enjoying pets.
- Talking to friends.
- Praying or meditating.
- Soaking in a warm, scented bath.
- Visiting a spa or beauty salon.

Balance and perspective
You may need to:
- Accept that you can change only your behavior, not that of others.
- Accept that you cannot have everything you want.
- Recognize what really matters.

- Challenge "shoulds," "oughts," and "musts" in your thinking.
- Forgive yourself and others.
- Try to see stressful situations as opportunities.
- Learn to say no.
- Reject perfectionism.
- Sift information to avoid overload.
- Resist negative thinking.
- Don't magnify or belittle problems.
- Accept the inevitable.

Self-management
Improve your ability to tackle stressful situations:
- Be assertive, rather than passive or aggressive. Take assertiveness training if you find this hard.
- Define problems, choose goals, and work out how to achieve them.
- Listen to your own needs and concerns.
- Try to stick with a decision once you've made it. Remember that every choice involves giving up something.

Time management
To feel more in control of your life, organize your time efficiently. Use such techniques as:
- Prioritizing.
- Setting realistic deadlines.
- Doing important or difficult tasks when you feel freshest.
- Anticipating stressful times and planning ahead.
- Making time for yourself daily.
- Not taking on too much.
- Delegating.
- Doing one thing at a time.

Relationships
Other people can reduce or bring on stress. Try to:
- Nurture intimate relationships.
- Improve your communication skills.
- Recognize other people's feelings and separate them from your own.
- Deal with relationship problems.
- Keep in touch with friends.
- Offer encouragement and support to those around you.

Help and support
Realize that you have resources both within yourself and outside of yourself:
- Every day, give yourself a metaphorical pat on the back for trying to manage stress more effectively.
- Ask for any support you need, whether from a member of your family, a friend, or a counselor.

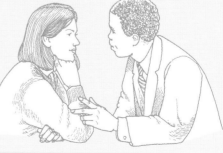

Reflexology for stress

Since the principal effect of reflexology is relaxation, you can relieve stress with a reflexology workout on your hands, or by asking a friend to do one on your feet (see pp. 52–53). The reflex points shown below are especially good to work on. Massage each of the areas shown two or three times in each direction. If any part is very sensitive, gently work the area again. (See "Giving Treatment," p. 52.)

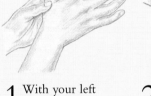

1 With your left thumb, work around the base of your right thumb.

2 Use your left thumb to work from the little finger side of the base of your right palm across to the thumb side, then up the outer margin of the thumb.

3 With your left thumb, work all over the area between halfway up the fleshy pad at the base of the right thumb, and the V formed by the thumb and index finger.

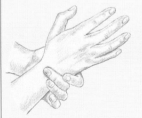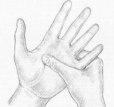

4 Use your left middle finger to work on the outside edge of your right hand, in front of the wrist bone.

5 Use your left thumb to work the top of the right thumb.

6 With your right thumb, work in horizontal lines from the little finger side over your left palm.

Flower essences: Choose a flower remedy whose description closely matches your state of mind and your personality (see p. 33). Relevant essences include:
- Rescue Remedy: for acute distress following a sudden shock.
- Olive: for exhaustion following a period of prolonged stress.

Other therapies: A counselor or psychotherapist can help you manage stress and examine the reasons why you may find coping with stress difficult. Acupuncture and many forms of therapy that involve exercise or physical manipulation (such as tai chi, massage, and yoga) can ease stress-related symptoms.

When to get medical help
- You feel overwhelmed by stress to the extent that your work or relationships are adversely affected.
- You have physical symptoms of stress, such as palpitations, breathlessness, or headaches.

See also:
ADDICTIONS, ANXIETY, APPETITE LOSS, CHRONIC FATIGUE SYNDROME, DEPRESSION, EATING DISORDERS, EMOTIONAL PROBLEMS, GRIEF, HEADACHE, HIGH BLOOD PRESSURE, INDIGESTION, IRRITABLE BOWEL SYNDROME, MIGRAINE, OVERWEIGHT, PAIN, PALPITATIONS, SHOCK, SLEEPING DIFFICULTIES

Styes

A small abscess in the eyelid, usually at the base of an eyelash, a stye makes the lid painful and swollen. Styes are most likely to occur when you are run-down or tired and therefore especially prone to infection. Home remedies can ease pain and speed up the healing process.

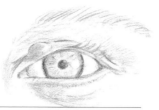

Styes, which are normally not serious, result from infection in an eyelash follicle. They generally heal either by bursting and releasing their pus or by slowly disappearing. Left untreated, a stye usually lasts 7 to 10 days. Most treatments aim to encourage a stye to diminish or burst, stop the infection from spreading, and build up immunity to further infection.

A soothing compress
Put cotton into the bowl of a wooden spoon, and wrap with a bandage. Dip the spoon in a suitable herbal tea (see "Herbal Remedies") or hot water, let cool, and apply to the eye for 5 to 10 minutes.

PREVENTION

Enhance resistance to infection with regular exercise, a healthy diet, and stress management. Styes are contagious, so anyone affected should not share towels or washcloths with other people, and they should change their washcloth daily. If you live with someone who has a bacterial infection of any kind, take care not to touch your eyes after touching the person; wash your hands first.

TREATMENT

Do not attempt to squeeze pus out of a stye. If it bursts spontaneously, carefully wipe away any discharge.

Herbal remedies

- Eat two cloves of raw garlic daily to boost immunity.
- Make a hot tea from one of the following: eyebright (which helps soothe any surrounding inflammation), burdock, or marigold (both counter infection). Prepare, let cool a bit, and apply a compress as described in the illustration. Repeat every two hours.
- In addition, drink two cups of tea daily made from echinacea, burdock, goldenseal, cleavers, and peppermint, to boost immunity.

Caution: For safety concerns, see pp. 34–37.

From the drugstore: Take daily supplements of vitamin C, flavonoids, and fish oil (for omega-3 fatty acids) to help overcome the infection.

Homeopathy

- Pulsatilla: for the onset of a stye, and for recurrent styes with yellow pus.
- Silica: to bring the stye to a head if Pulsatilla doesn't help.

When to get medical help

- The stye has not burst or diminished after three days.
- You suffer from recurrent styes.
- The stye grows large.
- The eye itself is red or has a discharge.

See also:
ABSCESSES AND BOILS

Sunburn

Although most common in fair-complected people, whose skin produces only small amounts of the protective pigment melanin, sunburn can affect anyone who has been excessively exposed to the sun's ultraviolet rays. Prevention is the best approach, especially for children, because severe childhood sunburns have been linked to malignant melanoma.

Safe in the sun
When you have to go out in strong sun, be sure to wear a wide-brimmed hat.

Repeated overexposure to ultraviolet A (UVA) rays leads to premature wrinkling and an increased risk of skin cancer. Overexposure to UVB rays causes sunburn, which damages the top layer of skin and also contributes to cancer risk. The redness and tenderness of sunburn usually increase for several hours after exposure and last for up to a week. The skin may blister.

PREVENTION

Limit exposure to strong sunlight to no more than 15 minutes a day at first, increasing the time gradually, if you must. Before going into the sun, apply a broad-spectrum sunscreen of factor 15 or higher, depending on your skin type. Reapply every few hours and after swimming. For further protection, wear tightly woven clothing. Try to avoid sun exposure from 10 A.M. to 3 P.M. Keep babies under six months out of the sun; use shading devices on strollers. When out in the sun, drink plenty of water to keep skin hydrated. Take the antioxidants beta-carotene, vitamins C and E, and selenium daily. After sun exposure, apply an antioxidant moisturizer.

TREATMENT

- Don't peel burned skin or prick blisters.
- Soothe sunburned skin with cool compresses or a cool bath or shower, or apply aloe vera gel or calamine lotion.
- Ease dryness and flaking with a moisturizer.
- Reduce the discomfort of mild sunburn with a dusting of cornstarch.
- Protect burned skin from further sun exposure.

Homeopathy

- Urtica, Calendula, or Hypercal cream: for stinging, unblistered skin.
- Urtica, Calendula, or Hypercal tincture (1 part diluted with 10 parts water): for any sunburn, applied to the skin liberally and immediately.
- Cantharis: for severe sunburn, taken hourly.

Flower essences: A cold compress made with a few drops of Rescue Remedy helps cool the skin.

When to get medical help

Get help right away if:
- You have severe redness and/or blistering.
- You experience fever, chills, dizziness, headaches, or vomiting.
- A young child is badly burned.

See also: BURNS

350

Swollen Ankles

A *n abnormal accumulation of fluid in the soft tissues can cause swelling, especially of the ankles. This condition, known as edema, may have an underlying cause that requires medical treatment, such as heart disease. Nevertheless, lifestyle changes and home remedies can often play an important role in reducing fluid retention and easing symptoms.*

Swelling begone!
Lie with your feet raised above your hips for at least 20 minutes twice daily to allow excess fluid to drain away from the ankles.

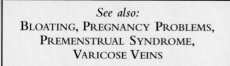

Ankle swelling unrelated to injury usually occurs when the normal balance between fluid levels in the blood and the body cells is disrupted. This can happen when higher than normal pressure in the small blood vessels, the capillaries, forces water into adjoining tissues. Long periods of standing or sitting, a high salt intake, and hormone fluctuations before menstruation and during pregnancy may all make swollen ankles more likely. The disorder sometimes indicates an underlying condition, such as varicose veins, a kidney problem, heart or other arterial disease, high blood pressure, or preeclampsia (high blood pressure and fluid retention during pregnancy).

TREATMENT
General measures
- Exercise daily for a half hour. This boosts circulation and discourages fluid from pooling in the lower limbs.
- To strengthen capillary walls, eat foods rich in vitamin C and flavonoids (see p. 12).
- Reduce your salt intake.
    - If you sit or stand still for a long time, contract your calf muscles frequently. This squeezes blood up through the calf veins, which helps prevent ankle swelling.

Aromatherapy
- Take a warm bath to which you have added six drops of geranium oil, six drops of lemon oil, or three of rosemary oil. (Avoid rosemary oil for the first 20 weeks of pregnancy.)

Herbal remedies
- Drink a daily cup or two of lukewarm-to-cool tea made from dandelion leaves and yarrow.
Caution: For safety concerns, see pp. 34–37.

When to get medical help
- Your symptoms worsen or fail to improve.
- Your symptoms begin after you take a new medication.
- The swelling is in only one ankle.
- You also have swelling or tenderness in the groin or lower abdomen.
- You are short of breath.
- You are pregnant.
- You experience numbness or tingling in the leg or foot.

See also:
BLOATING, PREGNANCY PROBLEMS,
PREMENSTRUAL SYNDROME,
VARICOSE VEINS

351

Swollen Glands

*T*he lymph nodes—commonly referred to as "glands"—are collections of cells along lymph vessels that play an important role in the body's defenses. Swollen glands are a sign that you are actively fighting an infection or other invasion by harmful organisms or cells. There's a lot that you can do to help the lymph nodes protect your body.

The lymph nodes manufacture infection-fighting antibodies and white cells. They also trap infecting microorganisms, cancer cells, and other invading particles. When they are swollen, you feel them as tender, painful, slightly warm lumps, usually under the skin of the neck, armpits, or groin. During a localized infection, as from an infected cut, lymph nodes near the affected area may become enlarged.

Swollen lymph nodes are most often caused by viral infections, such as colds, flu, and certain types of sore throats. They are one of the main symptoms of infectious mononucleosis, a viral disease. Swelling can also result from bacterial infection, as of the throat. In rare cases, swollen lymph nodes result from cancer of the blood or lymphatic system.

PREVENTION

You can take steps to reduce the likelihood of the infections that cause swollen lymph nodes.
- Eat plenty of immunity-enhancing foods—those rich in folic acid, flavonoids, copper, iodine, iron, magnesium, selenium, zinc, essential fatty acids, lecithin, and vitamins A, B complex, C, D, and E (see p. 12).
- Limit your intake of refined carbohydrates, such as sugar and white flour.
- Get regular exercise to boost immunity.
- Avoid alcohol and tobacco.

TREATMENT

Follow the advice given under "Prevention" and try these additional measures:
- Get enough rest and sleep.
- Eat some raw garlic daily.
- Take the herbal remedy echinacea and/or astragalus or shiitake mushrooms, all of which are immune-system boosters, and elderberry extract or goldenseal to fight infection. For safety concerns about the use of herbs, see pp. 34–37.
- Apply cold compresses (see p. 50) to the swelling for the first one to two days. Then apply heat, such as a covered hot-water bottle, at regular intervals until symptoms clear.

When to get medical help
- Mildly swollen lymph nodes remain swollen for more than one week.
- Your lymph nodes increase in size or become more tender after three days.
- You have a high or persistent fever.
- You have a headache, aching muscles, abdominal pain, jaundice, a rash, or a bacterial infection, such as tonsillitis.

See also:
ABDOMINAL PAIN, CHILDHOOD VIRAL INFECTIONS, COUGHS, EARACHE, FEVER, SORE THROAT

Toothache

An aching tooth (or teeth) is usually a sign of decay—possibly even an abscess—or inflammation inside the tooth or of the gum. These conditions always require treatment by a dentist, but you can use a variety of natural home remedies to relieve pain while dental treatment takes effect. You can also reduce the risk of future dental problems.

The main cause of tooth decay is plaque, a sticky film of food residue, saliva, and bacteria that accumulates on teeth. As the plaque bacteria consume sugars and starches from food particles, they produce an acid that can destroy enamel, the protective surface of the tooth. If your food contains added sugar, the amount of acid increases sharply, and its level stays high for about 25 minutes after eating unless removed, for example by brushing. If you eat sugary foods frequently, you run a high risk of suffering from tooth decay.

Advanced decay, with deep cavities that allow bacteria to enter the pulp well within the tooth, will eventually lead to a painful dental abscess.

PREVENTION

Keep your teeth healthy by brushing at least twice daily, and preferably after every meal. Use dental floss daily to remove food particles and plaque from between your teeth.

- Minimize your consumption of refined carbohydrates (such as added sugar and white flour). Such foods promote plaque formation and raise acid levels in the mouth.
- Reduce excess acidity in your mouth after eating by brushing your teeth or by ending your meal or snack with naturally antacid foods, such as nuts and cheese. Simply swilling water around in your mouth can also remove food residue and counter acidity.
- Drink tea, which is a good source of fluoride, a decay-fighting mineral. The tannins in tea also help combat bacterial activity.
- Discourage bacterial activity by rinsing your mouth daily with a solution of myrrh tincture or hydrogen peroxide.
- Have regular dental checkups.

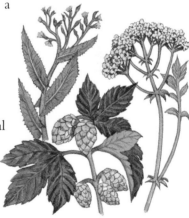

Pain-relieving herbs
Tea made from hops, valerian, or wild lettuce may ease toothache, because these herbs have a soothing effect on the nervous system.

➤ continued, p. 354

Teething pain

Many babies experience discomfort as their first teeth erupt through the gums, usually starting at about six months. Your child may cry more, have a "dribble rash" around the mouth, have difficulty sleeping, and be irritable or clingy. A teething ring to chew on may help. You can also try massaging the gum with your fingertip or using one of these homeopathic remedies:

- Chamomilla: for a cross, irritable child, who has one cheek redder than the other. Give this remedy as granules, which dissolve easily in the mouth.
- Pulsatilla: for a clingy child whose pain is helped by cool, fresh air.

TREATMENT

If you have a toothache or painful swollen gums, see your dentist as soon as possible. To reduce the pain of an abscess, apply a hot compress for five minutes every half hour and wash out your mouth with warm salt water afterward. This may help release the pus.

Aromatherapy: Rub a few drops of clove or cajuput oil on the gum above or beneath the aching tooth. Repeat several times daily. Avoid clove oil throughout pregnancy and cajuput oil in the first 20 weeks of pregnancy.

Herbal remedies

- Apply a cotton ball soaked in echinacea tincture to the affected tooth.
- Chew prickly ash bark, or apply a paste of powdered bark mixed with a little water.

Caution: For safety concerns, see pp. 34–37.

Homeopathy

- Belladonna: for an abscess that develops quickly and looks red, hot, and swollen. The tooth throbs and your mouth feels dry.
- Hepar sulphuris: for sharp, splinterlike pain that feels worse in cold air or when you touch the affected area. The abscess oozes thick, yellow pus with a foul smell; you feel cold and irritable.
- Mercurius solubilis: for sore, bleeding gums. The pain is worse at night; you feel thirsty; your mouth has more saliva than usual; and you have bad breath.
- Silica: for an abscess that is slow to burst or heal, or if you have many cavities.

Acupressure: With your thumb, press the point LI 4 on the back of your hand in the web of skin between your other thumb and your index finger (see p. 88). Apply pressure to the point for about two minutes. Do not use this point if you are pregnant.

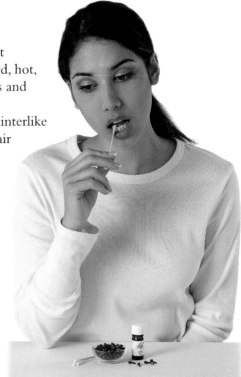

A natural anesthetic
Soak a cotton ball in clove oil and apply to the affected tooth, or chew a clove. Cloves contain eugenol, a local anesthetic often used by dentists.

Tooth-friendly foods
After meals, eat nuts or cheese, which counteract acidity, or a fibrous food, such as celery, which removes plaque because of its slightly abrasive effect.

When to get medical help

- See your dentist in all cases.

See also:
ABSCESSES AND BOILS, GUM PROBLEMS

Urinary Difficulties

*P*ain when urinating, frequent urination, and urinary retention (inability to empty the bladder properly) are the main difficulties of this type. These problems often require medical attention or even surgery. However, in many cases, self-care with natural remedies can support and enhance the effectiveness of the treatments prescribed by your doctor.

Most people pass urine between four and six times daily, depending on the amount of fluids they drink and how active they are. The problem of frequent urination may result from a large fluid intake, a urinary-tract infection, irritation from stones in the bladder, an enlarged prostate gland, urge or overflow incontinence (see p. 250), diabetes, or anxiety. Pain during urination, usually described as burning or scalding, may be caused by a urinary-tract infection, a vaginal yeast (candida) infection, inflammation of the penis, or kidney or bladder stones.

A slow or weak stream of urine is common in older men because of prostate enlargement. This symptom may also occur in older women, possibly because of weakness in the bladder-wall (detrusor) muscle. Inability to pass urine (urinary retention) most often affects men. It may result from an obstruction (such as a stone or a congenital anatomical abnormality) in the bladder or urethra, a tight foreskin, or an enlarged prostate. It occasionally happens in women because of pregnancy or fibroids in the uterus, both of which can put pressure on the urethra. Some urinary problems arise from long-standing nervous-system disorders, such as multiple sclerosis.

PREVENTION

- Drink plenty of water. Avoid caffeinated drinks, such as coffee, tea, and cola; these have a diuretic effect, creating large amounts of urine.
- Eat a healthy diet, with plenty of foods rich in flavonoids, selenium, zinc, plant hormones, and vitamins A, C, and E (see "The Right Nutrients," p. 356). These help boost your resistance to infection, ensure that your muscles, nerves, and other tissues are in good condition, and make prostate enlargement and fibroids less likely.

➤ continued, p. 356

Flush away problems
Drink plenty of water to keep your urinary tract in good health. For most people this means six to eight glasses of water a day.

- Eat ample fiber-rich foods, so as to prevent pressure on the bladder from constipation.
- Lose any excess weight, since deposits of fat in the abdomen can put pressure on the bladder.
- Empty your bladder regularly to prevent infection from developing in stagnant urine.
- To avoid anxiety, practice stress-management techniques, such as yoga, deep breathing, and other relaxation exercises (see p. 347).
- Women of all ages should practice Kegel exercises (see p. 251) to maintain the strength of the muscles that support the urinary and reproductive organs.
- Don't smoke, or at least cut down if you do, since cadmium from cigarette smoke can accumulate in the kidneys and encourage the formation of stones. Smoking is also a significant risk factor for certain types of bladder cancer.

TREATMENT

Appropriate treatment depends on the underlying problem. But anyone with urinary difficulties should follow the advice given under "Prevention" along with any prescribed treatment for an underlying disorder.

Herbal tonics for the urinary system
Take cleavers or couch grass in the form of a tea or tincture when a gentle diuretic effect is beneficial, as with cystitis or kidney stones.

The right nutrients
Brightly colored fruits, most vegetables, beans, whole grains, nuts, and seeds—all contain vitamins and other substances that help prevent urinary difficulties.

When to get medical help

- Urination is painful, or you have a discharge.
- Copious urination is accompanied by unusual thirst.
- Symptoms are severe or continue for more than a few days.
- Symptoms occur along with pain in the lower abdomen or, for men, the perineum.
- Urine is pink, cloudy, or bloody.
- A baby or child has urinary problems.

Get help right away if:
- You are unable to urinate.

See also:
ABDOMINAL PAIN, ANXIETY, CANDIDA
INFECTIONS, DIABETES, FIBROIDS,
INCONTINENCE, KIDNEY STONES,
OVERWEIGHT, PROSTATE PROBLEMS,
URINARY-TRACT INFECTIONS

Urinary-tract Infections

Inflammation and/or infection of the lower part of the urinary tract (bladder and urethra) affects one in five women at some time. Such infections are not usually a risk to general health. However, it is important to treat them promptly to avoid the risk of the kidneys becoming affected—a more serious problem. You can use natural remedies along with prescribed medication.

Most urinary-tract infections are caused by *Escherichia coli (E. coli)* bacteria. These are normally present in the large intestine, but they can spread from the anus to the urethral opening and up to the bladder. If conditions allow, the bacteria can settle into the bladder lining, multiply, and cause inflammation and infection. Conditions that make inflammation (and infection) more likely include urinary-tract injury, kidney stones, anatomical abnormality, concentrated or acidic urine, and certain food constituents.

SYMPTOMS

If your urinary tract is inflamed or infected, you may notice some of the following:

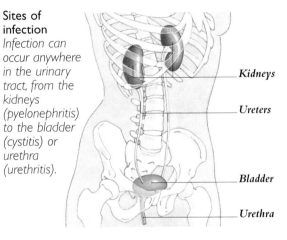

Sites of infection
Infection can occur anywhere in the urinary tract, from the kidneys (pyelonephritis) to the bladder (cystitis) or urethra (urethritis).

Kidneys

Ureters

Bladder

Urethra

- Burning or stinging before, during, or immediately after urination
- A frequent urge to urinate
- Low abdominal pain (from the bladder)
- Pain in the back above the waist (from one or both kidneys)
- Tenderness above the pubic bone
- Blood in the urine, making it pink or cloudy
- Pus in the urine, making it cloudy
- Strong—perhaps fishy—smelling urine
- A fever
- A sudden and irresistible urge to urinate

PREVENTION

- To flush out bacteria and other irritants, drink enough water to make the urine appear light in

---

Why women?

Several factors make infection more common in women than in men:
- The relatively short urethra in women allows bacteria easy access to the bladder.
- During intercourse the vagina, the urethra, and the base of the bladder may be bruised. Bacteria may also be pushed into the urethra.
- A tampon may press against the upper vaginal wall and irritate the base of the bladder.
- The rim of a diaphragm may press against the upper vaginal wall and irritate the bladder base.
- Spermicidal foams and gels may irritate the urethra.
- During pregnancy, the pressure of the enlarged uterus can make complete bladder emptying difficult, allowing infection to become established.
- After menopause, the urinary-tract lining may gradually become thinner, less elastic, and more vulnerable to irritation.

color at most times of the day. This is about six glasses a day for most people.

- Reduce intake of caffeine and alcohol, which can irritate the urinary tract.
- Stop or reduce smoking, since nicotine can irritate the urinary tract.
- Wash the genital area with water only to avoid irritation of the urethra.
- Never delay urinating unnecessarily—the longer urine remains in the bladder, the more likely are bacteria to take hold in the lining.
- Wash the genital area before intercourse. A woman should also urinate before and after sexual intercourse.
- Change sanitary pads or tampons frequently.
- Avoid bath salts, bubble baths, and such "feminine hygiene" products as vaginal deodorants, which may irritate the urethra.
- Don't wear tight or thick underwear if you suffer from recurrent cystitis.
- To help prevent bacteria from adhering to the bladder wall, drink cranberry juice daily for its anti-inflammatory properties.
- Eat plenty of foods rich in vitamin C and flavonoids (see p. 12) to increase your general resistance to infection.
- Drink a cup of echinacea tea (or take a few drops of tincture each day) and have some garlic (or garlic tablets) to boost your immunity.
- If cystitis occurs after swimming in a chlorinated pool, avoid chlorinated water, if possible, or drink plenty of water after swimming.

TREATMENT

Natural remedies are not a substitute for orthodox medical treatment. However, the measures

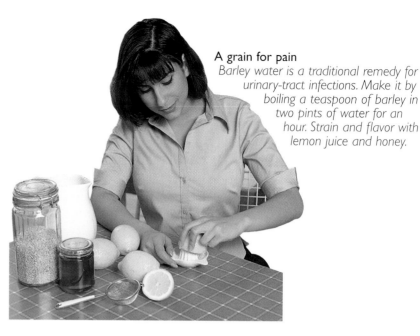

A grain for pain
Barley water is a traditional remedy for urinary-tract infections. Make it by boiling a teaspoon of barley in two pints of water for an hour. Strain and flavor with lemon juice and honey.

outlined under "Prevention" and the additional steps described below can be used alongside treatments prescribed by your doctor.

Kitchen cabinet remedies: Try one of the following barley-water remedies to reduce the burning pain on urination often associated with urinary-tract infections.

- Have two large cups of barley water (see photograph). Then drink one large cup every 20 minutes for three hours.
- To make the urine less acidic, every hour drink a cup of barley water with an added teaspoon of baking soda.

Herbal remedies

- Soothe symptoms with corn silk tea, up to three times a day.
- Benefit from buchu's antiseptic and diuretic

qualities by drinking buchu tea, but no more than three times a day.

- Drink a small cup of tea made from marshmallow leaf or sea holly (eryngo) root three times daily. This is soothing and mildly diuretic.
- Uva ursi can help reduce the growth of urinary-tract bacteria.
- If burning is severe, sit in a bath of strong chamomile tea.
- For a kidney infection, drink frequent cups of lukewarm echinacea, couch grass, and buchu tea.

Caution: For safety concerns, see pp. 34–37.

Aromatherapy: Essential oils can be of benefit because of their antiseptic effect.

- Sprinkle two drops each of juniper berry, eucalyptus, and sandalwood oils into a bathtub of warm water. Kneel and swish the water over your pelvic area. Repeat several times, then sit in the water for 10 minutes. Omit juniper berry oil if you are or might be pregnant.

Hydrotherapy: Warm and cold spraying of the pelvic area—three minutes using warm water, then one minute cold, repeated three or four times—may help combat urinary-tract infections. This boosts the local circulation and so brings more white cells and other infection-fighting agents to the area. Or take alternate hot and cold sitz baths (see p. 49).

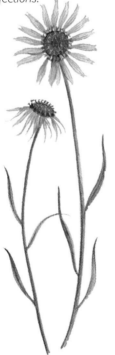

Marshmallow
This common herb is used to soothe inflammatory conditions of the urinary system, such as cystitis and urethritis.

Echinacea
The immunity-enhancing and antimicrobial properties of this herb may help urinary-tract infections.

Homeopathy

- Apis: for burning and soreness while urinating, with last drops particularly painful.
- Cantharis: for frequent urination with scalding pain, and when urine is hard to pass.
- Causticum: for burning pain while urinating.
- Sarsaparilla: for pain at the end of urination.

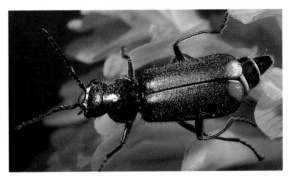

Spanish fly
This bug is the source of Cantharis, a homeopathic remedy for burning pains, such as those of cystitis.

When to get medical help

- You experience any of the symptoms of a urinary-tract infection (see p. 357).
- Your urine is bloody, pink, or cloudy.

Get help right away if:
- You have back pain in addition to any of the above symptoms.
- A baby or child is affected.

See also:
ABDOMINAL PAIN, INCONTINENCE, PROSTATE PROBLEMS, URINARY DIFFICULTIES

Vaginal Problems

Itching or inflammation of the vagina and vulva, abnormal vaginal discharge, and pain during intercourse are the most frequent problems affecting the female genital area. Such symptoms are usually a sign of a bacterial or yeast infection. Several home remedies and other self-help measures can help prevent or relieve these conditions.

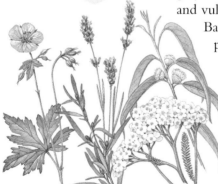

Itch relief
Geranium, tea tree, lavender, eucalyptus, and yarrow (shown from left to right) provide essential oils that can alleviate vaginal symptoms.

The vagina is normally kept free from infection by natural colorless secretions that keep the lining moist and produce a slightly acidic environment, which prevents excessive growth of any of the normal population of microorganisms. Any alteration to these conditions—for example, following a course of antibiotics—can cause an overgrowth of *Candida albicans*, a yeastlike fungus (see p. 118). Symptoms include itching, tenderness, soreness, and a thick, white discharge.

Other organisms may also multiply in the vagina. Bacterial vaginosis results from an overgrowth of one or more of the types of bacteria normally present in the vagina. It may cause a grayish discharge that has an odor. The vagina and vulva may itch, burn, and become inflamed. Bacterial vaginosis during pregnancy makes premature birth more likely. Microorganisms may also cause trichomoniasis, gonorrhea, or a chlamydial infection, any of which can be sexually transmitted. These disorders may produce a greenish-yellow discharge.

Possible causes of redness, itching, and soreness—vaginitis—include diabetes, changing hormone levels during pregnancy, and a reaction to chemicals in soaps, bubble baths and other toiletries, or laundry detergents. After menopause, the drop in estrogen may make the vaginal lining drier and thinner, leading to discomfort during sexual intercourse.

PREVENTION

- Wash the genital area regularly, and gently pat dry with a clean towel.
- Avoid hot baths and showers, and don't remain in the tub longer than 15 minutes.
- Don't use scented soaps, bubble bath, or other bath additives.
- Don't use feminine deodorants or douches (unless prescribed by your doctor).
- Wear cotton underwear, and stockings rather than panty hose. Avoid pants that are very tight.
- Avoid enzyme-containing laundry detergents.
- After using the lavatory, wipe from front to back to prevent the transfer of intestinal organisms to your vagina.
- Apply lubricating jelly or cream before intercourse, if necessary to avoid discomfort.
- Consider having your partner wear a condom. This will help prevent the transmission of infecting bacteria and other organisms.
- Change tampons every three to four hours.

TREATMENT
Herbal remedies

- To soothe irritation, sit in a shallow bath containing a cup of herbal tea made from a combination of chamomile, chickweed, goldenseal,

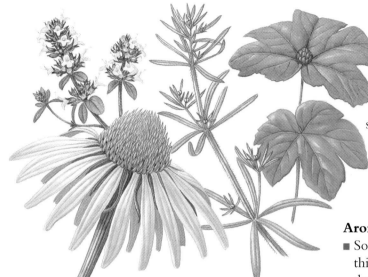

Helpful herbs
If you suffer from vaginal infections, improve immunity by drinking a daily cup of tea (or a few drops of tincture in half a cup of water) made from thyme, echinacea, cleavers, and goldenseal.

marigold, and thyme. Or bathe the area with a solution of witch hazel.

■ Relieve itching by bathing the genital area with chickweed tea, which has a gentle anti-inflammatory effect.

■ Try the teas suggested under "Helpful Herbs," above. The hormone-balancing herbs black cohosh and dong quai may also be beneficial.

Caution: For safety concerns, see pp. 34–37.

Diet

■ To counter infection, boost your immune system with a wholesome diet (see p. 9). Include plenty of foods rich in beta-carotene, folic acid, flavonoids, iron, magnesium, zinc, essential fatty acids, and vitamins B, C, and E.

■ Restrict your intake of saturated fats, sugar, meat, and caffeine (which stimulates insulin production, releasing sugar and encouraging candida). Include in your diet oils rich in monounsaturated fats, such as olive oil, which act against candida.

■ If you are postmenopausal, include soybeans and soy-based foods in your regular diet. These contain plant hormones that may counter vaginal dryness.

Aromatherapy

■ Soothe inflammation and irritation by applying this mixture to the external genital area: two drops of myrrh oil and four of lavender oil added to two and a half teaspoons of unscented lotion or jojoba oil.

■ Reduce itching by wearing a panty liner on which you have sprinkled a few drops of sweet thyme or tea tree oil diluted with two teaspoons of jojoba oil.

■ Lessen postmenopausal inflammation with chamomile, geranium, lavender, yarrow, tea tree, or eucalyptus oil. Add a total of six drops to a warm bath, and soak for 15 minutes.

When to get medical help

● You have an unusual vaginal discharge or unusual bleeding.
● Your symptoms last longer than three days.
● You are or might be pregnant.
● You have pain during or after intercourse.
● You have abdominal or pelvic pain.

See also:
CANDIDA INFECTIONS,
MENOPAUSAL PROBLEMS,
URINARY DIFFICULTIES,
URINARY-TRACT
INFECTIONS

Varicose Veins

Too much pressure inside veins can damage their valves and lead to a build-up of blood that makes them twisted and swollen, or varicose. This can happen to any vein, but superficial leg veins are those most frequently affected. Changing your lifestyle and using some natural remedies can help you avoid the need for surgery.

Improving blood flow
Make a half hour's daily exercise—such as walking, swimming, or cycling— a priority. This tones the veins and boosts circulation.

In a normal leg vein, valves stop blood from draining back down the leg under the force of gravity. When these valves no longer work efficiently, blood collects and dilates the veins, causing those just under the skin to turn blue and lumpy, especially on the backs of the calves and the insides of the legs. Some people have no additional symptoms, but others experience swelling of the feet and ankles, aching legs, itching, and in severe cases, eczema, skin discoloration, or ulceration.

One person in five develops varicose veins. Women are four times more likely to be affected than men, and the disorder tends to run in families. Other factors that increase your risk of developing varicose veins include a poor diet, too little exercise, standing or sitting still for long periods, and being overweight. Pregnancy also heightens the risk because of an increase in blood volume and because the enlarged uterus presses on the abdominal veins, causing more pressure in the leg veins.

PREVENTION
To reduce the risk of varicose veins:
- Whenever possible, avoid standing or sitting still for long periods.
- Lose excess weight.
- Improve your circulation with daily activity, such as walking.
- On long plane flights, get up and move around for 10 minutes every hour or two.
- When sitting, put your feet up, if possible.
- If your legs are tired or aching, rest them by raising them above hip level.
- Make sure panty hose, stockings, garter belts, and socks are not too tight.

TREATMENT
General measures: Take the precautions listed above. In addition:
- Don't stand still for too long, especially in hot weather. If you must stand for an extended time, tighten and relax your calf muscles frequently to prevent blood from collecting in your veins and making them swell further.
- When sitting, don't let the edge of your chair obstruct your blood flow by cutting into your thighs, and don't cross your legs.
- Consider wearing support stockings.

Diet: Eat at least five daily servings of vegetables and fruits. Citrus fruits are especially rich in nutrients that help maintain the strength and elasticity of the vein walls, including vitamin C, silica, and flavonoids (plant pigments). Berries and cherries, rich in red and purple flavonoids called proanthocyanidins, and buckwheat, rich in

another vein-strengthening flavonoid called rutin, are also valuable.

Eat plenty of fiber-rich foods, such as brown rice and whole-grain cereals. These help prevent constipation and the subsequent straining that increases pressure in the leg veins.

Kitchen cabinet remedy: Apple-cider vinegar has astringent properties and contains flavonoids,

which can ease vein swelling and inflammation. Apply over varicose veins morning and night.

From the drugstore: Take daily supplements of vitamins C and E, proanthocyanidins, rutin, silica, and zinc.

Herbal remedies: The astringent and anti-inflammatory properties of several herbs—some

---

Yoga to the rescue

Regular yoga exercises stimulate the circulation and improve the drainage of tissue fluid and lymph. They may prevent varicose veins from getting worse. Inverted yoga postures such as these are the most useful, but do not attempt them if you have untreated high blood pressure or if there is a possibility that you have blood clots in your legs.

Resting position

Try this position to ease your symptoms if you are new to yoga.

Lie on your back with your buttocks on a cushion about 18 inches from the wall.
Rest your feet against the wall, and breathe slowly and deeply. Hold the posture for about five minutes.

The shoulder stand

This posture can help reduce the pressure inside your leg veins. Do not attempt a shoulder stand if you are new to yoga, unless you are supervised by an experienced teacher.

1 Lie on your back with your legs together and hands palms-down by your sides. As you inhale, push down on your hands and slowly swing your legs up over your head. Raise your hips from the floor and support your lower back with your hands as far down as possible. This is the half shoulder stand.

2 As you exhale, bring your legs to a vertical position and straighten your spine into a full shoulder stand. Hold the pose for about 20 breaths, breathing slowly and deeply. Release the pose by bending your knees and slowly lowering your legs to the floor.

taken internally and some applied externally—lend themselves to alleviating the symptoms of varicose veins.

- To tone veins and reduce discomfort, bathe the affected area with one of the following: distilled witch hazel alone, four drops of calendula tincture in a tablespoon of distilled witch hazel, or cooled comfrey (if skin is not broken) or marigold tea.
- Soothe aching veins with a cold compress made with two teaspoons of calendula tincture in half a pint of cold water.
- To strengthen your vein walls and promote circulation, take a daily dose of gotu kola and/or ginkgo biloba. Bilberry and butcher's broom may also be effective.
- To relieve pain caused by varicose veins, apply comfrey ointment. Do not use this ointment on broken skin.

Caution: For safety concerns, see pp. 34–37.

Hydrotherapy

- Use alternate hot and cold compresses, leaving each one in place for 30 seconds and repeating the sequence three times. Always finish with a cold compress. Carry out this treatment once a day.
- Spray your legs and feet with cold water for two minutes twice daily to ease swelling and discomfort.

An astringent healer
Witch hazel (Hamamelis virginiana) is a native North American plant. Applied externally, its distilled extract promotes constriction of blood vessels, thereby reducing swelling.

Aromatherapy: Make a toning and soothing massage oil for varicose veins by adding three drops of cypress oil, two drops of sandalwood oil, and one drop of peppermint oil to five teaspoons of sweet almond oil or calendula lotion. Omit cypress oil if you are in the first 20 weeks of pregnancy. In the morning and evening, put your legs up and smooth the mixture over your veins with upward strokes.

Homeopathy

- Hamamelis: for veins that feel bruised and sore, with a bursting feeling. This remedy can also be used in the form of an ointment, massaged into the skin over the swollen veins.
- Vipera: for inflamed veins (phlebitis).

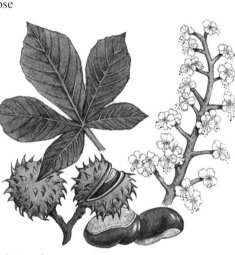

A circulatory tonic
Horse chestnut has anti-inflammatory properties and improves the tone of the vein walls. It should, however, be taken only under the supervision of a qualified practitioner.

When to get medical help

- Your varicose veins cause pain or bleed.
- Your leg becomes swollen, inflamed, or ulcerated.

Get help right away if:
- You have chest pain or sudden shortness of breath.

See also:
DERMATITIS, HEMORRHOIDS,
SKIN PROBLEMS

Voice Loss

Any disorder of the vocal cords can affect the ability to speak normally. Most temporary voice loss is caused by laryngitis—inflammation of the voice box (larynx) and the vocal cords within—as a result of infection. Another reason for the disorder is overuse of the voice. The condition is often painless and usually lasts only a few days. It responds well to home remedies.

DID YOU KNOW?
Clearing your throat can irritate the larynx. Try swallowing instead.

Voice loss occurs when the vocal cords, the fibrous bands of tissue inside the larynx that vibrate when we speak, are unable to move normally. This is frequently the result of a viral infection, such as a cold. Tobacco smoke and other irritants may also cause inflammation of the voice box. Singers and others, such as teachers, who use their voices a lot are susceptible to voice loss resulting from improper or excessive use. Persistent voice loss or hoarseness may be caused by polyps (benign growths) on the vocal cords, or, in rare cases, cancer.

TREATMENT

- If you have an infection, limit your activities, and treat as for a cold or sore throat.
- Rest your voice, but don't whisper.
- Keep the throat lining moist by humidifying the air with a humidifier, a boiling kettle of water, or bowls of water placed by radiators.
- Drink plenty of fluids, but avoid caffeine and alcohol, since they encourage dehydration by increasing urine production.
- Don't smoke or breathe polluted air.

Aromatherapy

- To bring swift relief, inhale steam scented with a total of four to six drops of antiseptic and anti-inflammatory oils, such as lavender, sandalwood, and chamomile.

- To reduce inflammation, gargle every two hours with two drops each of sandalwood and lemon oils in half a glass of warm water.

Herbal remedies

- Make a hot compress (see p. 37), using mullein, sage, thyme, or hyssop tea. Apply it to your throat. Wrap a dry towel around your neck to keep the heat in. Apply a new compress when the previous one has cooled.
- Gargle three to six times a day with a few drops of myrrh, sage, or tea tree tincture in half a glass of warm water.
- Every two hours, drink a cup of tea made from echinacea, mullein, catnip, coltsfoot, and thyme.

Caution: For safety concerns, see pp. 34–37.

Homeopathy

- Phosphorus: for all types of laryngitis.

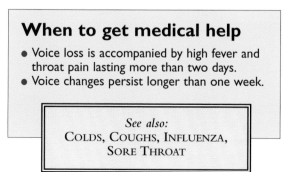

When to get medical help
- Voice loss is accompanied by high fever and throat pain lasting more than two days.
- Voice changes persist longer than one week.

See also:
COLDS, COUGHS, INFLUENZA,
SORE THROAT

Warts

Contagious growths consisting of dead skin cells, warts affect only the top layer of skin. These lumps have a rough surface and can appear almost anywhere, but most often they affect the hands and face. A wart on the sole of the foot, called a verruca or plantar wart, appears relatively flat because of pressure from the weight of the body.

Warts occur when viruses, usually the papilloma type, invade skin cells. They may be unsightly, and they occasionally itch. A plantar wart on the heel or ball of the foot can cause pain when you are walking, because the weight on the foot presses it inward. Most warts disappear within six months to two years without treatment.

PREVENTION
Wart viruses spread easily on moist floors, so cover your feet in public places, such as communal showers, hot tubs, and the area around swimming pools. Dry your feet well, and don't share washcloths or towels. Boost your resistance to infection with a healthy diet (see p. 9), two or three cloves of raw garlic each day, and daily supplements of vitamins A, C, and E.

TREATMENT
No treatment is entirely dependable, but several are worth trying.

Herbal remedies
- Paint the wart, morning and evening, with a few drops of thuja or marigold (calendula) tincture.
- In addition to external treatment, drink teas or tinctures of echinacea, burdock, dandelion root, or red clover.

Caution: For safety concerns, see pp. 34–37.

Backyard remedy
Squeeze a drop of juice from a dandelion stalk onto a wart each day.

Kitchen cabinet remedies
- Put lemon juice or the juice of crushed garlic on the wart morning and evening.
- Cover onion slices with salt, and leave overnight. Dab the juice on the wart twice daily.
- Every night, apply a bandage that has been soaked in apple-cider vinegar or that encloses a flat sliver of garlic.

Aromatherapy: Twice daily, apply lemon, tea tree, cypress, or lavender oil (for a young child, dilute one drop of oil in half a teaspoon of vegetable oil). Try not to touch the wart, and don't allow the oil to touch uninfected skin. Avoid cypress oil in the first 20 weeks of pregnancy.

Homeopathy
- Thuja, in pill form or as a cream or tincture.

When to get medical help
- Your wart hurts or looks or feels inflamed or infected.
- You have warts on the face or in the genital or rectal area.
- You develop a wart after age 45.

See also:
SKIN DISORDERS

366

Weight Loss

Everyone's weight fluctuates to some extent, generally because of varying levels of food intake, exercise, and hormones, or a change in the type of food in the diet. Although losing pounds may be beneficial if you are overweight, a sudden, unexplained weight loss can mean an underlying serious disorder, so it is important to discover the cause.

Unusual weight loss most often results from a restrictive diet or from being unable to eat—for example, after an operation or during a serious illness. Weight loss can also result from an eating disorder. However, there are other times when it is less easily explained, and your physician may need to exclude the possibility of a food sensitivity or an underlying disease, such as a peptic ulcer, inflammatory bowel disease, or irritable bowel syndrome. Depression and anxiety are also frequent causes of this problem.

PREVENTION

If you have a tendency to lose weight, make sure that you are eating a healthy, well-balanced diet. Opt for frequent, small, appetizing meals, and aid digestion by taking your time and chewing well. Don't skip meals, and plan the day's meals in advance. For example, if you won't be able to have a proper lunch, pack a nutritious meal and take it with you. Make a point of never going without a good breakfast. You may also want to take a multiple vitamin and mineral supplement to provide you with nutrients, such as vitamin B and zinc, that help maintain a good appetite.

TREATMENT

General measures: Try to increase your weight to the normal level for your height and build (see table, p. 302).

- Choosing items from all the food groups, eat more to provide more calories. Carbohydrates (such as bread and pasta) and monounsaturated fats (such as olive oil) are especially good. Liquid nutritional supplements between meals may also help.
- Get daily exercise, of both the aerobic and muscle-strengthening varieties, tailored to your own fitness level. Some people lose weight because they exercise too much, and a few seem to become addicted to excessive exercise levels, so don't overdo it.
- Make sure you get some sunlight on your bare skin on most days. Sunshine encourages your body to manufacture vitamin D, which helps keep your bones strong. This is important, because if you are underweight as a result of poor nutrition, your body "steals" calcium from the bones to maintain other vital functions, thereby weakening them. Do not overexpose your skin, however, and use a sunscreen in strong sunlight. If getting sun is a problem, ask your doctor about taking extra vitamin D.

Food sensitivity: By preventing the proper absorption of nutrients, a food sensitivity can cause weight loss. Symptoms of such a sensitivity —which may appear within minutes, hours, or even days of eating a particular food—include asthma, eczema, migraine, arthritis, depression,

diarrhea, fluid retention, food cravings, and recurrent abdominal pain. If you think your weight loss may be the result of a reaction to a food, track down the cause with help from a doctor. Advice from a naturopathic physician or nutritionist will help you correct your sensitivity while maintaining your intake of vital nutrients.

Emotional causes: If you are anxious or depressed, you may neglect your general health and lose weight. This is of particular concern if you are elderly, especially if you live alone.

It is important to address the underlying cause of anxiety or depression, to discover and use stress-management strategies (see p. 347), and to get expert advice, if necessary. The following measures may also help:

- Use lavender oil for its soothing properties. Sprinkle three or four drops into your bathwater. Also sprinkle a few drops onto a handkerchief so that you can inhale the vapor during moments of stress.
- Ask a friend to give you a massage using two drops each of lavender, geranium, and sandalwood oils, and one drop of ylang ylang oil, in two tablespoons of sweet almond oil.
- Try relaxation exercises and meditation. Yoga can also be a great help for stress relief; just 10 minutes a day will help you learn to relax. Join a class or practice at home.
- Drink a cup of herbal tea when you feel particularly pressured. Choose from yarrow, rosemary, nettle, and cinnamon.
- Try taking an appropriate flower essence, such as Olive, if you are physically and emotionally depleted by a period of stress.

Acupressure for calming the mind

Regular acupressure sessions can sometimes reverse loss of weight that is linked to emotional causes. Ask a friend or partner to do the following at least once a week:

1 Using only gentle pressure, move the palm over the point four thumb-widths above the navel. At the same time, using the other hand, apply gentle thumb pressure to the inner arm at the point two thumb-widths above the wrist crease. Treat each side for two minutes.

2 Using the same techniques as in step 1, apply simultaneous pressure to the point eight finger-widths above the navel and to the point on the outside edge of the little-finger side of the wrist crease.

When to get medical help

- Unwanted weight loss continues for four weeks or longer.
- You have other unexplained symptoms.
- You are more than 10 percent below your ideal body weight.

See also:
ANXIETY, APPETITE LOSS, DEPRESSION, EATING DISORDERS, IRRITABLE BOWEL SYNDROME, OVERWEIGHT

GLOSSARY OF TERMS

This glossary is intended to help you understand possibly unfamiliar terms related to natural medicine that you may encounter in this book or elsewhere. Words in capitals refer to entries defined elsewhere in this section.

Acidophilus
Lactobacillus acidophilus—beneficial BACTERIA found in yogurt with live (active) cultures or available in supplement form. These bacteria can help maintain a healthy balance of microorganisms in the intestine and counter any overgrowth of the YEAST *Candida albicans*, which causes thrush.

Adaptogens
Remedies, generally from plant sources, that help regulate the body's systems and restore a healthy balance. For example, ginseng helps balance the release of STRESS HORMONES.

Aerobic
Literally, "requiring oxygen." The term usually refers to forms of exercise that make you breathe hard and boost your heart rate, thereby increasing the capacity of your heart and lungs.

Allergen
A normally harmless substance that triggers an allergic reaction in the IMMUNE SYSTEM of a susceptible person. Most allergens are PROTEINS, and among the most common examples are pollen, dust-mite droppings, and animal dander.

Allergy
A condition in which the IMMUNE SYSTEM responds defensively to a normally harmless substance, causing symptoms, such as a skin rash, breathing difficulties, itchy eyes, and a runny nose.

Amino acids
The building blocks of PROTEIN, which the body needs to make and repair cells and to control metabolism. The body can manufacture some amino acids itself, but others must be obtained from food.

Antibodies
PROTEIN molecules that circulate in the bloodstream, latch on to potentially damaging particles (such as VIRUSES), and help destroy them. They are part of the IMMUNE SYSTEM.

Antioxidants
Compounds that help counteract the damage caused to the body by FREE RADICALS and thus offer some protection against diseases, such as infections and certain cancers. Vitamins C and E, beta-carotene, and the minerals selenium and zinc are antioxidants, as are some phytochemicals, substances found in berries, green tea, and other plant foods.

Antiseptic
A substance that disables or destroys BACTERIA and other microorganisms on the skin or on objects—for example, in the home—thereby preventing the spread of infection.

Astringent
A substance that dries out body tissues, reducing any secretion, discharge, or bleeding.

Atopy
An inherited tendency to develop an allergic condition, such as asthma, allergic rhinitis, or eczema (dermatitis).

Bacteria
Microscopic organisms. Some types usually live harmlessly in the body and may even be essential to such processes as digestion, while others are capable of causing a wide variety of illnesses, ranging from common ailments, such as gastroenteritis, to more unusual conditions, such as meningitis.

Blood sugar
Sugar that is produced when CARBOHYDRATES are digested, and that circulates in the blood so that it can be used by the body as fuel. Absorption into the cells is regulated by the HORMONE insulin, which is produced in the pancreas and released in response to an increased level of blood sugar. Eating sugary food causes a too-rapid surge in the blood-sugar level.

Carbohydrate
The energy-producing component of plant-based foods, comprising sugars and starches. Refined carbohydrates (from grains that have had their less digestible parts, such as the fiber, removed) and sugar are broken down and absorbed into the bloodstream quickly. Complex carbohydrates—from legumes and unrefined cereal grains, for example—take longer to digest and therefore release their sugar content more slowly.

Carcinogen
A substance that may promote the development of cancer. Well-known carcinogens include ultraviolet light, asbestos, and chemicals in cigarette smoke.

Cardiovascular system
The system, comprising the heart and blood vessels (arteries, veins, and capillaries), that circulates the blood to all parts of the body.

Collagen
A PROTEIN that is a major component of the connective tissue found throughout the body

in bones, cartilage, tendons, ligaments, and skin. It becomes less resilient with age.

Decoction
An herbal tea made by simmering the roots or the tough, woody parts of a plant in water.

Distension
Swelling or bloating, particularly of the abdomen. It can have a variety of causes, including INFLAMMATION, fluid retention, and excessive gas production.

Diuretic
A substance that stimulates an increase in the production of urine.

Electrolyte
An element essential for normal cellular function, such as sodium or potassium. Its levels may be depleted when excessive amounts of fluid are lost in sweat, urine, or feces.

Endorphins
A category of NEUROTRANSMITTER released in the brain that reduces the body's response to pain. Endorphins generate a feeling of well-being, as well as playing a role in other functions, such as temperature regulation.

Energy
For many complementary therapists, especially those influenced by Asian therapies, this is the "life force" (*chi*, *qi*, or *prana*), which is said to flow around the body in a network of channels called MERIDIANS in Chinese medicine and *nadis* in Indian medicine. Such therapies as yoga and acupressure aim to restore health by rebalancing this energy flow.

Enzymes
Chemicals whose task is to facilitate chemical reactions—for example, enzymes in the digestive system that break down food into simpler forms that can be absorbed by the body.

Esophagus
The tube from the back of the throat into the stomach. Reflux of acidic stomach contents into the esophagus can cause its lining to become inflamed.

Essential fatty acids
Fatty acids (see FATS) that are needed for growth and other processes but that cannot be manufactured by the body and must therefore be included in the diet. Omega-6 fatty acids, derived from the essential fatty acid linoleic acid (found in nuts, seeds, beans, avocados, cold-pressed safflower oil) are vital for healthy circulation and skin and for other bodily functions. Omega-3 fatty acids, derived from the essential fatty acid alpha-linolenic acid (found in highest quantities in oily fish but also present in beans, walnuts, flaxseeds, whole grains, and certain vegetable oils, such as canola), are also vitally important.

Essential oils
Aromatic oils derived from plants and used by aromatherapists in a variety of ways to try to heal, boost the IMMUNE SYSTEM, and rebalance the body's ENERGY.

Estrogen
A sex HORMONE released by the ovaries, adrenal glands, and fatty tissue that triggers female development at puberty and promotes the monthly buildup of the uterine lining. Its level changes during the menstrual cycle and tails off as menopause begins. Men produce small amounts of estrogen as well.

Eustachian tubes
Fine tubes that link the air-filled middle ears with the throat, equalizing the pressure within the ear with that in the throat.

Fats
The most concentrated food source of energy. Certain fats (ESSENTIAL FATTY ACIDS) must come from the diet. Others circulate in the

blood or are stored in the body. Dietary fats are divided into two broad groupings: saturated and unsaturated. Saturated fats are mostly solid at room temperature and are derived mainly from animal sources. Foods containing large amounts include fatty cuts of meat, butter, and most cheeses. Excessive consumption of these fats can lead to serious health problems, such as heart disease, stroke, and obesity. Unsaturated fats are further subdivided into polyunsaturated and mono-unsaturated forms. Both types are usually liquid at room temperature. Most vegetable, seed, and nut oils are unsaturated. Oily fish also contain unsaturated fats. In general, eaten in moderation, unsaturated fats pose fewer health risks than saturated fats.

Fiber
Sometimes called nonstarch polysaccharides or roughage, this is the indigestible part of edible plant matter, which provides bulk in the feces. Fiber helps keep the digestive system working properly and may offer some protection against certain bowel diseases, breast cancer, and heart disease. There are two types: soluble and insoluble. Soluble fiber, which is softened by water, is found mainly in legumes, fruits, and vegetables. Insoluble fiber, found mainly in the husks of cereal grains and present in the diet in whole-grain bread, brown rice, and bran, passes through the digestive system largely unchanged.

Flavonoids
Pigments responsible for most of the bright colors of fruits and vegetables. Flavonoids (sometimes called bioflavonoids) act as important ANTIOXIDANTS. Their action is enhanced by vitamin C.

Food sensitivity
A reaction provoked by eating a food, or a constituent of food, which causes no problem for most people. The reaction may appear hours or even days afterward.

Free radicals
Unstable particles created during oxidation reactions in the body and encouraged by a variety of physical stressors, including a diet lacking in ANTIOXIDANTS, pollutants such as cigarette smoke, and excessive exercise. They play a role in the aging process and in triggering certain diseases, such as arterial disease and cancer.

Gluten
A PROTEIN that is present in most cereals, especially wheat, barley, rye, and oats, and thus in many foods made with cereal flour, such as bread, cakes, pies, and pasta. People with gluten intolerance cannot digest it and must follow a gluten-free diet to prevent damage to the intestines. Such damage may lead to celiac disease, fertility problems, and anemia.

Hormones
Chemical secretions released into the bloodstream by the endocrine glands to stimulate cells or tissues to perform certain actions. They control an enormous range of bodily processes—from growth to reproduction. Any improper hormone level can lead to disease.

Immune system
A complex armory, including different types of white blood cells and ANTIBODIES, designed to resist and fight infection or invasion by foreign particles or—in the case of auto-immune diseases—by particles perceived as foreign. A wide range of conditions and symptoms can result from malfunction of the immune system.

Inflammation
Swelling, redness, heat, and tenderness around a damaged or diseased area of the body. These changes are produced by the response of the IMMUNE SYSTEM to injury and infection as it acts to protect and repair affected tissues.

Infusion
An herbal tea made by steeping the leaves or flowers of a plant in boiling water.

Legumes
Peas, beans, and lentils. Legumes contain complex CARBOHYDRATES that are broken down slowly into glucose by the digestive system. They are also good sources of PROTEIN and PHYTOESTROGENS, and they are high in soluble FIBER.

Lymphatic system
A complex system of one-way drainage vessels (lymph vessels) and capsules, called lymph nodes, that contain white blood cells and ANTIBODY-producing lymphoid tissue. This system drains fluid from the tissues, traps foreign particles, microorganisms, and cancer cells, and carries infection-fighting cells to wherever they are needed.

Mantra
A word or short phrase repeated silently during meditation to help focus the mind and eliminate distracting thoughts and anxieties.

Melatonin
A HORMONE produced by the pineal gland in the brain in response to diminishing levels of daylight. Melatonin is made from a NEUROTRANSMITTER called serotonin. It induces drowsiness and sleep, and the cyclical fluctuation in its levels is disrupted by jet lag.

Meridians
The 14 channels through which ENERGY, or *qi*, is said by practitioners of Asian healing techniques to run in the body.

Metabolism
The process by which your body's cells turn food into energy. The rate at which this happens varies between individuals but is increased by regular exercise and decreased by eating a very low-calorie diet. Certain conditions, such as an underactive thyroid gland, can also depress the metabolic rate.

Micronutrients
Compounds, such as some VITAMINS and MINERALS, that are needed by the body only in very small amounts and for most people are supplied by a varied diet.

Minerals
Nonorganic substances that are required as NUTRIENTS for good health. Some minerals, such as calcium, are found in the body in large amounts. Others, such as chromium, are present in only trace amounts.

Monosodium glutamate (MSG)
A flavor enhancer commonly used in Chinese cuisine. It may cause bloating and headaches in sensitive individuals.

Mucous membrane
A layer of cells that line the openings of the body to the "outside," such as the mouth, nose, urethra, and vagina. Protective secretions from these cells form part of the body's outer defenses against infection.

Neurotransmitters
Chemical messengers released by nerve cells that enable an electrical signal to cross the gap between one nerve cell and the next.

Nutrients
Chemical compounds vital for the maintenance of life that are usually obtained from the diet. These include PROTEINS, CARBOHYDRATES, FATS, VITAMINS, and MINERALS.

Organic
Any food, whether from plants or animals, that is grown in natural conditions, without the use of pesticides, fungicides, HORMONES, or chemical fertilizers.

Phobia
An often disabling fear of things or activities that offer no genuine threat. The reasons for this fear lie in the unconscious mind. Common triggers include heights, enclosed spaces, public speaking, thunderstorms, mice, snakes, and spiders. Controlled exposure therapy, alongside cognitive therapy to aid understanding, is often successful.

Phytoestrogens
Compounds naturally present in plant foods that can mimic in a mild way the action of certain HORMONES (such as ESTROGEN) in the body, or counteract the effect of an overly high level of certain hormones in the body. Good sources include soybeans and other beans, rhubarb, fennel, and celery.

Pituitary gland
Situated in the brain behind the nose cavity, the pituitary produces important HORMONES, such as growth hormone, and also controls the hormone production of certain other endocrine glands.

Poultice
A paste—usually warm—of herbs or other ingredients that is spread on a cloth or gauze and applied to the skin to treat such conditions as boils.

Platelets
Tiny cells manufactured in the bone marrow and carried in the bloodstream. Their role is to help seal any injury to the blood vessels and enable a blood clot to form over the site to halt loss of blood.

Progesterone
A sex HORMONE produced by the ovaries during the second half of the menstrual cycle. It helps build and maintain the uterine lining after ovulation. Production ceases if the egg is not fertilized, triggering menstrual bleeding. Progesterone is produced by the placenta during pregnancy, helping to maintain the pregnancy. Production falls after menopause.

Proteins
A group of NUTRIENTS made of AMINO ACIDS that are essential for growth and body maintenance as well as for the manufacture of many important body parts, including cell membranes, HORMONES, NEUROTRANS-MITTERS, ENZYMES, and the blood pigment hemoglobin. Animal protein in the diet comes from meat, poultry, dairy foods, eggs, and fish. Vegetable sources include grains, LEGUMES, nuts, and seeds.

Sinuses
The air-filled spaces in the bones in the cheeks and forehead. The MUCOUS MEMBRANES lining them may become inflamed as a result of infection or ALLERGY, and their openings may become blocked, causing pain, as fluid accumulates inside.

Stress hormones
The HORMONES epinephrine (adrenaline) and cortisol, which are secreted by the adrenal glands when the brain signals danger from physical or psychological stress. They shut down nonessential body processes, such as digestion, and boost those, such as respiration and heart rate, needed for "fight or flight."

Toxin
A substance that may have a harmful effect on the body. Examples in the environment include pesticide residues, lead, atmospheric pollutants, such as those in cigarette smoke, and industrial chemicals, such as dioxins. Certain disease-producing BACTERIA may also produce toxins that are responsible for the symptoms of infection.

Virus
An infection-causing agent that can invade living cells and make use of their structure to reproduce, causing damage and the symptoms of disease. Viral illnesses include the common cold, influenza, chicken pox, and the various types of herpes infection.

Vitamins
NUTRIENTS required in varying quantities by the body. All except vitamin D (mostly manufactured by the action of sunlight on the skin) and vitamin K (made by bacteria in the intestines) must be obtained from the diet. Vitamins are divided into two groups: water soluble and fat soluble. Water-soluble vitamins (B and C) are not stored in the body and so have to be consumed on a frequent basis. Fat-soluble vitamins (A, D, E, and K) are stored in fatty tissue. Deficiency of any vitamin can cause disease; however, consumption of excessive amounts, especially of fat-soluble vitamins, can also be harmful.

Whole grains
Unrefined cereal grains, which include the germ and husks and retain more of the original grain's nutritional value as well as the natural FIBER, which is largely lost when the grain is refined. Whole grains are digested more slowly than refined cereals and therefore release their CARBOHYDRATES over a longer period, which helps prevent excessive fluctuations in BLOOD SUGAR. Common food sources of whole grains include brown rice and whole-grain bread and pasta.

Yeast
An ingredient of many bakery foods and alcoholic drinks, which may provoke a wide range of symptoms of FOOD SENSITIVITY in susceptible people. A diet high in yeast may also make a candida infection more difficult to eradicate. Brewer's yeast, used in beer-making, is a useful source of a variety of B vitamins and the MINERALS chromium and selenium.

RESOURCE GUIDE

GENERAL

American Holistic Health Association
P. O. Box 17400
Anaheim, CA 92817-7400
Phone: 714-779-6152
E-mail: ahha@healthy.net
Web: http://ahha.org

American Holistic Medical Health Association
6728 Old McLean Village Drive
McLean, VA 22101
Phone: 919-787-0116
Web: www.holisticmedicine.org

National Center for Complementary and
Alternative Medicine
P. O. Box 8218
Silver Spring, MD 20907-8218
Phone: 888-644-6226
Fax: 301-495-4957
Web: http://altmed.od.nih.gov

American Holistic Nurses Association
P. O. Box 2130
Flagstaff, AZ 86003-2130
Phone: 800-278-AHNA
Web: http://www.ahna.org

American Preventive Medical Association
459 Walker Road
Great Falls, VA 22066
Phone: 800-230-2762
E-mail: apma@healthy.net
Web: http://www.apma.net

American College for Advancement
in Medicine
23121 Verdugo Drive, Suite 204
Laguna Hills, CA 92653
E-mail: acam@acam.org
Web: http://www.acam.org

ACUPUNCTURE

American Academy of Medical Acupuncture
5820 Wilshire Blvd, Suite 500
Los Angeles, CA 90036
Phone: 323-937-5514
E-mail: webmaster@medicalacupuncture.org
Web: http://www.medicalacupuncture.org

American College of Acupuncture and
Oriental Medicine
9100 Park West Drive
Houston, TX 77063
Phone: 713-780-9777 and 800-729-4456
Fax: 713-781-5781
Web: http://www.acaom.edu

American Association of Oriental Medicine
433 Front Street
Catasauqua, PA 18032
Phone: 610-266-1433
Fax: 610-264-2768
E-mail: aaoml@aol.com
Web: http://www.aaom.org

ALEXANDER TECHNIQUE

North American Society of Teachers
of the Alexander Technique
P. O. Box 517
Urbana, IL 61801
Phone: 217-367-6956 and 800-473-0620
E-mail: nastat@ix.netcom.com
Web: http://www.alexandertech.com

Alexander Technique International
1692 Massachusetts Avenue, 3rd Floor
Cambridge, MA 02138
Phone: 617-497-2242
Fax: 617-876-2709

AROMATHERAPY

American Alliance of Aromatherapy
P. O. Box 309
Depoe Bay, OR 97341
Phone: 800-809-9850
Web: http://205.180.229.2/aaoa

National Association for Holistic
Aromatherapy
P. O. Box 17622
Boulder, CO 80308
Phone: 888-ASK-NAHA
E-mail: info@naha.org
Web: http://www.naha.org

AYURVEDA

The National Institute of Ayurvedic Medicine
584 Milltown Road

Brewster, NY 10509
Phone/fax: 914-278-8700
E-mail: drgerson@erols.com
Web: http://www.niam.com

BATES METHOD

Natural Vision Center of San Francisco
P. O. Box 16403
San Francisco, CA 94116-0403
Phone: 415-665-2010
Fax: 415-664-2121
E-mail: RELRN2SEE@aol.com
Web: http://www.nvcsf.com

BIOFEEDBACK

Association for Applied Psychophysiology
and Biofeedback
10200 W. 44th Avenue, Suite 304
Wheat Ridge, CO 80033-2840
Phone: 800-477-8892/303-422-8436
Fax: 303-422-8894
E-mail: AAPB@resourcenter.com
Web: http://www.aapb.org

CHIROPRACTIC

American Chiropractic Association
1701 Clarendon Boulevard
Arlington, VA 22209
Phone: 800-986-4636
Fax: 703-243-2593
Web: http://www.amerchiro.org

National Association for Chiropractic
Medicine
15427 Baybrook Drive
Houston, TX 77062
Phone/fax: 281-280-8262
E-mail: r_slaughter@msn.com
Web: http://www.chiromed.org

CRANIOSACRAL THERAPY

The Upledger Institute, Inc.
11211 Prosperity Farms Road
Palm Beach Gardens, FL 33410-3487
Phone: 561-622-4334 and 800-233-5880
Fax: 561-622-4741
E-mail: upledger@upledger.com
Web: http://upledger.com

FLOWER ESSENCES
Flower Essence Society
P. O. Box 459
Nevada City, CA 95959
Phone: 530-265-9163 and 800-736-9222
Fax: 530-265-0584
E-mail: mail@flowersociety.org
Web: http://www.flowersociety.org

The World Wide Essence Society
P. O. Box 285
Concord, MA 01742
Phone: 978-369-8454
E-mail: wwes@essences.com
Web: http://www.essences.com/wwes

HERBAL MEDICINE
American Herbalists Guild
P. O. Box 70
Roosevelt, UT 84066
Phone: 435-722-8434
Fax: 435-722-8452
E-mail: ahgoffice@earthlink.net

American Botanical Council
P. O. Box 144345
Austin, TX 78714-4345
Phone: 512-926-4900
Fax: 512-926-2345
E-mail: abc@herbalgram.org
Web: http://www.herbalgram.org

American Herbal Products Association
8484 Georgia Avenue, Suite 370
Silver Spring, MD 20910
Phone: 301-588-1171
Fax: 301-588-1174
E-mail: AHPA@ix.netcom.com
Web: http://www.ahpa.org

HOMEOPATHY
National Center for Homeopathy
801 North Fairfax Street, Suite 306
Alexandria, VA 22314
Web: http://www.healthy.net/nch

North American Society of Homeopaths
1122 East Pike Street, Suite 1122
Seattle, WA 98122
Phone: 541-345-9815
E-mail: nash@homeopathy.org
Web: http://www.homeopathy.org

MASSAGE
American Massage Therapy Association
820 Davis Street, Suite 100
Evanston, IL 60201-4444
Phone: 847-864-0123
Fax: 847-864-1178
Web: http://www.amtamassage.org

Associated Bodywork and Massage
 Professionals
28677 Buffalo Park Road
Evergreen, CO 80439-7347
Phone: 800-458-ABMP (2267)
Fax: 303-674-0859
E-mail: expectmore@abmp.com
Web: http://www.abmp.com

MEDITATION
American Meditation Institute
P. O. Box 430
Averill Park, NY 12018
Phone: 518-674-8714
E-mail: postmaster@americanmeditation.org
Web: http://www.americanmeditation.org

NATUROPATHY
American Association of Naturopathic
 Physicians
601 Valley Street, Suite 105
Seattle, WA 98109
Phone: 206-298-0126
Fax: 206-298-0129
Web: http://www.naturopathic.org

American Naturopathic Medical Association
P. O. Box 96273
Las Vegas, NV 89193
Phone: 702-897-7053
E-mail: webmaster@anma.com

Bastyr University
14500 Juanita Drive NE
Kenmore, WA 98028-4966
Phone: 425-823-1300
Fax: 425-823-6222
Web: http://www.bastyr.edu

NUTRITION
American College of Nutrition
301 E. 17th Street
New York, NY 10003
Phone: 212-777-1037
E-mail: office@am-coll-nutr.org
Web: http://www.am-coll-nutr.org

Center for Science in the Public Interest
1875 Connecticut Avenue NW, Suite 300
Washington, DC 20009
Phone: 202-332-9110
Fax: 202-265-4954
E-mail: cspi@cspinet.org
Web: http://www.cspinet.org

OSTEOPATHY
American Osteopathic Association
142 E. Ontario Street
Chicago, IL 60611
Phone: 800-621-1773
Fax: 312-202-800
E-mail: info@aoa-net.org
Web: http://www.aoa-net.org

REFLEXOLOGY
International Institute of Reflexology
P. O. Box 12642
St. Petersburg, FL 33733-2642
Web: http://www.reflexology.org

THERAPEUTIC TOUCH
Healing Touch International, Inc.
12477 W. Cedar Drive, Suite 202
Lakewood, CO 80228
Phone: 303-989-7982
Fax: 303-980-8683
E-mail: htiheal@aol.com
Web: http://www.healingtouch.net

YOGA
The American Yoga Association
P. O. Box 19986
Sarasota, FL 34276
Phone: 941-927-4977
Fax: 941-921-9844
E-mail: YOGAmerica@aol.com
Web: http://members.aol.com/amyogaassn

Index

The pages for the main entry or information on a subject are in **bold** type.

Acknowledgments

Photographic credits
p. 8 The Stock Market; p. 35 The Geffrye Museum, London; p. 48
Telegraph Picture Library; p. 81 Science Photo Library; p. 102
Science Photo Library; p. 114 Mother & Baby Picture
Library/Emap élan; p. 123 Mother & Baby Picture Library/Emap
élan; p. 129 (all) Science Photo Library; p. 170 Frank
Murphy/Rosie McCormick; p. 232 Science Photo Library; p. 270
The Stock Market; p. 288 (left) National Medical Slide Bank;
p. 359 NHPA.

Color origination by Mullis Morgan plc

The publishers would also like to thank the following individuals
and organizations for their help in the preparation of this book:
Aleph One; the British Diabetic Association; Amy Godfrey-
Smythe; Freddie Godfrey-Smythe; Lorie Gould; Katie Greenhalgh;
Morgan Kilgallen; Jon Meakin; Anna Moture; Neal Street East;
Kevin Owen; Mehmet Oz, M.D., New York–Presbyterian
Hospital, New York; Eljay Yildirim. Special thanks are also due to
the Marquess Research Trustees: Ray Coventry, John Clutton,
William Greaves, Kil Hamilton, John Pearson, Mickie Steinmann,
Roger Stong, and Associates; Dennis Bergkamp, Iain Carson, and
Nwanko Kanu.